The Complete
Aromatherapy
& Essential Oils
Sourcebook

A PRACTICAL APPROACH TO THE USE OF ESSENTIAL OILS AND AROMATHERAPY FOR HEALTH, BEAUTY, AND WELL-BEING

JULIA LAWLESS

The Complete
Aromatherapy
& Essential Oils
Sourcebook

A PRACTICAL APPROACH TO THE USE OF ESSENTIAL OILS AND AROMATHERAPY FOR HEALTH, BEAUTY, AND WELL-BEING

HARPER
thorsons

Thorsons is an imprint of HarperCollins*Publishers*

HarperCollins*Publishers*
1 London Bridge Street
London SE1 9GF

www.harpercollins.co.uk

First published as *The Complete Illustrated Guide to Aromatherapy*
by Harper Element in 1997.

This revised edition published by HarperCollins*Publishers* in 2017.

1 3 5 7 9 10 8 6 4 2

Text © Julia Lawless 1997, 2001, 2016, 2017

Cover and interior photographs © iStock except as credited on page 409

Cover and interior design by Rosamund Saunders

A catalogue record of this book is available from the British Library

ISBN 978-0-00-828146-5

Printed and bound in China

Note from the Publisher
Any information given in this book is not intended to be taken as a
replacement for medical advice. Any person with a condition requiring
medical attention should consult a qualified practitioner or therapist.

Contents

Part one: Aspects of Aromatherapy

Part Two: Aromatherapy Massage

Part Three: Aromatic Remedies

Part Four: Index of Essential Oils

Part Five: Index of Carrier Oils

Part Six: Safety Guidelines

Further Reference

Rose.

io.nature. f. m. c. f. m. z. melior ereis. de iumat persia re
ceptes. iuuamentu cerebro calido. nocumentis effiat quibdaz
meschaicremotio noci. ci camphora.

.82.

Preface

Returning to nature is in vogue! Having worked in the field of aromatherapy for over forty years I have seen the popularity of natural botanical products go from strength to strength. Pure essential oils can now be purchased on every high street and downtown center, and the use of natural aromatics in commercial toiletries has both expanded and diversified. This is because the remarkable therapeutic potency of these botanical oils has been increasingly validated by scientific research and by clinical tests, verifying their healing potential. This is especially true in the field of skin care, particularly in helping to combat aging skin, as well as in the treatment of common infections and viruses.

This trend is matched by the ever-growing interest in eating organic food, using botanically based cosmetics on our skin and utilizing 100 percent natural products in our homes. In short, we have become tired (and ill) from being surrounded by synthetic and chemical products for decades. Now we are collectively realizing we have mistreated "mother nature" for too long and it is time to start respecting our planet and all living things, including the plant kingdom, by valuing the gifts it has to offer. This is especially true of the attitudes among young people in the West, who are taking upon themselves the responsibility for living an ethical and ecologically conscious lifestyle.

I am delighted to introduce this new updated and beautifully designed edition of *The Complete Aromatherapy & Essential Oils Sourcebook*. It is now over twenty years since I started to research and write the original material for the first edition of this book … yet it has stood the test of time. Far from becoming outmoded, the theme of this book … that of living in harmony with nature and learning how to use and create our own 100 percent pure botanical products, is becoming ever more important and valid. In the words of Jennifer Peace Rhind:

ABOVE *Melissa (lemon balm) is a plant much used by herbalists which also yields a valuable essential oil.*

"We live in exciting and enlightening times: the future of aromatherapy is very bright indeed if we embrace traditional aromatic knowledge in the light of contemporary understanding."

LEFT *This early 15th-century manuscript shows the cultivation of the rose, already long-established at that time.*

Introduction

The 21st century has witnessed a remarkable renaissance of interest in, and practice of, natural healing methods. In recent years, such forms of treatment as medical herbalism, osteopathy, shiatsu, reflexology, acupuncture, and aromatherapy have all attained varying degrees of credibility in the eyes of health professionals, as well as among the general public. Of these, aromatherapy is amongst the most popular alternative or complementary forms of treatment available in the United States and other Western countries. Yet only half a century ago the therapeutic use of herbs and essential oils was frowned upon or even officially banned. Plant medicines were seen as something archaic and outmoded in comparison to the new pharmaceutical drugs, and in 1941 herbal medicine was even made illegal in the United Kingdom. Barely more than fifty years later, the scientific world is reappraising the value of natural remedies: as the limited effectiveness, and unwanted side effects, of aggressively synthesized medications are being recognized, aromatic essences are coming back into their own once again.

However, the current popularity of aromatherapy is not just another fashion or fad … it's part of a larger sociological and cultural movement. Firstly, many of the so-called "alternative" therapies, including aromatherapy, are not new or modern techniques. They are based on ancient medical systems that have been built up over thousands of years from accumulated empirical evidence. Medical herbalism, and the use of aromatic remedies in particular, are very much older forms of treatment than Western allopathic, or orthodox, medicine. Unlike many modern drugs, plant remedies have been tried and tested over generations, and any side effects or environmental consequences carefully noted. Herbal medicine and aromatherapy consequently represent "a return to nature," being based on principles requiring ecological awareness. This corresponds with many people's interest in "green" issues, and a widespread concern regarding the unknown effects of certain chemicals on the whole ecosystem and the long-term consequences of our exploitation of natural resources and global warming.

Secondly, alternative forms of therapy embrace a holistic approach to health. They focus on the well-being of the individual as a whole, including that person's emotional or mental disposition. They are thus able to fulfill society's need for some kind of psychological support during an era of instability. An aromatherapy massage, for example, can provide a valuable antidote to the fast pace of 21st-century life and help relieve many of the stress-related problems that are so widespread today.

Thirdly, with regard to aromatherapy massage at least, it is a very comforting yet multifaceted form of treatment. During a treatment, the pleasingly scented aromatic oils produce both psychological and physiological effects as they are rubbed into the skin and absorbed into the bloodstream. In addition, the essential oils themselves are highly concentrated and easy to use, and require little or no preparation. This means that they can readily be employed by all kinds of people in a variety of ways to enhance their health and the overall quality of their lifestyle, rather than being limited to the hands of health professionals.

This book concerns itself with their therapeutic and cosmetic applications and concentrates on the diversity within the aromatherapy tradition as it is practiced today. It is above all a practical handbook, both for the practicing therapist and for more general use. Special emphasis is placed in the book on what I call

BELOW Perhaps the most feminine of all scents, roses have been used in perfumes and healing remedies since ancient times. The Ancient Romans used the wild rose as a remedy for the bites of rabid dogs. Roses are still highly valued today and rose essential oil is very expensive.

"simple" aromatherapy—a basic, practical approach to self-treatment. It has always struck me as being a great pity that the whole realm of self-help using folk medicine, which was once a natural part of family life, has been largely lost in Western culture. It is in this middle ground that aromatic remedies have such a lot to offer—playing their part in the home treatment of common everyday conditions such as period pains, headaches, eczema, and other skin complaints.

Accepting responsibility for one's own health and condition is also an affirmative statement. It encourages individual responsibility and opens a door to self-knowledge as well as a window into the natural world, for all essential oils are derived directly from plants. In fact the whole field of fragrant plants and natural medicine is a vast area. I have also found that, like gardening, aromatherapy has an addictive quality—once hooked, you will find it is hard to let go, for there is always more to learn and discover.

The reality of climate change, as well as the impact of environmental and ecological issues, has also taken on a greater sense of urgency over these past two decades, largely as a direct result of our consumer culture. The need to pay attention to the type of products we choose to buy, their method of production, and their overall impact on the world in which we live now needs to be of paramount concern to anyone who cares about future generations.

Since essential oils are 100 percent naturally derived agents, functioning in a positive, holistic manner both within our own bodies and within our larger environment, their utilization represents an authentic route towards demonstrating a greater caring for our planet. However, it is important to source essential oils from companies that uphold responsible environmental policies, such as supporting reforestation, avoiding the exploitation of endangered botanical species (such as Amazonian rosewood), and employing ecological packaging materials (p. 395).

This philosophy goes hand in hand with adopting a lifestyle that respects and works together with nature, and in doing so, helps to preserve the beautiful globe on which we live.

ABOVE *The art of herbal distillation has been perfected over the centuries.*

PETITGRAIN

THYME

How to use this book

THIS BOOK IS FOR EVERYONE interested in the art and science of aromatherapy, from the professional practitioner to any newcomers to the subject. The book is divided into four main parts, covering every aspect of aromatherapy as practiced today.

The first part of the book introduces aromatherapy to the reader. It outlines the various aspects of aromatherapy, and focuses in detail on simple household uses of essential oils, skin and body treatments, and perfumery. Containing simple recipes and step-by-step instructions, Part 1 is designed to help the reader practice aromatherapy at home.

The second part of the book describes the approaches to, and techniques of, aromatherapy massage, and gives detailed, step-by-step descriptions with clear illustrations on how to give a full-body massage, therapeutic massage for local areas, and massage for special circumstances, such as sports massage.

Aspects of Aromatherapy provides a thorough introduction to the many uses of essential oils and describes simple home aromatherapy and perfumery. *Aromatherapy Massage* explains the massage techniques, while *Aromatic Remedies* focuses on the medical uses of essential oils. The *Index of Essential Oils* and the *Index of Carrier Oils* are comprehensive guides to all the aromatherapy oils referred to in the book, with clear, at-a-glance information about the uses and qualities of each oil.

In the appendix, notes on safety data show how to use the oils safely, and the chemical analysis is given for each oil. A nutrition sheet provides a quick source of dietary advice, a glossary explains all the medical and scientific terms used in the book, and there is a list of useful addresses telling the reader where to find the oils and further information about aromatherapy. Finally, there is an extensive list of books for further reference.

The third part of the book describes the ways in which aromatherapy is used in the field of medicine. The science of essential oils and the ways in which the oils are tested in the laboratory are explained, and the links between the chemical constituents of the various oils and their effects on the body are shown. It also shows how essential oils can be used safely and efficiently for medical treatment in the home. Remedies are divided into the different body systems, with clear instructions on the use of oils in treatment.

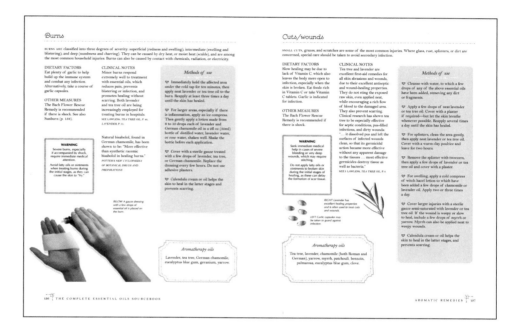

The fourth part of the book is an index of essential oils, followed by an index of carrier oils, listed in botanical name order. Each oil is described in detail, including its characteristics, actions, method of extraction, use in aromatherapy, nutritional value, scent qualities, and physiological and psychological effects.

PART ONE

♡

Aspects of
Aromatherapy

Aspects of aromatherapy

Interest in aromatherapy is growing year by year. As more and more brands of essential oils and aromatherapy products are to be found in the shops there is a steady increase in the home use of aromatic essential oils. Professional aromatherapy treatment is now available in beauty salons, fitness clubs, and hairdressers, while essential oils are used therapeutically in modern hospitals as well as complementary health centers.

Aromatherapy involves using pure essential oils, derived from plants, in a huge range of health and beauty treatments, as well as for pleasure. In offering us a "natural" way of caring for our health, it is just one aspect of the growth of interest in all forms of alternative or complementary medicine and traditional home remedies. Modern (or allopathic) medicine is spectacularly successful in many ways, but increasing numbers of people feel that they would like to know about ways of preventing illness in the first place, and to be able to use simple, safe, and drug-free home remedies for ordinary, everyday ailments. There is also a growing feeling that in modern medicine we are treated as a collection of parts, some of which may have problems, rather than as a whole organism, and least of all as a person. In contrast, complementary medicine, of which aromatherapy forms a part, offers a way of being treated holistically—as a whole being in whom there are many aspects of a disease or illness and for whom individually tailored treatment is required.

In our search for ways of keeping fit and healthy without needing to use synthetic drugs, aromatherapy oils offer the advantage of their complete naturalness and their general safety and simplicity of use. They offer ways of preventing illness and treating ourselves at home, and in the hands of professional practitioners they can be used as part of a multifaceted holistic treatment.

In fact, of course, things are never quite as simple as they seem. Aromatherapy is complex in many ways. Firstly, it means different things to different people, and secondly the oils used, although simple in that each is the pure, natural product of a single plant, are complex and potent substances that need to be used with care, knowledge, and experience.

The oils can be used simply for their fragrance and its effect on mood and emotion, but in professional practice their physiological effect is central. This is generally obtained through the oils being used in massage treatment, but some practitioners (with full medical qualifications) also use essential oils clinically in the tradition of the French pioneer, René-Maurice Gattefossé, in minutely prescribed oral doses and through inhalation.

The word "aromatherapy" literally means therapy through aroma or scent, without specifying the source of the scent. But aromatherapy in practice uses only essential oils, and no other form of scent. Its richness is that it has so many aspects, which are complementary to each other, and which may also overlap, but which are nevertheless distinct. In professional medical practice, it is the substances or oils themselves and their biochemical effects that are central, while in many home uses of essential oils it is the aroma that counts, and the pleasure of the scent is the main reason for using the oils. Between these two extremes are cosmetic aromatherapy and massage, where the scent and the beneficial physiological effects of essential oils go hand in hand, and simple medical aromatherapy, which uses the oils' many curative effects. Aromatherapy must be unique in having so many facets, and in offering such a wealth of pleasurable, practical, and therapeutic uses.

"VOLATILE ESSENCES HAVE HEALED PEOPLE SINCE THE DAWN OF TIME."
RENÉ-MAURICE GATTEFOSSÉ

Aromatherapy basics

"WHEN WE PEEL AN ORANGE, walk through a rose garden or rub a sprig of lavender between our fingers, we are all aware of the special scent of that plant.
But what exactly is it that we can smell? Generally speaking, it is essential oils which give spices and herbs their specific scent and flavor, flowers and fruit their perfume."

(THE ENCYCLOPEDIA OF ESSENTIAL OILS, JULIA LAWLESS)

All essential oils are extracted from the plant kingdom, from flowers, herbs, trees, vegetables, or spices. They are organic compounds that occur naturally in a wide variety of different species, and can be found in leaves (rosemary), bark (cinnamon), blossoms (neroli), fruit (orange), wood (cedar), resin (pine), roots (vetivert), or buds (clove). They are called "essential" because they not only capture the plant's fragrance, but also its healing properties in a very concentrated way.

The main method of extracting an essential oil from a plant is by steam distillation. This applies to the majority of herbal essences including lavender, thyme, rosemary, and marjoram. Most citrus oils such as bergamot and orange are extracted by simple expression or pressure to the peel of the fruit. The more delicate perfume essences require a more complicated technique—jasmine, neroli, and rose for example, are extracted using volatile solvents. Essential oils are the tools of the modern healing practice known as aromatherapy.

The term "aromatherapy" was first used in the 1920s, but the knowledge of how to extract and apply essential oils is a very ancient art. Aromatic plants and oils have been used for thousands of years as perfumes, incense, and cosmetics as well as for their medicinal and culinary applications. The ancient Egyptian, Persian, Indian,

Chinese, and Arab cultures made use of many aromatic oils, as did the early Greek and Roman civilizations. The distillation of essential oils is thought to date back to as early as 3500 BCE based on primitive clay apparatus found in Mesopotamia. However, it was not until the 11th century CE that the Arab physician and alchemist Avicenna perfected the art of distilling aromatic oils from botanical raw materials in the purest form.

At one time, most large houses in Europe had a "still-room"—literally a distillation room where essential oils were prepared. Even small cottages and farms had fragrant herbs hanging from their rafters, and shelves were lined with rows of aromatics contained in pots for scenting linen, sweet bags, and clothes. The herbs and oils were of course also employed as household remedies and used to maintain a fragrant and hygienic environment. This is because in the past, all perfumes, toiletries, and soaps were made using essential oils from plants, which were generally sourced locally. With the development of biochemical advances, gradually essential oils were replaced by synthetic substitutes in cosmetics, perfumes, and remedies for commercial purposes. Now in the 21st century essential oils from all over the planet have become widely available due to the global economy. Oils from the Mediterranean region as well as from India, China, and Australia form the majority of the items found in a professional therapist's collection.

Today, scientific research is also confirming many of the traditional usages of essential oils, as well as making new and valuable discoveries. For example, the bactericidal, antiseptic, and fungicidal qualities of tea tree oil have been shown through trials to be even more effective than many of its synthetic substitutes; while the use of lavender essential oil has been adopted by some hospital wards to help patients sleep and overcome feelings of anxiety, due to its natural sedative effects. It is also now being found that essential oils interact with our own biological activity in such a way that makes them very effective skin-care agents on a basic molecular level.

Massage is the most popular method utilized in the practice of aromatherapy in the West. In this case, the topical application of essential oils is combined with

CHAMOMILE

Absorption through the skin was observed by Jager:
"When a 2 percent solution of lavender was applied to the abdomen,
10 percent of the lavender was absorbed into the general blood circulation
with plasma levels peaking after 20 minutes. Levels of linalool and
linalyl acetate, active constituents of lavender oil, dropped to zero
after 90 minutes. During this period after application, the lavender oil
constituents were circulated to tissue via capillaries. Potentially higher
levels of absorption are likely across the highly vascular cribiform plate in
the nose with a direct pathway to the brain."
(Jager 1992)

In aromatherapy practice, when essential oils are applied externally they are transported via the blood to various parts of the body and are able to influence the internal systems of the organism not just the surface skin. Indeed, it is now well accepted that essential oil components can be absorbed through the skin to reach internal organs—in fact, the use of skin patches has become a common mechanism for dispensing pharmaceuticals.

But perhaps an aspect of aromatherapy that is less understood is that the inhaled aromatic molecules absorbed via the lungs acts provide a fast-acting pathway by which the chemical constituents of essential oils reach internal tissues. In this way they are absorbed into the blood stream by thin membranes of the nose, bronchioles, and lungs, much more rapidly than through the skin. Whenever essentials are inhaled, such as during massage, in the bath or shower, or as a steam inhalation or room fragrance, the effect of the particular essential oil influences us on a chemical level almost instantly!

At the same time, the inhaled molecules also react with nerves in the olfactory bulb and relay nerve messages to the limbic system, which controls factors such as mood and memory. This explains why certain fragrances or perfumes can have such an immediate effect on our emotional state. Essential oils can consequently have a direct effect both psychologically and physically simply when they are inhaled, not only by lifting or improving our mood as with a perfume or room spray, but also on a molecular level when they are absorbed via our lungs.

Essential oils are therefore effective for both physical and emotional complaints—the two being intimately connected. Thus the fragrance of each essential oil plays a vital role in its overall healing quality, which acts upon the individual in a unique and subtle manner. Nowadays our sense of smell is often undervalued or unappreciated, but this does not mean that it has no effect. Since smell is intimately connected with mood and memory, modern research has shown that the scent of certain essential oils can help combat conditions such as insomnia, anxiety, depression, and mental fatigue, which are so often the result of today's stressful lifestyle.

Recent studies have also shown how scent can alter our brain wave patterns, regulate the systems within our body, and influence our moods. One of the most effective ways to alter our attitude from a negative one into a positive one is through the use of natural fragrances: this is because our sense of smell connects directly to the part of our brain that processes our emotions.

the beneficial effects of touch and physical massage techniques to make a potent healing method, especially when applied to many of our modern stress-related conditions. But how do the essential oils contribute to the therapeutic process in this case? Scientific research has confirmed that a proportion of the constituents in each essential oil are absorbed into the body when applied to the skin.

In aromatherapy, the use of massage is an important aspect of the treatment due to the healing effects of touch, which has been found to have particular value in the treatment of emotional or nervous disorders, including stress-related conditions. Massage therapy is of course also beneficial for a wide range of physical conditions such as arthritis, high blood pressure, muscular pain, or sports injuries. Aromatherapy massage and the application of aromatic body or facial oils has also proved to be one of the most effective ways of rejuvenating the skin and dealing with many common skin complaints, such as acne or dermatitis.

In summary, in modern-day aromatherapy practice, essential oils as well as other aromatic products such as those shown opposite, are used in combination with massage as a form of natural holistic treatment. In a treatment, several essential oils are generally blended together in a vegetable carrier oil, such as sweet almond oil, to suit the specific needs of the individual, before being applied to the skin. In this way the skin is nourished by the application of the vegetable oil, while the essential oils interact chemically with the systems of the body as well as exerting an emotional effect through their scent.

"*Scent, even in hard materialistic times like these, still offers a direct route to the unconscious... Perfume is one of the last territories of the irrational. The deep aim of perfumery is to find ingredients that will open new doors.*"

Maurice Rogers

A guide to aromatic raw materials

Essential oils are mostly produced by steam distillation, which is by far the most widespread method used for extracting natural fragrances today. Some citrus oils, such as lemon, are produced by simple expression from the peel of the fruit. Essential oils can be extracted from a wide range of plant species and parts including their leaves, roots, seeds, wood, and flowers: many of the most commonly used essential oils are from the Mediterranean, such as lavender, rosemary, marjoram, and basil.

Flower waters are a natural by-product of the steam distillation process. A flower water or "aromatic hydrosol" is the actual water used in the distilling process, which retains the natural aroma of the plant processed. For example, rose flower water is produced in vast quantities as a by-product in the distillation of rose otto. It is also possible to make flower waters by using a special aqua-emersion technique using natural spring water.

Concretes are traditionally made when the heat from steam distillation will adversely affect the odor, as is the case with jasmine or tuberose and other delicate florals. Instead, the plant material is macerated in a volatile solvent, which causes the absolute and much of the wax (stearoptene) to dissolve. After filtration, the solvent is removed by gentle warmth, which causes it to evaporate. The concrete left behind is a mixture of absolute and wax.

Absolutes are produced from the concrete by separating out the wax from the compound. Pure alcohol is used to turn a concrete into an absolute, as the wax does not dissolve in the alcohol. An absolute is closer to nature in scent than an essential oil but is generally more costly; it is also often more difficult to handle as many absolutes are viscous at room temperature.

Gum-resins are the starting point for the extraction of several well-known aromatics including myrrh and frankincense. Gum-resins are often used in their crude form as incense materials. Elemi (*Canarium luzonicum*) occurs in nature as a gum-resin that exudes from a tree found in the Philippines; it is then steam distilled from the crude gum-resin to produce an essential oil.

Balsams are oily or gummy oleoresins, usually containing benzoic acid or cinnamic acid, obtained from the exudates of various trees and shrubs and used as a base for the production of certain essential oils. Examples of botanical balsams include: Balsam fir (*Abies balsamea*) and Peruvian balsam (*Myroxylon pereirae*). Crude balsam of Peru is a dark brown, thick liquid, which is traditionally soaked up by rags wrapped around the tree, which then are boiled in water.

Approaches to aromatherapy

THE THERAPEUTIC USE of essential oils covers a very wide spectrum. This is part of their charm and uniqueness. At their simplest, oils can be worn as natural perfumes, made into aromatic bath preparations or used in many ways as home remedies. They can also be combined with both home and professional massage to provide a very effective treatment for stress-relief. At the other end of the scale, specific botanical essences can be used by clinically trained therapists or doctors for the treatment of serious medical conditions.

ABOVE Rose petals are a traditional ingredient in potpourri.

The ways in which aromatherapy can be practiced can be separated into five areas of specialization. Although it is impossible to draw hard and fast lines between these various aspects, classifications of this kind are helpful, at least in the short term, for the process of clarification and understanding. These different areas are: simple aromatherapy for home use, cosmetic aromatherapy, perfumery and the psychotherapeutic use of oils for the effects of their odors on the mind, massage using essential oils, and medical and clinical aromatherapy, where essential oils are used to treat medical complaints.

SIMPLE AROMATHERAPY

A basic approach uses aromatic oils in a wide range of methods, including vaporization, aromatic bathing, local massage, cosmetic creams, and steam inhalation, for first-aid purposes and in the treatment of common complaints. This approach is in the ancient tradition of herbal "simples"—home remedies or household secrets, originally passed on from generation to generation. It can be adapted by nurses and other professionals and used as an adjunct to medical treatment. As a type of preventive medicine, it can help to ward off infectious illness and promote general health and well-being.

COSMETIC AROMATHERAPY

The use of essential oils for skin and beauty care is an ancient and specialized aspect of aromatherapy. There are records that show that many primitive cultures used natural aromatics as a means of adornment and as a way of enhancing their beauty. Indeed, many indigenous peoples still do so today. However, the earliest and richest associations concerning the cosmetic use of aromatic materials are to be found in the practices of the Ancient Egyptian civilization, some 5,000 years ago. Aromatic herbs, gums, and oils were incorporated into carefully formulated cosmetic ointments and other beauty preparations, as well as being employed in the embalming process. Seen in this light, the Ancient Egyptians were the original precursors of modern beauty therapists, especially those who use aromatic oils as part of their cosmetic treatments.

PSYCHO-AROMATHERAPY AND PERFUMERY

The term psycho-aromatherapy is used to describe the use of the psychotherapeutic benefits of essential oils, effected mainly by inhalation but also by other methods of application. In the practice of psycho-aromatherapy, the ways in which botanically derived aromas can influence moods and emotions and help to induce certain states of mind are studied. This can be by bringing about a state of relaxation or through their energizing and stimulating effects. This contrasts with aromachology, in which both natural and artificial scents are studied for their therapeutic value, but principally for purely commercial purposes in the perfume industry. Nevertheless, psycho-aromatherapy does have a great deal in common with the art of perfumery, especially since all perfumes were originally made using natural aromatics, and since they both focus on the psychological effects of scent and require a high degree of olfactory discrimination and knowledge.

ABOVE "The Roses of Heliogabalus" by Sir Lawrence Alma-Tadema, 1836–1912.

AROMATHERAPY MASSAGE

There are many benefits to be derived from combining massage with the use of essential oils. It is the main method adopted by professional aromatherapists working in the field of alternative health care. Aromatherapy massage has been largely influenced by the French pioneer, Marguerite Maury, whose research work was directly aimed at utilizing the healing and revitalizing properties of aromatics, especially through application to the skin. This approach is notably beneficial for the treatment of stress-related disorders and requires a substantial degree of training, both in acquiring massage techniques and in understanding the many and varied properties of the essential oils that may be used.

MEDICAL AROMATHERAPY

Medical aromatherapy includes the systematic use of essential oils in the treatment of clinically diagnosed medical conditions. It adopts a wide range of methods, including oral prescription. It should only be practiced by suitably trained medical doctors or by clinical therapists, who, like qualified medical herbalists, have undergone a training period of at least four years. This is the approach of the 20th-century founder of aromatherapy, René-Maurice Gattefossé, and his scientific and medical successors.

Simple aromatherapy

THE PRACTICE OF AROMATHERAPY benefits from being placed within the context of holistic health care as a whole. Whereas the emphasis in modern allopathic or orthodox medicine is to target a given complaint with a specific remedy, from a holistic point of view, the best form of treatment is always a multifaceted one. The air we breathe, our nutrition, exercise, relaxation, and, above all, our emotional or mental disposition, are all essential factors that need to be taken into account.

Holistic health care is more concerned with cultivating an understanding of healthy living and of preventive techniques than with providing symptomatic relief. In any case of "disease," it is vital to assess the overall health of the person, both physically and mentally, and then to try and ease the problem at its source, while at the same time building up the body's natural immunity. It is preferable to prevent the problem from occurring in the first place.

Preventive medicine is not given enough value or emphasis in Western society today. It is all too easy to let health slide, then reach for a bottle of pills when something goes wrong. Yet most people are prepared to service their car regularly, rather than wait for the inevitable breakdown to occur. Why do we not seem to take the same precautions to nurture both our bodies and minds as in the East? There, many patients traditionally receive acupuncture treatment at each change of season to ensure that the body and mind remain in optimum health for the following quarter. It is also still traditional for Chinese people of all ages to gather outside in the mornings to practice tai chi, an ancient martial art form that combines gentle exercise with moving meditation to promote good health and longevity.

From the perspective of holistic health care, a wholesome diet, fresh air, and sufficient exercise, together with a sense of emotional security, intellectual satisfaction, and some form of daily spiritual or psychological nourishment, are all factors that can help to preserve a sense of well-being. Herbal tonics and natural aromatics have also held a traditional place in the preventive medicinal practices of many cultures, both ancient and modern. It is certainly true that people who are exposed to the beneficial effects of essential oils on a daily basis tend to have a greater resistance to disease in general.

"People who use essential oils all the time, as part of their daily bathing, skincare and household routines … have a high level of resistance to illness, 'catching' fewer colds … than average and recovering quickly if they do."[1]

Essential oils exert a psychological lift (called their "cephalic effects") and help to promote a positive mental state, while, on a more physiological level, they stimulate the immune system and exhibit all types of preventive and curative properties. In the words of the French medical aromatherapist, Dr. Daniel Penoël:

"Aromatic medicine is a preventive healing focusing on the evolutionary side of all living beings in the Biosphere, be it in the animal or the vegetable kingdom."[2]

The pressures of Western society place many stresses and strains upon the individual. If these are not recognized, they can lead to more serious health problems. Aromatherapy, with its holistic approach to health and well-being, can be used to intervene and prevent long-term problems occurring.

> "CONSCIOUSLY OR UNCONSCIOUSLY, EVERY BEING IS CAPABLE OF HEALING HIMSELF OR OTHERS …"
>
> INAYAT KHAN

For more information about the emotional and mental
benefits of aromatherapy, see page 62.

A holistic approach

APART FROM AROMATHERAPY and medical herbalism, there are many other types of alternative treatment that can be used in holistic medicine to complement and enhance one another. A condition such as osteoarthritis, for example, benefits from a multifaceted approach that would include specific herbal remedies, dietary changes, gentle exercise, aromatic baths, and massage treatments, as well as osteopathy, and possibly even pyschotherapeutic advice. On the other hand, it is possible to treat a condition such as a boil or bruise more simply at home with a combination of dietary nutrients and local aromatic applications. This book refers to the related treatments wherever possible.

In the section on aromatic remedies (pp. 133–237), each complaint is defined and a number of different methods of treating the problem are suggested, both with the use of essential oils in a variety of ways and with supportive techniques. "We are what we eat" is perhaps overused as a slogan, yet its truth remains. In holistic health care, and in the field of preventive medicine in particular, diet, together with a positive mental attitude, is very influential in maintaining well-being. Details of the specific vitamins that are required by the body, and their dietary sources, are given at the end of the book in Vitamins and dietary sources (p. 380).

Other types of treatment that are raised and given emphasis in this book are the use of Bach flower remedies, allergy testing, osteopathy, psychotherapy, counseling, yoga and relaxation, and meditation and prayer. Despite this emphasis upon alternative medicine as prevention and treatment, orthodox and alternative approaches should not be seen as necessarily working in opposition. Each has its own value: what is required today is an integration of modern scientific techniques and traditional knowledge. In India and China, for example, traditional forms of medicine are being used alongside the newly adopted surgical skills and other modern innovations, while in the West there has been a surge of interest in the medicinal potential of aromatic materials and herbal medicine.

Body and mind

Aromatherapy treats mind and body together. The scent of the essential oils used can have a powerful effect on the emotions while the oils' chemistry affects the body.

LEFT A wholesome and balanced diet, with plenty of fresh fruit, plays an important part in maintaining health.

ABOVE Borage is used to make a base oil and is very beneficial to the skin.

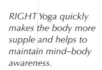

RIGHT Yoga quickly makes the body more supple and helps to maintain mind–body awareness.

The aromatic medicine chest

LIKE TRADITIONAL HERBAL remedies, essential oils are very valuable self-help tools because they are effective in the prevention and treatment of many common conditions, yet are simple and easy to use. It is wise to build up a collection of the most useful essential oils, together with a small selection of vegetable base or carrier oils and creams for use in the home medicine chest. The most important of these are arnica ointment, calendula cream or oil, grapeseed oil, sweet almond oil, jojoba oil, and wheat germ oil.

Many essential oils, apart from being used for first aid or for the treatment of common complaints, are also ideal as bath oils, perfumes, or room fresheners. Even when they are used purely for esthetic purposes, they are still fulfilling a positive preventive and therapeutic role. A small essential aromatic oil kit can prove to be an extremely valuable asset at home, in the workplace, or while on vacation, and when traveling. There is a group of five invaluable oils to keep in the home medicine cabinet, or to take with you when traveling: lavender, tea tree, rosemary, Roman chamomile, and peppermint.

The chart on the next page gives an overview of 100 essential oils, broken down by commonality. In the section on specific remedies (p. 133), several essential oils are usually mentioned for each illness, including some from all of these groups (see overleaf). It is not, however, necessary to buy all the oils listed, as it is possible to treat many common illnesses by using up to five oils, especially when the oils are mixed or blended together in various combinations. The recommended blends, which are highlighted in the section on the treatment of specific problems, are always made up from a selection of the essential oils listed overleaf.

blending dish

absorbent cotton

dropper top

large jar for base oil

dark, well-sealed bottle

ROSMARINUS LAVANDULA MELALEUCA CHAMAEMELUM CITRUS EUCALYPTUS MENTHA

Essential oils for a "make-your-own" home kit

GROUP 1
Invaluable oils

Lavender is extremely versatile, especially for stress-related disorders and for skin complaints.

Tea tree is invaluable for its antiviral, antiseptic, fungicidal, and immune-stimulant properties.

Rosemary has stimulant properties, and is an expectorant as well as being a tonic to the entire system.

Roman chamomile is a mild relaxant and anti-inflammatory agent, especially as a children's remedy.

Peppermint is good for digestive complaints such as nausea or indigestion, and for respiratory problems, and for treating fever.

GROUP 2
Commonly used oils

Atlas cedarwood
Bay
Bergamot
Black pepper
Carrot seed
Citronella
Clary sage
Clove bud
Cypress eucalyptus blue gum
Frankincense
German (blue) chamomile
Ginger
Grapefruit
Jasmine
Juniper
Lemon
Lemon eucalyptus
Lemongrass
Lime
Mandarin
Myrrh
Myrtle
Neroli
Palmarosa
Patchouli
Petitgrain
Rose geranium
Rose
Sandalwood
Scotch pine needle
Spanish sage
Sweet basil (basil)
Sweet fennel (fennel)
Sweet marjoram (marjoram)
Sweet orange (orange)
White thyme (thyme)
Valerian
Ylang ylang

PEPPERMINT

ROSEMARY

FRANKINCENSE

GROUP 3
Specialist oils

Amyris
Angelica
Aniseed
Balsam Peru
Benzoin
Cajeput
Camphor
Caraway
Cardamom
Celery seed
Cinnamon leaf
Citronella
Coriander
Cumin
Dill
Elecampane
Elemi
Fir needle (silver)
Fragonia
Galbanum
Ho wood
Hyssop
Laurel
Lavandin
Linaloe
Manuka
May chang (*Litsea cubeba*)
Melissa
Niaouli
Nutmeg
Parsley seed
Pine (longleaf)
Plai
Ravensara
Rosewood
Spearmint
Spruce
Tagetes
Virginian cedarwood
Vetivert
West Indian bay
Yarrow

GROUP 4
Rare/Perfumery oils

Champaca
Fenugreek
Frangipani
Immortelle
Labdanum
Lotus
Lovage
Mimosa
Oakmoss
Rose damask (otto)
Styrax
Tuberose
Turmeric
Vanilla
Verbena (lemon)
Violet

CELERY SEED

ANISEED

Aromatic bathing

ONE OF THE SIMPLEST and most pleasant ways to use essential oils is in the bathtub, where the oils enhance the relaxing effect of a long warm bath, or the stimulating effect of a brisk hot bath or cold dip. The therapeutic effects of bathing have been recognized for centuries. The sophistication of many of the Ancient Roman spa bath houses can still be seen, with their hot and cold compartments, steam rooms, and aromatic massage quarters. Very hot baths stimulate perspiration, which is valuable in cases of infectious illness and for encouraging elimination of wastes and detoxification. However, they can also be draining and, in the long run, can cause the skin to lose its elasticity. A medium-hot or warm bath has a soothing and relaxing effect on both the mind and body, while cool or cold water has a more invigorating and stimulating effect. Lukewarm baths are good for lowering the temperature in cases of fever.

PURE ESSENCES

This is the easiest and most popular way of using essential oils for bathing. Simply add 5 to 10 drops of your chosen essential oil (or a blend of oils) to the bathtub when it is full, and relax in the aromatic vapors. Use lavender oil for promoting relaxation, rosemary as an invigorating tonic, or marjoram for soothing tired muscles.

LEFT Rosemary invigorates.

BATH BAGS

Gather a selection of fresh herbs or aromatic flowers together, such as lavender sprigs, rose petals, lemon balm leaves, and chamomile flowers, and tie them loosely in a muslin bag with a piece of string or ribbon. Choose specific herbs both for their therapeutic properties and for their scent. If you wish, add a few drops of a chosen essential oil to the bundle to enhance the fragrance. Then tie the bag to the faucets and let it hang in the stream of hot water while the bathtub is filling.

BATH SALTS

Epsom salt (magnesium sulphate) or Dead Sea salts are healing substances in themselves, and make an excellent medium for combining with essential oils. Salt contains precious minerals, has an alkalizing effect on the body, promotes the elimination of acidic wastes from the muscles and joints, and induces copious perspiration—good for infectious illness, rheumatism, arthritis, and for promoting relaxation. Dissolve one or two handfuls of Epsom salt in boiling water, add a few drops of essential oil, and pour into the bathtub. Alternatively, simply add 5 drops of essential oil to every handful of Epsom salt or Dead Sea salts, pour directly into the bathtub and agitate the water before getting in.

MOISTURIZING BATH OILS

A few drops of an essential oil can also be mixed in a teaspoonful of vegetable oil, such as sweet almond oil, before being added to the bathtub. This helps to moisturize the skin and ensures an even distribution of the essential oil, which is especially

WARNING
Always check with specific safety data before using a new oil in the bathtub, to avoid possible irritation. Details are given for each oil in the information on pp. 239–343. Increase the dilution during pregnancy and for babies or infants to at least half the recommended amount. For babies, avoid the possibly toxic or irritant oils altogether.

LEFT Marjoram relieves aching muscles.

important in the case of babies and young children.

To make a larger quantity, mix 200 drops of an essential oil (or blend) with 3½fl oz (100ml) jojoba oil or another base or carrier oil (pp. 345–371) containing 5 percent wheat germ oil and store in a tinted glass bottle. Add a teaspoonful of this mixture to the bath water when required.

FOOT AND HAND BATHS

Valuable for warding off chills, for easing arthritic or rheumatic pain, and for the treatment of specific foot complaints, a hot aromatic foot bath can also be very effective for relieving stress and over-exhaustion (use lavender and sweet marjoram), and is a quick aid to combating excessive perspiration (use tea tree and rosemary). Simply sprinkle 5 or 6 drops of essential oil into a bowl or basin of warm or hot water and soak feet or hands for about ten minutes. Alternatively, dilute the essential oils in a teaspoonful of cider vinegar, honey, or a moisturizing vegetable oil beforehand.

THERAPEUTIC HIP BATH OR DOUCHE

This method can be helpful in the treatment of urinary or genital conditions, such as pruritus (itching), thrush, or cystitis. The area can be bathed in a hip or sitz bath or a bowl of warm water to which 3 to 5 drops of a suitable essential oil have been added—a mixture of cypress and lavender, for example, can help to heal the perineum after childbirth. Alternatively, an enema pot or plastic douche can be bought from some pharmacies. Mix 3 to 5 drops of a suitable essential oil with warm water before inserting—bergamot and tea tree mixture is effective for the treatment of thrush.

THE SAUNA

In Scandinavia, the sauna is the traditional method of cleansing and toning the whole system. Dry heat and steam are used to open the pores and promote the elimination of waste products. This is followed by a plunge into very cold water that closes the pores, and tones and refreshes the skin. In Finland, where the tradition of the sauna originates, bundles of fresh birch twigs are slapped on the skin, stimulating the circulation and imparting a delicious fragrance. Essential oils that are most suitable for use in the traditional sauna include fresh-scented oils such as pine, juniper, myrtle, eucalyptus, and cedarwood. (Very rich or floral oils such as lavender, ylang ylang, or patchouli are too heady and should not be used.) Add 2 or 3 drops to 17fl oz (500ml) of warm water and throw on the heat source for an aromatic and refreshing steam bath.

LEFT Valerian produces an oil used to relieve nervous tension and insomnia.

ABOVE Two or three drops of soothing oil can be used in a baby's bedtime bath and this may lead to a more restful night for everyone.

Therapeutic massage and body oils

THERAPEUTIC AROMATIC MASSAGE is the main method used by professional aromatherapists, but it can also be practiced at home—either on oneself, or on a friend or partner. Body oils are best applied after a warm bath, when the pores of the skin are still open, to encourage rapid absorption.

For the purpose of massage or general application to the skin, a few drops of essential oil are always mixed with a larger measure of base or carrier oil, usually a light vegetable oil such as sweet almond oil or grapeseed oil. When preparing a body oil or massage oil, the dilution should be in the region of 5 to 30 drops of essential oil in a bottle of 2fl oz (50ml) of base oil, depending upon the type of essential oil used and its specific purpose. For general massage purposes, a dilution of 2.5 percent (see below) is suitable for adult use. To calculate how much essential oil to add to a base oil, assess the amount of base oil in fluid ounces/milliliters and add half the number of drops of essential oil.

Special dilutions

For 2fl oz (50ml) of base oil:

BLEND PERCENTAGE	ESSENTIAL OIL IN DROPS
0.5%	5
1%	10
1.5%	15
2%	20
2.5%	25
3%	30

Standard dilution (2.5%)

BASE OIL AMOUNT	ESSENTIAL OIL IN DROPS
1 tsp (5ml)	2–3
1 tbsp (15ml)	6–7
1fl oz (25ml)	12–13
2fl oz (50ml)	25
3½fl oz (100ml)	50

Vaporized oils and steam inhalation

ALL ESSENTIAL OILS are highly volatile, and evaporate or vaporize on exposure to air, giving off their aroma. In inhaling these aromas we absorb the essence in two ways: while the scent itself directly affects receptors in the brain, molecules of substances from the oils are absorbed into the blood stream and circulated around the body. Many oils have a medicinal effect in the air itself as well as on the person breathing them, as they are powerful antiseptics that can kill airborne bacteria. Heating the oils speeds up their evaporation rate. Vaporized essential oils can be used for various purposes: a penetrating oil such as sweet basil to scent a room and dispel unwanted odors; an antiseptic oil such as eucalyptus to rid a room of germs in cases of infectious illness; insecticides such as citronella to repel mosquitoes and other insects; steam inhalation, using an oil such as rosemary, for respiratory disorders. The five main methods of assisting the vaporization of essential oils are described in detail below.

VAPORIZER

Purpose-made ceramic or metal vaporizers are now readily available in specialty shops and some health stores. A few drops of essential oil are put in the bowl of the burner and a night-light is then placed underneath, causing the oil to heat up and evaporate. A little water can be mixed with the oil in the bowl to slow down the evaporation rate if required. Because they have a naked flame, vaporizers of this type should be kept well out of reach of children or pets.

LEFT This traditional vaporizer uses a night light.

CITRONELLA

Useful oils for vaporizers

To disinfect a sickroom: eucalyptus, myrrh, thyme, pine, tea tree. To freshen the air and cheer the spirits: basil, bergamot, lavender. To keep insects at bay: citronella, geranium. For sensual perfume: black pepper, clary sage. To clear the head and mind: hyssop, marjoram, peppermint.

BASIL

LIGHT BULB RING

A very easy and cheap way of vaporizing essential oils is to use a ceramic or metal light bulb ring. Simply put a few drops of essential oil into the ring, place on top of a light bulb, then switch the light on. Please see the warning, right, for safety.

ELECTRIC DIFFUSER

An electric diffuser is more expensive to buy than a ceramic or metal vaporizer, but has the advantage of not needing a naked flame to generate heat. This makes it more suitable for night use, especially in children's bedrooms. Also, many electric diffusers have a variety of settings to adjust the rate of evaporation.

WARNING
Do not apply essential oils directly to a light bulb, as this can cause the bulb to explode.

STEAM INHALATION

Vaporizing an essential oil using hot water as a medium is especially valuable for respiratory conditions, such as whooping cough. It can also be used to help to keep up the humidity levels in centrally heated rooms. For environmental purposes, simply add a few drops of essential oil to a bowl of hot water placed on a radiator or any other source of heat.

Direct steam inhalation is especially suited to congested sinus, throat, and chest infections. Soaking in a steaming hot bath to which have been added 5 or 6 drops of expectorant oils such as myrtle or rosemary, which are both nonirritating to the skin, helps to clear congestion. This method also acts as a kind of facial steam or sauna: the use of cleansing antiseptic oils such as tea tree can help unblock the pores and clear the complexion of minor blemishes.

SCENTED FABRICS

A simple technique to help combat coughs and colds is to apply a few drops of an expectorant essential oil such as myrtle to the pillow, pajamas, night clothes, or handkerchief. If you wish to keep insects at bay, applying a few drops of an essential oil such as geranium to hanging ribbons or sprinkling the oil onto your clothing can be a very effective way of doing this. Because essential oils are volatile, unlike vegetable oils, they will not leave a stain on linen or clothing.

ABOVE Inhaling vaporized essential oils, such as peppermint, from a bowl of steaming-hot water is a simple way to treat respiratory infections.

Inhalation for a cold

Add about 5 drops of a decongestant essential oil such as peppermint to a bowl of steaming water, cover the head with a towel, and breathe deeply for three minutes, keeping the eyes closed.

LEFT Oils sprinkled onto a handkerchief can be inhaled throughout the day.

Simple medicinal and household uses

THERE ARE MANY other beneficial and pleasurable ways in which to use essential oils in the home, many of them closely allied to uses of herbs in medicine, or linked to well-established, longstanding household traditions of using flowers and herbs. The five quintessential oils for the medicine chest (p. 32) are all good standbys for simple first-aid treatments and straightforward medical care for common complaints, while for perfumery and fragrance the choice is largely a question of personal preference.

HOT AND COLD COMPRESSES

This method is suited to a variety of first-aid cases—use a hot compress for abscesses, muscular aches, pains, and severe tension; a cold compress for bumps and bruises, headaches, migraine, and sprains.

GARGLES AND MOUTHWASHES

For the treatment of mouth ulcers, sore throat, bad breath, or other mouth or gum infections, simply add 3 to 5 drops of an essential oil such as fennel or thyme to a glass of warm boiled water and mix well. Then swill the mouth out well and/or gargle.

NEAT APPLICATION

In general, essential oils should not be applied neat to the skin as they are highly concentrated. Some oils can cause irritation or a burning or tingling sensation when they are applied in an undiluted form. However, there are exceptions to this rule. (See First aid, p. 40; Perfumes and household fragrance, p. 40.)

WARNING
Essential oils should never be used undiluted or taken internally except as specified in this book or on the advice of a trained physician. Always follow the instructions carefully.

RIGHT Gargling with water and a few drops of thyme oil soothes a sore throat and is a useful treatment for a range of mouth infections.

THYME

LEFT Hot and cold compresses can be used with appropriate oils for injuries, aches and pains, headaches, abscesses, and indigestion.

Preparing a compress

Prepare a hot compress by dipping a clean facecloth or piece of absorbent cotton in a small bowl containing about 17fl oz (500ml) of steaming water to which has been added 5 or 6 drops of an essential oil such as lavender. Squeeze out any excess water, and then apply to the affected area. Apply a bandage if required and repeat as necessary.

Make a cold compress by dipping a clean facecloth or cotton pad in a bowl of cold water to which has been added 5 or 6 drops of a cooling oil such as peppermint, squeezing out any excess water. Alternatively, wrap the cloth round an ice cube before applying to the affected area. Refresh the compress regularly and apply until the swelling or pain subsides.

FIRST AID

Lavender oil is very soothing and rapidly helps the skin to heal, usually without even leaving a scar. It can be applied directly to burns, insect bites, cuts, and spots as first-aid treatment. Tea tree is another oil which can be used neat for first-aid purposes. However, before applying any oil neat to the skin, always do a patch test as described on p. 375.

DISINFECTANTS

Such oils as tea tree or lavender can be used for disinfecting clothes and diapers. For washing by hand, add up to 50 drops of essential oil to a bowl of warm water; otherwise add the same quantity to a liquid detergent and use in the washing machine. For washing floors and kitchen and bathroom surfaces, add up to 50 drops of essential oil to a bucket or bowl of water.

PERFUMES AND HOUSEHOLD FRAGRANCE

Some essential oils can be applied undiluted to the skin in minute amounts as perfume. Several essential oils are ideal natural perfumes—either on their own or combined with others. Ylang ylang is renowned as a well-balanced fragrance in its own right; others, such as rose, jasmine, neroli, and sandalwood, are well-known traditional perfume ingredients. Such oils can be dabbed on the wrists or behind the ears, either neat or diluted to 5 percent in jojoba or a bland base oil. Always carry out a patch test on the skin before using a new oil as a perfume (see p. 375).

Aromatic oils can be used to scent the hair, linen or clothes, paper, ink, potpourris or other items, directly from the bottle. Pure essential oils have a totally different quality to synthetic perfumes, since they are derived from natural sources. Artificially made perfumes do not have the subtle balance of constituents and the therapeutic qualities of real essential oils.

OILS FOR FURNITURE AND WOOD

A few drops of an essential oil such as cedarwood or rosemary can be used to perfume wooden items such as beads or boxes, or added to furniture polishes. Freshly scented oils such as these can also be sprinkled on logs before they are burned on an open fire.

AROMATIC SACHETS AND PILLOWS

As well as having a pleasing fragrance, lavender oil makes an excellent insect repellent. Lavender has been used for centuries to protect clothes and linen from moths. It imparts a lovely scent when used in aromatic sachets kept in the linen closet or in drawers. Use dried herbs impregnated with a few drops of oil as the stuffing and seal them in small linen or lace sachets, which can be tied at the top with ribbon. Scented pillows can be made for the bedroom in similar fashion.

SCENTED PAPER AND INK

An easy way to scent writing paper is to put a few drops of a chosen essential oil onto a ball of absorbent cotton and store this in a sealed box together with the sheets of paper. After about ten days, the paper will have absorbed a good deal of the fragrance. A few drops of aromatic oil can also be dropped into writing ink. Many household items can be scented in a similar manner.

POTPOURRIS

Essential oils can be used in making potpourri or used to revive them. Making dry potpourri is quick and straightforward. The principles and basic method for making dry potpourri are given on p. 42, together with a sample recipe for a traditional floral potpourri.

ABOVE *Bee stings can be soothed with a cold compress.*

LAVENDER

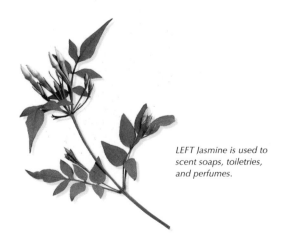

LEFT *Jasmine is used to scent soaps, toiletries, and perfumes.*

Making a potpourri

MANY TRADITIONAL DRY potpourri mixes displayed in open ceramic bowls in the bedroom or living room are based on rose petals, often with the addition of lavender flowers. However, a great deal of flexibility and individual creativity can be used in choosing plant material and other ingredients. A fresh citrus blend based on herbs such as lemon balm and lemon-scented geraniums together with dried lemon peel and marigold petals can make a refreshing bathroom blend. Spicy mixtures, which are suitable for the kitchen or for festive occasions, may include ingredients such as lemon or orange peel, cinnamon sticks, vanilla beans, whole cloves and other spices, bay leaves, and sprigs of dried rosemary.

TRADITIONAL POTPOURRI RECIPE

INGREDIENTS

♡

2 cups (25g) dried rose petals
½ cup (6g) dried lavender flowers
½ cup (6g) dried mint leaves
½ tbsp (7.5ml) orris root powder
half a nutmeg, grated
20 to 30 drops rose oil
20 to 30 drops lavender oil
decorative rosebuds
small glass mixing bottle
mortar and pestle
small spoon for mixing
glass or ceramic storage jar
decorative bowl

1 Measure out the essential oils and blend them together in a glass bottle. Put on the lid securely and set aside.

2 Grind the grated nutmeg and orris root powder together, using the mortar and pestle. Add half the total quantity of essential oils and mix with a spoon.

3 Place the main ingredients in the storage container and add the remaining essential oils, mixing well.

4 Add the powdered material from the mortar and mix gently, so as not to damage the plant materials. Seal the container and leave to mature for two to six weeks in a dark place.

5 Transfer the potpourri mixture into a decorative bowl or jar and arrange a few tiny rosebuds on top. Later, as the aroma starts to fade, more essential oils can be added to revive the mixture and prolong its life.

Potpourri inspiration

Experiment with your favorite scents to create potpourris for every occasion. The traditional recipe on the previous page is soothing and relaxing—try blending citrusy scents like lemon verbena, lemon balm, and lemon thyme with marjoram to create an invigorating alternative.

Cosmetic aromatherapy

COSMETIC AROMATHERAPY aims to rejuvenate and beautify the body through the use of aromatic oils, and generally to improve our outward appearance. Much of this section focuses on the different methods by which essential oils can be used to improve the complexion or to treat specific skin conditions. Beauty, however, is not just skin-deep. The condition of the skin expresses the overall health of an individual. A relaxed attitude, together with a well-balanced diet, enough exercise, and a daily intake of plenty of spring water or herbal teas, all help to keep the system in top condition.

Our outward appearance is certainly kept high on the cultural agenda today, with health and beauty issues attracting a wide audience among the general public. New weight-control programs, fitness plans, and nutritional regimes are emerging all the time. But the emphasis that our culture places on the body and the importance of beauty, like all things, has both a positive and a negative side. On the positive side, it can encourage a sense of well-being, self-confidence, self-awareness, and self-motivation. On the negative side, it can foster addictions, narcissism, or a lack of self-worth by holding up a concept of perfection or beauty that is ultimately unattainable. Taken to the extreme, an over-materialistic attachment to the beauty of the body can lead to a youth-oriented society in which people have an exaggerated fear of growing old.

LEFT Women wearing perfume cones on their heads as depicted in an Ancient Egyptian wall painting.

Essential oils have themselves been linked to the old alchemical tradition of the search for physical immortality—but, as the medieval alchemists discovered for themselves, ultimately it is not possible to transmute base matter into gold. What they did discover through their laborious experimentation was how to perceive an "inner map" for the transformation of the psyche or nature of the soul. In the end, as Paracelsus realized, the material body is only a receptacle or instrument for the transcendental soul.

However, before considering the contribution or limits of an aromatherapeutic approach to rejuvenation, and the value of essential oils in beauty and cosmetic preparations, it may be helpful to take a look at the structure of skin itself and the types of physical problems to which it is exposed.

> "*WHY NOT TAKE CARE OF THIS BODY, WHICH IS THE RECEPTACLE OF OUR SOUL, SO THAT IT MAY REMAIN AS HEALTHY, STRONG, AND PERFECT AS POSSIBLE ...*"
> PARACELSUS

ROSE PETALS

The skin and its health

THE SKIN IS the largest organ of the human body, consisting of over three million cells. Like the heart or liver, the skin is a very active organ and is responsible for all kinds of bodily processes, including temperature regulation, elimination of metabolic waste, and the manufacture of vitamin D, as well as protecting the body from external invasion.

The skin is divided into three main layers:

♡ **The subcutaneous or bottom layer**: this contains muscles and fatty tissue that help to keep the skin toned and firm.

♡ **The dermis or middle layer**: this contains sensory nerve endings, blood and lymph vessels, hair follicles, and the sebaceous and sweat glands. This is also the place where new living skin cells are manufactured before emerging on the surface.

♡ **The epidermis or top layer**, known as the "stratum corneum": this is the visible surface of the skin, which is composed of flat, essentially dead cells.

LEFT Massage and dry skin brushing help to improve the circulation and discourage toxic wastes from accumulating in the thigh area.

The more rapidly the dead surface cells are replaced by new ones from beneath, the softer and smoother the skin looks. A mass of lifeless cells clinging to the surface of the skin creates a tired and dull-looking complexion. On the other hand, an excessive turnover of epidermal cells, due to a dysfunction of skin enzymes, gives rise to psoriasis. Since the natural process of renewal slows down as we age, rejuvenating aromatherapeutic skin products are largely aimed at stimulating rapid cell regeneration in the dermal layer, thus protecting the health of the skin from within.

LEFT This diagram shows the three layers of the skin.

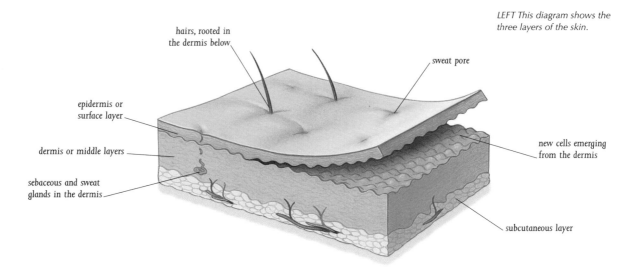

hairs, rooted in the dermis below

sweat pore

epidermis or surface layer

dermis or middle layers

sebaceous and sweat glands in the dermis

new cells emerging from the dermis

subcutaneous layer

ALLERGIC REACTIONS

As the body's first line of defense from external invasion, the skin is prone to attack from pathological organisms such as bacteria or viruses, as well as from other external dangers through injury or potential allergens. Many common skin complaints are due to an allergic reaction, or hypersensitivity to certain conditions or substances. Allergies are associated with the level of histamine, a protein that is released in response to injury or tissue damage. Histamine causes the capillaries to dilate in the affected area, bringing extra blood to the damaged cells to help in their repair. When fluids seep out of the dilated blood vessels this can also cause local redness, swelling, and irritation. Other actions of histamine include contraction of the bronchi (this is the cause of asthma attacks).

The release of histamine is a normal defense mechanism, but in allergic reaction the level produced becomes excessive. For example, an excess of histamine can quickly build up after insect bites or plant stings, since histamine is also present in their poisons. Excessive amounts of histamine may also be released in response to inhaling pollen, animal hair, or other irritants, as is the case with hay fever.

Why such reactions arise is not known, but there is often a hereditary pattern involved in such conditions, with a tendency for one allergy to lead on to another. Alternatively, there may be a sudden breakdown in the body's resistance to potential irritants which were previously tolerated. Stress, and psychological or emotional factors, often trigger an attack.

Allergies are said to be on the increase, due to higher stress levels and the general over-exposure to food additives, insecticides, and other synthetic chemicals to which we are subjected on a daily basis. Essential oils such as chamomile, melissa, tea tree, or lavender can be very helpful for many types of allergic skin conditions, although it is vital to carry out a patch test beforehand to check for individual sensitization levels, as described on p. 375.

Antihistamines are used in the treatment of allergic reactions, Vitamin C being a good natural example. Pantothenic acid (Vitamin B5) is also valuable in treating allergies, as it builds up the adrenal glands, which produce cortisone, a substance known to have protective qualities against allergies. Infantile eczema usually responds to treatment with gamma linoleic acid (GLA) in the form of evening primrose oil capsules. Allergic skin conditions most commonly affect those with dry or sensitive skins.

WARNING

Cinnamon leaf oil is an irritant to the skin and thus can only be used in low dilutions, whether used singly or in combination with other oils.

FUNGAL INFECTIONS

Fungal or viral organisms are another common cause of skin irritation. Tinea, for example, which manifests in several forms, all characterized by red, flaky skin and itching, is caused by a microscopic fungal mold. Forms of tinea are athlete's foot (*tinea pedis*), ringworm (*tinea capitis*), dhobi itch (*tinea cruris*), which affects the groin, especially in hot climates, and *tinea barbae*, sometimes known as barber's rash, which affects the face and neck. Candida is another fungus that causes infection, and it thrives in moist, warm conditions. It is often found in the vagina, where it can cause thrush, with irritation, itching, and sometimes severe redness and discomfort. However, thrush also occurs in the mouth, where it erupts in a white speckled rash, and is also seen in some forms of the irritating childhood complaint known as "diaper (nappy) rash." Like viral infections such as herpes, which in its various forms can cause cold sores, shingles, genital herpes, and chicken pox, fungal infections tend to attack the body when it is run down.

Essential oils that have a powerful fungicidal and antiviral action include tea tree oil, lemon-scented eucalyptus, and cinnamon leaf.

BACTERIAL INFECTIONS

Other forms of skin infection are bacterial, and may be caused by a wide range of invading organisms such as types of Streptococci or Staphylococci. Tea tree, cinnamon leaf, clove, rosemary, marjoram, thyme, lemon, oregano, and savory are all effective bactericidal agents—but some of the most powerful antibacterial oils also have high toxicity levels or are skin irritants or skin sensitizers.

A condition such as acne often involves bacterial infection—so an oil such as tea tree, which is mild on the skin yet has powerful antiseptic qualities, is very valuable in such cases. Congested skin conditions such as acne, boils, and blemished skin tend to affect those with oily or greasy complexions, since the pores of the skin are already blocked by sebum, a greasy substance formed around the base of hairs.

GRAPEFRUIT

MELISSA

LEFT Fungal infections can cause a form of "diaper rash" in babies.

EVENING PRIMROSE CAPSULES

Beauty and rejuvenation

APART FROM THEIR role in preventive medicine, and in the treatment of common disorders and skin complaints, essential oils have been utilized for thousands of years purely for their cosmetic potential. The Ancient Egyptians were renowned for their expertise in this field, successfully using aromatic essences and herbs in the embalming process for their preservative qualities. Recent research has confirmed that certain essential oils, such as rose, neroli, lavender, frankincense, and myrrh, can indeed stimulate cellular granulation, which is the first stage of healing after an injury, and keep the skin looking youthful. Many traditional preservative herbs, such as rosemary and sage (but not their essential oils), have also been found to have potent antioxidant properties that prevent the decomposition of organic material.

The pioneering French aromatherapist Marguerite Maury spent many years researching the specific ways in which essential oils could be used to preserve the youth of the skin, and the best ways in which oils could be utilized for their rejuvenating properties on the body and spirit as a whole. She summed up her findings as follows:

"Passionately interested by works dealing with the essential oils, perfumes and aromatics we have discovered their vast possibilities—particularly with regard to the problem of regeneration."[3]

According to Mme. Maury, certain essential oils can rejuvenate the skin by regulating the activity of the capillaries and restoring vitality to the tissues—in her own words "they make the flesh more succulent." She used individually formulated aromatic treatments or prescriptions (IPs) which were specifically adapted to the physical and emotional disposition of her clients in order to bring about a transformation in both their physical health and mental attitude. This aromatic mixture complemented exactly the needs of the patient, and was compared to the negative of a film, with its reversed shadows and light. It was made up using essential oils of different densities. She also found that in the course of a treatment, it was often necessary to modify the mixture as the client's condition changed.

Mme. Maury did not use an alcoholic base for her prescription, as would a perfumer, but mixed the essences with a vegetable oil carrier for direct application to the skin. She noted that essential oils were rapidly absorbed in this way, but that different essences passed through the skin at different rates according to their viscosity. Although the heavy, resin-bearing essences often had the greatest influence on the quality of the tissues on a deep cellular level, they were the slowest to be assimilated, while the very light and fluid essences penetrated easily into the extra cellular fluids[4] that play a key role in maintaining the body's state of balance. When preparing aromatic remedies for rejuvenation, it is therefore valuable to incorporate several essences of various densities so as to create a synergy, or, to use the language of perfumery, a perfect accord of top, middle, and base notes.

Further information on the blending of oils, and the principles of perfumery can be found on pp. 62–73.

MYRRH

RIGHT The Ancient Egyptians used plants for their cosmetic value, and also knew about their powers as preservatives.

Essential oils for the skin and hair

THERE ARE MANY ESSENTIAL oils that are useful skin-care agents: oils such as sandalwood, geranium, palmarosa, bergamot (which should be bergapten-free), myrrh, and frankincense. These are all very valuable additions to the beauty therapist's list of ingredients, or an aromatherapist's collection of massage oils. There are also many essential oils that make excellent conditioning treatments for the hair and scalp due to their pleasing scent, gentle action, and powerful antiseptic properties. These include rosemary, West Indian bay, and sage, which can help to regulate the activity of the sebaceous glands, cleanse the scalp of bacterial infection, and disperse dead skin cells. Lavender oil is also said to smooth knots and tangles and encourage hair growth.

However, there are five essential oils (p. 50) that stand out as being especially valuable for general skin and hair care because of their skin compatibility. They are all mild on the skin (nonirritant, nonphototoxic, and generally nonsensitizing), yet they possess powerful medicinal properties, being bactericidal, antiseptic, cytophylactic (healing), or anti-inflammatory, and all have a long history of use as cosmetic aids. These five oils are indispensable for all who wish to take an interest in the overall health and beauty of their skin.

Skin-care oils

For a guide to the properties of essential oils see pp. 239–343, and for details of base oils used in skin care see pp. 345–371.

BELOW Sources for some of the best oils for the skin and hair. From left to right: palmarosa, rosemary, geranium, and lavender.

LEFT Essential oils can be used for hair, scalp, and face in many ways.

Valuable oils for the skin

♡ ROSE

Rose has long been used as a favorite perfume ingredient and cosmetic oil. It is one of the most useful skin-care oils because, apart from its rich, feminine scent, it has good wound-healing properties that help in the daily process of skin repair. Rose oil and rose water have been used as ingredients in cosmetics for centuries, and their effects have been well tried and tested. Rose oil can help to keep the skin healthy, lubricated, and elastic, making it less prone to wrinkles. For general skin care, it is suited to all types of complexion, particularly dry, sensitive, and aging or mature skin.

♡ LAVENDER

Lavender is perhaps the most versatile skin-care oil of all because, although it has excellent antiseptic properties, it is very mild on the skin. It is also an excellent cicatrizant or wound-healing oil, which promotes tissue regeneration in everyday use and prevents scarring when used to treat damaged or injured skin. It is a valuable oil for all types of skin injury, but also for the treatment of a wide range of specific skin conditions. It is suited to all types of complexion, particularly oily and blemished skin. This gentle oil can safely be used neat if required.

♡ CHAMOMILE

Chamomile oil is a well-known soothing remedy, and particularly well suited to children. Because of its sedative and relaxant properties it is especially good for all types of skin complaints that have a nervous or stress-related element, such as the many types of dermatitis or eczema. It is also the best anti-inflammatory herb. Like rose oil it is good for sensitive skin, but it is especially indicated for all types of swelling, irritation, rashes, red or sore skin, including allergic skin conditions. Both Roman and German chamomile can be used in skin care.

♡ NEROLI

Neroli (derived from orange blossom) and the similar petitgrain (from the leaves of the bitter orange tree) are powerful bactericidal and antiseptic agents with excellent cytophylactic properties (encouraging the formation of new skin cells). Like rose and lavender, they have a most beautiful, classic scent, which is uplifting, fresh, and citrus-like. Orange flower water is traditionally used to soften the skin and it also has a gentle toning and astringent action. Neroli, petitgrain, and orange flower water are beneficial for all skin types, including normal or combination skin.

♡ TEA TREE

Tea tree is a valuable skin-care agent because it has excellent antiseptic, fungicidal, and antiviral properties, yet is very mild on the skin. It can be used for a wide range of specific skin conditions and for more general disinfectant purposes. In a theoretical comparison between tea tree and other antiseptics used for skin care, tea tree oil came closest to having all the properties of an ideal skin disinfectant.[‡] Although this oil is generally used medicinally, it is a useful addition to a collection of oils for cosmetic use.

RIGHT Roses have been cultivated for use in beauty and therapeutic products for centuries.

Tea tree oil and its uses

Tea tree oil is particularly indicated for infected skin conditions, including injuries (especially where there is pus or dirt), and for combating fungal diseases such as tinea or candida. It is also excellent for treating problems of viral origin such as cold sores, genital herpes, warts, and veruccas. It is especially recommended for use by those with blemished skin, acne, and greasy complexions.

BELOW In massage tea tree is diluted, and usually combined with other oils.

♡ It acts swiftly and effectively against a wide range of bacterial and fungal organisms, has good persistence, and the added benefit of excellent absorption into the skin.
♡ It possesses powerful cleansing properties noted repeatedly in the clinical literature.
♡ It does not irritate the skin, is not poisonous, does not harm tissue cells, and has no significant side effects.

♡ It is not easily contaminated.
♡ It is cosmetically very suitable, being colorless and having a pleasant, clean odor.
♡ It is nearly neutral in pH.
♡ It is notably effective where there is organic detritus (pus).
♡ It can be used to treat viral complaints with success.

Basic skin care

In skin care, most essential oils are used diluted. In the simplest treatments an essential oil is mixed with a suitable base oil (pp. 345–371) or with spring water. Basic creams and moisturizers for both cosmetic and medical use can also be made very simply. When making healing ointments, choose the oils you use for their therapeutic value, following the guide to aromatherapy use in the index of essential oils (pp. 238–343) and specific remedies on pp. 133–237. For cosmetic use, choose oils by reference to skin type, or by their scents.

SIMPLE HEALING OINTMENTS

♡ Ointments for treating specific skin complaints can be made by blending essential oils with a ready-made nonallergenic cream base, a herbal cream such as calendula cream, or homemade cold cream (see p. 55). Dilute to between 0.5 and 2.5 percent depending on the type of disorder and the area of the body (see p. 36). For a small quantity mix 2 to 3 drops of essential oil to a teaspoonful of cream base in a small container.

SIMPLE MOISTURIZER

♡ To make an aromatic facial moisturizer mix 8 to 10 drops of an essential oil (according to skin type) with a ready-made hypoallergenic, unscented cream or lotion (3½fl oz/100ml tube or 3½ oz/100g jar). In a glass or ceramic container, mix the essential oils into the cream, using a spoon. This blend can be used therapeutically and cosmetically for the face, neck, and hands, but also for body massage. Store in a sealed container away from light and heat.

Skin-care routine

MAINTAINING A HEALTHY, youthful-looking skin depends on everyday skin care as well as on general health. Products containing mineral oil are not absorbed into the lower dermal layers where the newly emerging cells require optimum nourishment. Mineral oil is also known to leach fat-soluble vitamins, especially A, D, and E, from the body. Most commercial toners contain alcohol, which has a drying effect on the skin and can cause irritation, as can many other synthetic ingredients found in creams and lotions. Even lanolin, though natural, is heavy, animal-derived and rather unpleasantly scented, and can cause allergic reactions. In contrast, natural vegetable oils, waxes, and creams, with selected essential oils, are ideal cosmetic aids because they are highly penetrative and can reach the small blood capillaries in the deeper dermal layers, thus rejuvenating the skin from within, while gentle flower waters tone without dehydrating the skin, and have a mild bactericidal action.

Many beauticians and body therapists now regularly use essential oils as part of their cosmetic treatments. It is also possible to carry out many effective beauty treatments at home, as part of a regular skin-care routine. Simply by using a selection of vegetable oils and essential oils together with other natural ingredients such as yogurt, clay, honey, oatmeal, and distilled water, it is possible to achieve and preserve a youthful-looking skin.

A basic skin-care routine

Different skin types require individual treatment but a good basic skin-care routine, which takes very little time, involves cleaning, toning, and moisturizing every morning and evening, and giving the skin extra-special nourishing, cleansing, and revitalizing treatments once a week. Recipes for basic oils, gels, and creams are given on pp. 54–56, recipes for masks and moisturizers are on p. 57, and recipes for simple fresheners and toner/cleansers on p. 58.

EVERY NIGHT

♥ Remove grime and make-up with a light vegetable oil (such as coconut, sweet almond, or apricot kernel oil) or a mild cleansing cream (such as the cold cream made as described on p. 55) with a cotton pad.
♥ Wipe away any excess oil using a cloth or pad dipped in warm water.

♥ Refresh the face and neck by applying flower water or a toner or cleanser (see p. 58) suited to your skin type.
♥ Apply moisturizing oil or night cream as suited to your skin type.
♥ Sparingly apply a moisturizing eye oil, cream, or gel (as shown, right). Wheat germ or rosehip seed oil is ideal.

EVERY MORNING

♡ Cleanse with a light cream or oil, then remove any excess with a cloth or pad and warm water.
♡ Refresh the face and neck with a flower water or toner/cleanser suited to your skin type.
♡ Apply a light moisturizing oil or cream (with sun protection if wished). Let it be absorbed by the skin before applying make-up, if worn.

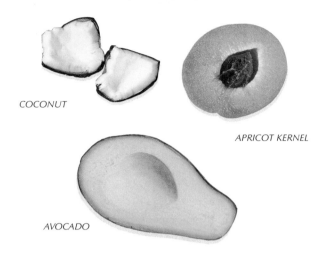

Sources of ingredients

COCONUT

APRICOT KERNEL

AVOCADO

Oils derived from fruits are nourishing and beneficial to the skin in many ways. Research has shown that they encourage the formation of fresh cells.

ONCE A WEEK

♡ To remove dead cells and debris from the skin surface, use dry skin brushing, a skin scrub, or an exfoliant.
♡ Give the face a nourishing massage (or receive a professional facial treatment) using rich oils, such as evening primrose, avocado, or borage. Massage with upward strokes.
♡ Give your face a steam treatment or facial sauna as described on p. 59. This opens the pores and deep-cleans the skin, to get rid of accumulated grime or dirt as well as detoxifying and bringing fresh blood to the surface.
♡ Apply a mask made from natural ingredients, as shown right. The ingredients of the mask should be chosen according to skin type. For instructions on making a mask and choosing ingredients see p. 57.

Oils and creams

BEAUTY, ESPECIALLY SKIN and hair care, is central to the practice of aromatherapy. But while receiving a full body massage from a professional aromatherapist or having an aromatic facial in a beauty clinic is certainly a treat, it is not essential for maintaining a clear and healthy complexion. Many aromatic recipes are simple to make, and regular treatment can easily be carried out at home.

FACIAL OILS

Facial oils are made up in the same way as general massage or body oils (p. 36), except that the base or carrier oil, as well as the essential oils, can be adapted to the type of skin which is to be treated. Suitable carrier oils include avocado, olive, wheat germ, hazelnut, apricot kernel, peach kernel, borage seed, carrot, and evening primrose, as well as the more basic carrier oils such as sweet almond, grapeseed, jojoba, or sunflower oil. Apart from nourishing and toning the skin, facial oils can also be used for facial massage and local self-massage.

TAPIOCA GEL RECIPE

Use 3½fl oz (100ml) water to 1½ tsp (7.5ml) tapioca. Mix and simmer until the tapioca is dissolved. Strain off the liquid and let it cool to form a transparent gel. Stir in a few drops of essential oil just before it sets.

FACIAL CREAMS

An aromatic facial cream should moisturize, heal, and nourish the skin, trapping the moisture in, but also letting the skin breathe. To make up a basic cream at home, use the instructions on p. 55, based on what is traditionally known as Galen's cold cream recipe.

ABOVE Apart from nourishing and toning the skin, facial oils can be used for massage.

GRAPES

HAZELNUTS

AVOCADO

BELOW Making your own beauty treatment oils and creams enables you to choose ingredients best suited to your skin, and a fragrance to your liking.

Facial oil recipe

Mix two parts of a basic carrier oil and one part of a specific carrier oil suited to the skin type, with 0.5 to 1% of an essential oil (or a blend of oils).

BASE OIL	PERCENTAGE	DROPS
1 tsp (5ml)	0.5–1%	1
1 tbsp (15ml)	0.5–1%	1–3
1fl oz (25ml)	0.5–1%	3–5
2fl oz (50ml)	0.5–1%	5–10
3½fl oz (100ml)	0.5–1%	10–20

Cold cream recipe

INGREDIENTS

4fl oz (120ml) almond oil ♥ ½oz (15g) beeswax beads or grated wax ♥ 2fl oz (50ml) rose water ♥ 6–10 drops rose essential oil or other essential oil according to skin type

BEESWAX

1 Put the beeswax beads into a toughened glass bowl and pour in the almond oil.

2 Place the bowl in a pan of water over a gentle heat, and mix until the ingredients are melted together.

3 Warm the rose water in a second bowl or jar, then add to the wax and oil mixture bit by bit, beating all the time.

4 Finally, stir in the essential oil, transfer the mixture to a pot, and put the pot into the refrigerator to set.

GELS

Water-based gels provide a useful, nonoily medium for the application of essential oils, as an alternative to oils and creams when required. A gel can be used to dilute any essential oils for irritating skin conditions such as eczema or athlete's foot, particularly if the skin is broken or sensitive. Gels are also suitable as a substitute for base or carrier oils for general skin care, especially if the skin is apt to be greasy. The percentage of essential oil to add to the gel base depends on where it will be used and for what purpose. Healing gels may include up to 2.5 percent of an essential oil when applied to the feet, whereas 0.5 percent is enough for application to the face or for general skin-care purposes. A natural soothing and cooling gel can be made with tapioca and water.

LEFT Water-based gels are a good means of applying essential oils to treat skin conditions. This is especially useful for oily skin.

MASKS

Face masks or packs have many benefits—they can nourish, rejuvenate, stimulate, cleanse, or soothe the skin, and generally improve its texture and quality. Masks can be made from a wide range of natural ingredients, including fruit pulp, oatmeal (for allergic and irritated skin conditions), egg yolk (for all skin types), yogurt, honey, and clay. Fruits such as avocado (for dry skin) or strawberry (for oily skin) are extremely nutritious. Powdered oatmeal is also very nourishing and gives the skin a smooth, silken appearance, and brewer's yeast is good for all types of skin. Egg yolks are rich in lecithin, an invaluable skin aid. Natural yogurt contains lactic acid, which is good for large-pored, oily, and blemished skin and to balance combination skin. Honey is moisturizing and slightly antiseptic and can be incorporated into masks to soothe, soften, and nourish the skin—especially dry, sensitive, and mature complexions.

Clay is a useful ingredient for making masks, and is suitable for all but very dry skins. An aromatic clay mask is excellent for the treatment of acne and congested skin conditions, and can nourish dry or mature complexions and help to balance combination skin. However, those with dry, sensitive, or mature complexions should not use a clay-based mask more than once a week because they do have an overall drying effect. Masks are best applied after a bath or shower, when the pores are open and the skin is still warm and slightly damp.

Clay cleanses and draws out toxins. It also aids skin regeneration, stimulates the circulation, and soothes inflammation. There are many different kinds of clay available, but green clay is the most versatile, being rich in minerals and a good antiseptic. Fuller's earth is also a good neutral clay base, which is more readily available.

ALTERNATIVE CLAY MASK

To make a more elaborate mask first mix 2oz (50g) green clay powder with 2 tsp (10ml) colloidal oatmeal and keep in a jar. To make the mask, mix 1 tbsp (15ml) of the basic mixture with 1 tbsp (15ml) runny honey or plain live yogurt, one egg yolk, 2 to 3 drops of an essential oil suited to your skin type, and enough water to give a smooth consistency. Apply to the skin and leave for 10 to 30 minutes—less for dry skin and longer for greasy/blemished skin. Rinse off with warm water. Finish by patting on a floral water.

Simple clay mask

To make a simple mask just add 2 to 3 drops of an essential oil to 2 tbsp (30ml) of wet clay paste, and apply to the skin. Leave in place for 10 to 30 minutes while you relax. Rinse off with warm water.

FLORAL WATER

Flower waters and steams

IT IS EASY to make flower (or floral) waters at home, and they are beneficial for all types of skin. Simply add 10 to 30 drops of essential oil (or a blend) to a 3½fl oz (100ml) bottle of spring or distilled water, leave it to stand for up to a month, and then filter the liquid using a coffee filter paper. (A more basic preparation can be made without filtering, but this must be shaken before each use.) Even a few drops of essential oil will impart their scent to this amount of water, making it very lightly fragranced. These delicately scented waters can be used to freshen and hydrate the skin, either dabbed on with absorbent cotton or sprayed from a small plant spray. This can be helpful during pregnancy, when traveling by air, in hot, dry climates, or simply to help counter the drying effects of central heating.

REFRESHING TOILET WATERS

A variety of essential oils can be diluted in a minute proportion with alcohol, cider vinegar, or witch hazel to make toilet waters, eau-de-Cologne, or after-shave lotions. For example, a traditional toilet water called eau-de-Portugal can be made as follows:

INGREDIENTS

20 drops sweet orange ♥ 5 drops bergamot ♥ 2 drops lemon ♥ 2 drops benzoin ♥ 1 drop geranium ♥ 1 tbsp (15ml) vodka ♥ 3½fl oz (100ml) spring water

METHOD

Dissolve the oils in the vodka, then add to the water, shaking well. Leave the mixture to mature for a month at least, then filter and bottle.

TONER/CLEANSERS

Using a flower water as the base, add a little witch hazel, which increases the overall astringency for a greater toning action. For additional moisturizing and cleansing properties, add up to 25 percent of natural glycerine to the mixture. Flower waters that contain a proportion of witch hazel and glycerine will remove oily residues from the skin as well as acting as an astringent and antiseptic. If no make-up (or very light make-up) is worn, they can be used for simple one-step cleansing and toning.

BELOW A few drops of essential oil can be added to spring water for the simplest toilet water.

ORANGE PEEL

LEMON LEAF

FACIAL TREATMENT

Used once a week, steaming can help to hydrate the skin, cleanse the pores, and eliminate deep-seated grime and toxins. It is possible to buy a special facial sauna or steamer, but the same result can be achieved by simply filling a basin with boiling water, covering your head with a towel, and letting the steam work for five minutes on your face.

To make the steam treatment even more effective, add to the water 6 to 10 drops of an essential oil (or a blend) suited to your skin type. Soaking in a steaming hot bathtub containing a few drops of aromatic oil can also help clear skin congestion.

After steaming, the skin should be cooled and balanced with a flower water to close the pores. This should be allowed to dry naturally. When the skin is completely dry, a light moisturizer should be applied.

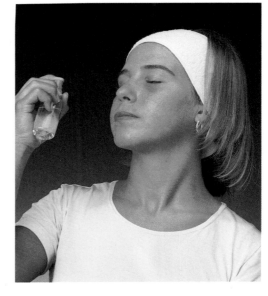

ABOVE Spray the face with fragrant flower waters to hydrate and freshen the skin.

WARNING
Avoid steam treatments if your skin is prone to thread veins. This type of skin reacts adversely to extremes of heat and cold and should be treated gently at all times.

RIGHT Eau-de-Cologne and toilet waters should be decanted into decorative glass bottles and kept well stoppered.

RIGHT Rose oil is one of the best skin treatments.

RIGHT Chamomile water soothes the skin.

Toiletries and treatments

FACE SCRUB OR EXFOLIANT

To remove dead cells from the surface of the skin and stimulate the circulation, moisten a little medium-ground oatmeal (or colloidal oatmeal—available from pharmacists) in the palm of your hand using a suitable aromatic flower water (see p. 58), and rub gently all over the face. For dry or sensitive skins, use ground almonds.

DRY AND WET BODY-BRUSHING

Rub one or two drops of a chosen essential oil into a dry loofah or a natural-bristle brush to make it smell fragrant. Start by rubbing the feet firmly with the brush, then gradually work your way up the body, concentrating on any congested or fatty areas, such as the hips or thighs. Work up the arms, paying special attention to the backs of the upper arms, up the back from the waist, up over the abdomen, and down the front from the shoulders.

Popular in Scandinavia, this technique stimulates the circulation, helps break down fatty deposits, and brings a glow to the skin. Used in combination with other approaches, it is helpful for removing cellulite. For a milder effect, the same technique can also be used in the shower or bath, using a few drops of essential oil on a wet brush, loofah, or sponge.

AROMATIC SCALP OIL PREPARATIONS

Local massage is very effective for conditions such as hair loss and brittle or dry hair, if it is carried out on a regular basis. Massage also stimulates scalp circulation and nourishes the deeper layers of the skin, bringing more nutrients to the follicles and improving the hair. To make a scalp massage oil, mix 8 tsp/40ml coconut oil and 2 tsp (10ml) wheat germ oil with between 10 and 25 drops of essential oil depending on hair and skin type.

BELOW Massage oil into the scalp to nourish the scalp. Lavender oil is good for dandruff.

LAVENDER

OATMEAL

ABOVE Body-brushing or an oatmeal scrub improves the circulation and acts as an exfoliant to remove dull-looking dead cells.

Body powders

Aromatic body powders can be made by mixing about 4 tbsp (30g) unperfumed talc or cornstarch with 5 to 6 drops of essential oils. Seal the mixture in a closed container and let the base absorb the oils for at least 24 hours before use.

HAIR CONDITIONER

To make a good hair conditioner to encourage hair growth and improve the quality of the hair structure, mix 10 drops of essential oil with 5 tsp (25ml) of slightly warmed jojoba oil, castor oil, or extra virgin olive oil, and rub this thoroughly into the scalp. Cover the hair with a layer of waxed paper, wrap in warm towels, and leave for an hour. Wash out, applying shampoo before the water, otherwise the hair will remain oily. Repeat weekly.

HAIR TONIC

Aromatic hair tonics are especially recommended for oily or thinning hair, because they can help to balance sebum levels (the oil produced at the base of the hair) and promote hair growth. Dissolve about 10 drops of essential oils suited to your hair type in one tablespoon of cider vinegar and add to 3½fl oz (100ml) of lavender water. Shake well and massage into the scalp.

QUICK SCALP RUB

A quick method to use for treating the scalp between washes, if required, is to rub about 10 drops of pure tea tree or lavender oil into the scalp using the fingertips. This is beneficial for the treatment of dandruff and as a general conditioner.

DRY SHAMPOO

It is not beneficial to wash the hair too often, as this can strip the hair of its protective acid mantle. When short of time, or between shampoos, simply add a drop of rosemary essential oil, or an oil chosen for its fragrance, to one tablespoon of orris root powder or fuller's earth. Part the hair in sections and sprinkle the mixture on. Leave for five minutes, then brush out thoroughly.

AROMATIC SHAMPOO

Buy a neutral pH shampoo (this is marked on the label) and add your own choice of essential oils to it. Add one or two drops of essential oil to a capful of shampoo at each wash, or add 30 to 50 drops of your chosen essential oil (or a blend) to a 3½fl oz/100ml bottle of shampoo, and shake well before using.

AROMATIC RINSE

Add a few drops of a suitable aromatherapy oil, such as chamomile, lavender, or rosemary, to the final rinse water together with one tablespoon of cider vinegar. This very effective, yet simple, procedure gives the hair a wonderful shine and maintains the acid mantle of the scalp. It also imparts a delicious fragrance and new vitality to the hair.

LEFT Powdered orris root can be used as the basis of an effective dry shampoo.

RIGHT Fuller's earth is used for scalp treatment.

WARNING

Some oils, including ylang ylang, cedarwood, cypress, lemon, lime, juniper, mandarin, and pine, are not stable in shampoo or detergent and should therefore not be used.

Aromatherapy and perfumery

THE PSYCHOLOGICAL EFFECTS of fragrance have long been recognized, while herbs have probably been used for their specific effects by so-called "primitive" peoples since the dawn of time. It is certain that in the past natural aromatic substances were often employed successfully for their hallucinogenic, sedative, stimulating, sexually arousing, or anesthetizing effects on the mind, but a proper study of the action of scents, and specifically of essential oils, on the mind and behavior has never been completed.

Psycho-aromatherapy

Psycho-aromatherapy, which focuses primarily on the psychological potential of essential oils, consists of two separate but interrelated fields—aromatic medicine and perfumery. In psycho-aromatherapy, the physiological effect of specific essential oils on the systems of the body is combined with the individual's emotional or psychological reaction to their fragrance—with both aspects working together in a psychosomatic unity. It could be said that there are three different dimensions involved:

♥ **the physiochemical dimension:** the chemical structure of the odor, its quality and concentration or intensity

♥ **the physiological dimension:** the primary and secondary biological processes that are initiated upon contact with the oil

♥ **the psychological dimension:** the subjective individual response to an odor—how the individual describes and is affected by it.

Some fragrances are generally experienced as pleasing, while others are widely perceived as repugnant, yet it is difficult to make hard and fast rules about how any individual will react to a particular smell. This is because the physiological effect of a given odor can be overridden by an individual's specific emotional associations and psychological preferences. Sometimes even an unpleasant smell can have beneficial results if the associations are positive.

The close connection between the sense of smell and the experience of emotion has often been noted. It is suggested that, physiologically, molecules of odor in some way stimulate the same brain centers that signal the drives toward or away, which underlie almost all human emotion.[5]

> "HE SAW THAT THERE WAS NO MOOD OF THE MIND THAT HAD NOT ITS COUNTERPART IN THE SENSUOUS LIFE ..."
>
> OSCAR WILDE

ABOVE Responses to scents vary, but the rose has a perfume that is universally appreciated.

Our sense of smell influences our moods, emotions, and memories. In view of the idiosyncratic quality of smell, it is virtually impossible to assess accurately in advance an individual's reaction to a particular odor, or to prescribe a fragrance for therapeutic purposes without taking all the following considerations into account:

♡ **biological:** the effect the odor is likely to have physiologically on the systems of the body—whether it is stimulating or sedating

♡ **archetypal associations:** any universal associations the odor may have—the scent of the rose, for example, suggests femininity, love, divinity, and sweetness in all cultures

♡ **cultural connotations:** certain scents take on a specific meaning according to the environmental, social, and cultural factors involved—the odor of frankincense, for example, will be especially significant in a culture that is Roman Catholic

♡ **individual responses:** personal associations and preferences due to first-hand experience, which may be either positive or negative.

Since our response to scent is so individualistic, to what extent is it possible to use odors to bring about a predictable response? The writer Michael Stoddard asserts that although there is no odor capable of systematically inducing a given reaction in human beings, it is nevertheless possible that we are still subconsciously manipulated by odors. Since the sexual and social instincts of human beings are no longer controlled by scent-signals as they are in other mammals, odors do not bring about overt changes in human sexual or emotional behavior; rather, they create changes in mood or feeling states, often at a subliminal level. Such changed states, as studies have shown, can subtly color and redirect our thoughts, often without our noticing.[6]

Scents largely influence us unwittingly. This is what endows them with such great psychological potential, for better or for worse. At present, there is a great deal of scientific interest in the potential psychological effects of aromas, and the Fragrance Research Foundation in New York has in recent years coined the term "aromachology" to describe the study and use of natural or synthetic odors in this field. The current commercial trend is also moving toward a rapid increase in the utilization of fragrance as a marketing agent. For example, in a trial test using fragranced shoes, it was shown that customers were attracted to the scented items in preference to nonscented items—even if they did not know why.

For exactly the same reasons that scent can sell shoes, fragrance can also be used as a very powerful therapeutic tool, especially for psychological or psychosomatic complaints. Fragrance has been found to be an ideal candidate for use in relaxation work, because it directly targets the inner mind, and bypasses any critical interference by the verbal, conscious mind.

ABOVE Masked Venetian ladies buying perfume in "The Perfume Seller" by Pietro Longhi, 1702–1785.

ABOVE Strong odors such as frankincense are thought to affect mood and emotion through a physiological effect on the brain.

CARDAMOM

LEMON

The word "osmotherapy" has been suggested specifically to describe the utilization of scents, both natural and artificial, for therapeutic purposes.[7]

This approach, however, is quite distinct from psycho-aromatherapy, in that the latter employs only natural fragrances derived from botanical sources, and also combines inhalation with other methods of treatment. In aromatherapy, therapeutic massage forms a large part of the individual's treatment. Aromatherapy massage is particularly beneficial because it combines inhalation with the healing effects of touch. Aromatic bathing also harmonizes scent with relaxation, as well as promoting absorption of the essential oils through the skin.

Thus, the practice of psycho-aromatherapy, while concentrating on the power of smell, actually embraces a variety of methods and techniques. In this respect it is a truly psychosomatic type of treatment for it operates on the body, mind, and emotions.

GERANIUM

LAVENDER

SCENT AND STRESS

The sense of smell is intimately connected with, and influences the functioning of, the central nervous system. Moreover, many illnesses could be said to be rooted in the mind—in a person's negative outlook or underlying fears. It is well known that mental states such as anxiety, irritation, or anger cause physical changes in the body, including an increase in heart rate, and change in breathing pattern and muscle tone. Stress and mental unrest, which are thought to be at the root of so much of our 20th-century "disease," eventually produce a degenerative effect on the entire organism.

There is also a reciprocal relationship between stress and scent, in that certain smells, especially those with pheromonal potential (the potential to influence others of their species), can cause stress reactions and vice versa. Animals are particularly sensitive to this phenomenon, but the smell of fear or the smell of disease can sometimes be picked up by humans with a trained nose. Happiness and good health have their characteristic scents, too.

A person's subconscious attitudes are related to the limbic system, the most primitive part of the brain concerned with basic emotions and mood. Since the body and mind are intrinsically related, a change in the mental or psychological disposition of an individual can have dramatic results on the person's physical health.

And, since the limbic system is especially susceptible to the effects of fragrance, it is possible to heighten or influence a person's underlying dispositions and attitudes by subjecting him or her to certain scents.

While scents have a chemical effect as they are absorbed by the bloodstream via the nose, they also work at a psychobiological level: for example, when we savor a pleasant fragrance, we take perceptibly deeper and slower breaths, relaxing our respiratory pattern much as we do in meditation. A scent can also serve to distract us, by becoming the focus for our attention, or by inducing positive memories and emotions.[8]

Mood and fragrance

Some negative emotional states that can be altered by fragrance are:

PASSIVE	ACTIVE
Depression	Anxiety ♥ Nervous
♥ Apathy ♥	tension ♥ Anger ♥
Melancholy ♥	Impatience ♥ Panic
Indecision ♥	
Despair	

RIGHT Scents rapidly affect our mood and emotions via the brain.

olfactory bulb

molecules of scent

scent enters nasal cavity

brain

thalamus

receptor cells

supporting cells

Aromatherapy massage treatment can take advantage of the fact that the benefits of the massage are reinforced by the scent of the oils used, and that the scent comes to be associated quickly with the beneficial, pleasure-giving and relaxing effects of the treatment. The odors of the oils used thus carry a positive association that makes the recipient more receptive and reinforces the effect of subsequent treatments, by causing positive anticipation. The subtle choice of oils to match a person's emotional make-up can open the door to helping that person to re-experience pleasure or joy.

This is similar to the use of incense in ritual and religious practices, where the familiar scent of the incense helps to bring about, through repetition as well as in its own right, a receptive and uplifting state of mind.

In a recent research trial, J.R. King found that some fragrances were normally very effective in promoting relaxation through association, despite individual variations. He has utilized a seaside fragrance in his relaxation work, because of its widespread positive associations, although he points out that if it is then used to counteract negative moods in stressful situations, such a fragrance would be best used sparingly and for brief periods, to preserve its value as a conditioned stimulus. Judiciously chosen and employed, however, essential oils, used in conjunction with massage in aromatherapy, can form a counter-vibration to that of the negative mood, and help to restore harmony.

Different attempts have been made to structure the relation between mood and scent. In *Essential Oils as Psychotherapeutic Agents*, Robert Tisserand proposes eight mood categories, in which essential oil can be used to help counteract or balance extremes of emotion (as illustrated on facing page). The essential oils are highlighted in terms of the mood which they generally evoke. Ylang ylang generally inspires passion and also helps combat anger, and can be used to help frigidity and introversion. Jasmine may be used as a valuable oil for a person who is uninspired, dull, and in need of new ideas.

There can be a danger in linking particular essential oils too closely with specific emotions, because of the idiosyncratic nature of smell. When using natural aromatics for psychotherapeutic purposes, it is important to assess the personality or temperament of each person and to take his or her odor associations and preferences into account. In choosing fragrances that may correspond to the needs of an individual, personal preferences can often be of value as a therapeutic guide. Much as at times we crave certain foods that can supply nutritional elements which our body is lacking, so we may be emotionally drawn toward particular fragrances that have a balancing effect on our psychic disposition as a whole. Even a disagreeable reaction to a particular scent may give the aromatherapist an indication of a hidden or repressed area of psyche that needs attention.

Aromatherapists will frequently observe that their clients are instinctively drawn toward the essential oil that is right for their needs, and that as the client's emotional state alters, so, often, does their aroma preference.

ABOVE Scents function at the psychobiological level.

BELOW The Tisserand wheel illustrates the links between some common emotional states and specific oils. Personality type is shown in the outer wheel, then the "emotional" quality of the perfume and name of the oil, next the emotional state the oil can act on, and finally the type of action that the oil has.

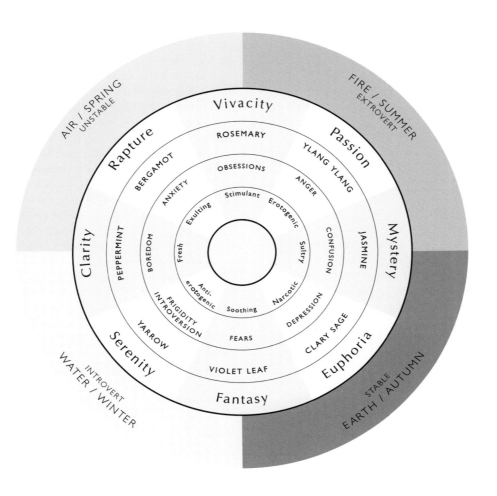

Wheel labels (outer ring, clockwise):
- AIR / SPRING UNSTABLE
- FIRE / SUMMER EXTROVERT
- EARTH / AUTUMN STABLE
- WATER / WINTER INTROVERT

Emotional qualities (outer): Vivacity, Passion, Mystery, Euphoria, Fantasy, Serenity, Clarity, Rapture

Oils and emotional states (inner rings):
- Rapture — BERGAMOT — ANXIETY — Exulting
- ROSEMARY — OBSESSIONS — Stimulant
- YLANG YLANG — ANGER — Erotogenic
- JASMINE — CONFUSION — Sultry
- Mystery
- CLARY SAGE — DEPRESSION — Narcotic
- VIOLET LEAF — FEARS — Soothing
- YARROW — FRIGIDITY INTROVERSION — Anti-erotogenic
- PEPPERMINT — BOREDOM — Fresh
- Clarity

Center ring actions: Exulting, Stimulant, Erotogenic, Sultry, Narcotic, Soothing, Anti-erotogenic, Fresh

YARROW

JASMINE

YLANG YLANG

Perfume and personality

CHOOSING A PERFUME to suit their mood and personality is one way in which most women—and, increasingly, many men—practice a form of aromatherapy on themselves. We can all observe that choice of perfume, just like color preference, is highly individual, despite prevailing fashions, and moreover that there is a distinct link between personality types and the type of perfume worn.

Why does a person like or dislike a particular scent or choose one perfume rather than another? The relationship between perfume and personality, between the "essence" of a person and the "essence" of a perfume, is an area that has intrigued the perfumery industry for centuries. The correlation between personality and fragrance was initially a supposition based on observation, but research into the psychophysiological factors involved in this field now supports the truth of the theory. Whatever the scientific explanation, the perfume chosen can highlight the personality of the wearer, and a personalized perfume, made as a unique blend for the person alone, can do this even more perfectly. An English physician of the 19th century stated that, in his opinion, a perfume should correspond to the personality, physical, emotional, and mental characteristics of its wearer, and should be as specific to each woman as the sound of her voice.[9]

PERSONALITY TYPES AND COLOR AND PERFUME PREFERENCE

A specific correlation of different scent types with personality types was made by the scientist and perfume expert R.W. Moncrieff. He noted that extroverts were less finely tuned in their odor preferences than introverts, and that they preferred lighter fragrances while introverts tended to be drawn to heavier, oriental scents.

The researchers Mensing and Beck have developed these notions further, showing a link between color and perfume preferences. They produced a series of eight circles, each with eight different overlapping color segments. The colors within each circle were chosen to match the preferences of the eight most common personality types, as shown below.

Orange/yellow/red/green: "extroverted mood tendency" — readiness to take risks, sociable, like stimulation. Fragrance has fresh (green) notes.

Purple/violet/white: "introverted mood tendency" — need inner tranquility, less need for stimulation, individual/alternative lifestyle, younger age group. Fragrance has oriental notes.

Black and white: "emotionally ambivalent mood tendency" — highly sensitive, moody, romantic, fashion-oriented. Fragrance has floral, powdery notes.

Bright pastels: "emotionally ambivalent with extroverted mood tendency" — idealistic, cheerful, impulsive, satisfied, and content. Fragrance has floral fruity notes.

Dark violet/warm colors: "emotionally ambivalent with introverted mood tendency" — materialistic, need security, avoid conflicts, like stability. Fragrance has oriental floral notes.

Dark red/green/orange: "emotionally stable with extroverted mood tendency" — conservative, socially active, family-oriented, radiate warmth and strength, appreciate quality. Fragrance has chypre (sandalwood) notes.

Bright blue/yellow: "emotionally stable with introverted mood tendency" — well-mannered, self-controlled, do not overstep others' boundaries. Fragrance has aldehydic (almost overpowering) floral notes.

Brown/green/yellow: "indefinable" — straightforward, uncomplicated people with very stable moods. These people do not have a typical preferred fragrance.

Formulating an individual blend

A MORE ELABORATE version of Mensing and Beck's color chart is still used widely in the perfume industry to create new scents and to help target specific markets. It has also been adapted for psycho-aromatherapeutic purposes, where it can be employed to help aromatherapists select an essence from the range of natural aromatics. An introverted individual, for example, is likely to be attracted to oriental oils and incense materials, such as frankincense, patchouli, sandalwood, or galbanum—while an extroverted type will prefer fresh, fruity oils such as bergamot, lemon, or grapefruit.

When we move into the therapeutic use of essences, there are other factors to be considered apart from the esthetic appeal. While in perfumery the esthetic consideration is paramount, in therapeutic work the efficacy of the remedy is of prime importance. When dealing with the therapeutic application of essences, there are two separate dynamics to consider:

♥ a fragrance that corresponds to the physical, emotional, and mental characteristics of the wearer

♥ ingredients that are needed to balance what is absent in the health or personality of the wearer.

The need to choose a fragrance specifically tailored to the requirements of each individual client was the conclusion reached by the aromatherapist Marguerite Maury in her therapeutic work. She found that, of all the aspects of plant oils and their fragrances, "the greatest interest lies in the effect of fragrance on the psychic and mental state of the individual. Powers of perception become clearer and [events] are seen more objectively, and therefore in truer perspective."[10]

In devising her individual prescriptions, Mme. Maury assessed the physical, mental, and emotional disposition of each patient so that the remedy perfectly mirrored the patient. There is, for example, the case of the sad and anxious elderly man suffering from stress and insomnia, with a heart and kidney weakness. The individual mixture for this client was made up from rose, sandalwood, lavender, geranium, and benzoin. Benzoin dispels anxiety and interposes "a padded zone between us and events. Rose and sandalwood oil compensate for renal and cardiac deficiencies; lavender and geranium normalize…"[11]

Since remedies are so allied to the patient's state, blends evolve and change during the course of treatment in a subtle interaction between oils, blender, and patient.

MAKING A PERSONAL PERFUME

You will need:

A selection of essential oils with dropper tops ♥ jojoba oil or fractionated coconut oil ♥ small, clean glass bottle with a tight stopper or lid ♥ note pad and pen ♥ blotting paper strips

Before beginning, lay out all the ingredients and materials needed on a clean surface in an odor-free environment. Using the blotting strips to assess the scent is described in detail on p. 72.

1 Select the oils that you think will be required to constitute the dominant notes in the blend (p. 70), including base note, middle note, and top note oils. Measure out the base oils in drops into a small glass bottle containing 1 tsp (5ml) jojoba or fractionated coconut oil, following your intuition as to proportions. Record the name and exact quantity of each oil used.

3 Add the top notes, measuring and recording as before. Shake well and test.

2 Shake the bottle and assess the scent with a blotting paper strip. Add the middle note oils, measuring and recording carefully. Shake the bottle again and assess the effect as before.

4 Fine-tune, either by adding more drops of some ingredients, or by incorporating a new element. Add these oils a drop at a time, as one drop can radically affect the overall balance. Test the revised mixture on a new blotter strip.

5 When satisfied, seal the mixing bottle. Store it in a dark place for several weeks to mature. Check again to ensure the scent is rounded and well balanced.

The art of perfume blending

PERFUMERY IS BOTH a science and an art—it requires precision and sensitivity, but above all the ability to translate an intangible emotional experience or idea into a tangible composition.

In blending a perfume, the "rules of composition" have to be obeyed, as in music or painting, but the blender's creative skills transcend these rules to produce an indefinable blend that stirs the emotions and echoes a mood. A professional perfumer has to have a thorough knowledge of the properties of a huge range of ingredients, and how they interact, but it is nevertheless possible to make successful perfumes for one's own use, and as gifts for other people, using essential oils.

People generally prefer a many-layered fragrance, since a combination of different aromas tends to be more interesting and intriguing. When natural aromatic oils are combined, the effect is a chemical reaction that breaks up their original molecular structure and they recombine to form entirely new molecules. The final quality of the blend is always an unknown factor. The aim is to make a "bouquet" or a "seamless scent," where the whole adds up to more than just a sum of its parts. The famous French perfumer Pierre Dhumez declared that the ideal perfume

LEFT Many of the spicy and more exotic essential oils come from the East.

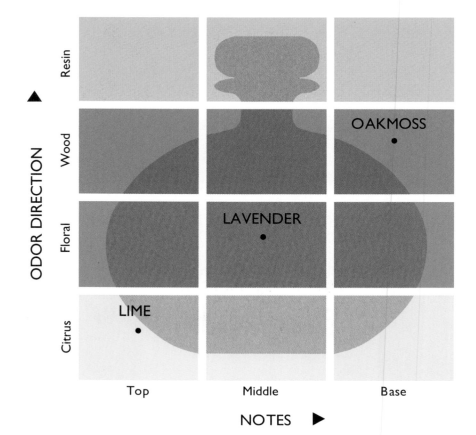

LEFT A good perfume has a range of top, middle, and base notes.

ODOR DIRECTION ▲

Resin
Wood
Floral
Citrus

OAKMOSS

LAVENDER

LIME

Top   Middle   Base

NOTES ▶

consisted of a basic harmonious blend of just three or four dominant "bodies." When combined in "inspired" proportions they form a whole in which it is impossible to distinguish one odor from the other. The scent is a perfectly balanced mixture which smells as a separate entity. This basic harmony, once it has been achieved, is enhanced by the addition of tiny amounts of other fragrances.

In the art of blending, balance is everything. In his book *The Art of Perfumery*, Charles Piesse was the first to draw an analogy between odors and sounds. To create a perfect "bouquet" of odors, he chose scents that combined to create a harmonious chord and added other scents to act as half-notes.

Modern perfumery still uses Piesse's terms to describe the art of blending, although in a simplified form. The perfume should be a perfect balance between the top, middle, and base notes. The top notes are immediately apparent—the ones that are light and fresh—and are the most volatile ingredients. Typical top notes include lime, lemon, and bergamot. The middle note lies at the heart of the fragrance, and usually forms the bulk of the blend—typical middle notes are florals such as lavender, rose, or geranium. The base note gives depth to the fragrance and acts as a fixative for the more volatile components—typical base notes include oakmoss, benzoin, or patchouli.

Another simple way of blending oils is to put them into families. Fragrances from the same family tend to mix together well, as do those from neighboring families. A small proportion of a scent from an opposed or diverse family can add interest or piquancy to an otherwise dull blend.

NEROLI

PETITGRAIN

LEFT A fine perfume is worthy of a fine container.

ABOVE The art of perfumery is as old as civilization.

Fragrance families

THE BIRTH OF modern Western perfumery as we know it today occurred during the 14th century with the discovery of alcoholic extraction techniques. Before that time, perfumes had been based on fatty or oily materials which did not allow the finesse afforded by alcohol or synthetics. Many modern perfumers consider that it is impossible to make a good perfume without the use of synthetics or alcohol. This is because these ingredients can impart lift, radiance, and diffusion to an accord. In their view, only eau-de-Colognes can be made wholly from simple, natural ingredients (known as naturals).

On the other hand, synthetics can have a flat and two-dimensional quality, whereas natural essences are more full-bodied and complex. In addition, many people are sensitive to certain chemicals used in modern perfumes and toiletries, which can cause skin allergies, headaches, or other side effects in sensitive individuals. Some modern perfumes contain well over 100 different ingredients or compounds, but for the purpose of aromatherapy it is enough to blend as few as three oils to produce an interesting result. This is because pure essential oils, unlike synthetic chemical fragrances used in modern perfumery, already contain many different components, each being made up, in some cases, of hundreds of different constituents, including trace elements. Rose oil, for example, contains over 300 constituents, which is why it is so difficult to imitate it or to construct a "nature identical" rose scent.

To gain familiarity with the different essences and to develop your sense of discrimination, test oils individually. Do not smell essential oils directly from the bottle. Always use a strip of blotting paper. Ideally, dilute the oil to 50 percent, using a bland base. Dip the paper into the essence, then study the odor immediately. After a few minutes smell it again, then periodically over several hours. You will see that the most volatile components will rise quickly up the blotting paper and disperse, while the more viscous elements will remain at the tip. Mark the strip clearly at the other end and record your results on the perfumery dial shown opposite, starting at the top with the floral notes and then moving round the face. For example, if floral notes are absent, put a dot in the center; if predominant, put a dot in the outer circle. Continue around the circle, trying to detect each note in turn, to complete the profile.

Trying to identify or verbalize a particular scent is difficult, yet odor classification is most important for developing scent discrimination and perfecting the art of blending. In modern perfumery work, this discrimination includes knowledge of all the synthetic fragrances now available. Indol, for example, is a natural component of jasmine absolute, now produced chemically. In concentration, it smells strongly camphoraceous, but in minute proportions it adds sweetness and volume to heavy, floral-based accords. In psycho-aromatherapy, however, the groups of aromas are wholly natural in origin, as in original perfumery classifications.

MANDARIN

RIGHT Many essential oils are a complex blend of fragrances in their own right. Using this perfumery dial helps in analyzing the individual elements and building up a fragrance profile for a particular oil. The dial is shown marked up for rose oil.

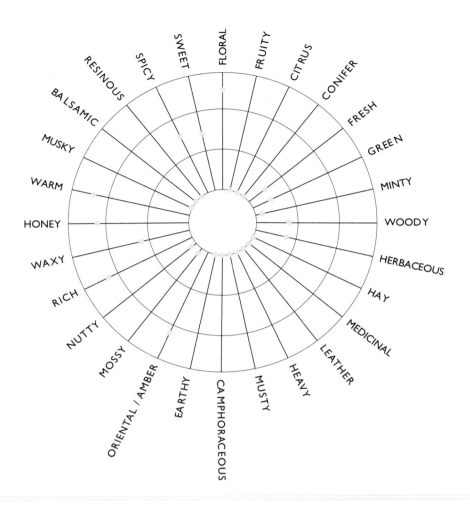

The labels around the wheel (clockwise from top):

FLORAL, FRUITY, CITRUS, CONIFER, FRESH, GREEN, MINTY, WOODY, HERBACEOUS, HAY, MEDICINAL, LEATHER, HEAVY, MUSTY, CAMPHORACEOUS, EARTHY, ORIENTAL / AMBER, MOSSY, NUTTY, RICH, WAXY, HONEY, WARM, MUSKY, BALSAMIC, RESINOUS, SPICY, SWEET

Fragrance families and their effects

The following table is based on the Austrian perfumer, Jellinek's concept of relating perfumes to skin and hair type.

FRESH (BLOND)

GREEN ♥ Reviving (e.g. thyme)
HERBACEOUS ♥ Stimulating (e.g. basil)
MEDICINAL ♥ Clearing (e.g. eucalyptus)

SOOTHING (BRUNETTE)

SPICY ♥ Warming (e.g. nutmeg)
WOODY ♥ Appeasing (e.g. sandalwood)
EARTHY ♥ Grounding (e.g. vetivert)

SULTRY (BLACK)

MUSKY ♥ Aphrodisiac (e.g. patchouli)
ORIENTAL ♥ Comforting (e.g. benzoin)
HONEY ♥ Heady (e.g. ylang ylang)

EXALTING (RED)

FLORAL ♥ Uplifting (e.g. geranium)
FRUITY ♥ Enlivening (e.g. petitgrain)
CITRUS ♥ Refreshing (e.g. lemon)

PART TWO

Aromatherapy
Massage

Aromatherapy massage

MASSAGE IS ONE of the most fundamental forms of therapy, and has been utilized by many diverse cultures for thousands of years. The need to be touched is itself an essential and primitive human instinct, for without physical contact, the overall health of the individual suffers. Recent research has shown that a lack of tactile contact is associated with immune depression, and positive touch with immune stimulation.

Over the course of time, many different massage techniques have been developed, each having its own individual therapeutic approach. The oriental art of shiatsu massage, for example, works primarily with specific pressure points along the lines of the meridians or channels of energy in the body, to influence the overall balance of energy within the body, much like acupuncture. In contrast, the Western style of Swedish massage concentrates more on releasing areas of tension trapped within the muscles, joints, and connective tissues of the body. Even performing the same stroke in different ways can produce different effects. A single movement performed vigorously can stimulate the body, while a similar movement performed slowly can promote relaxation.

Massage not only improves circulation and relaxes muscles, but also has psychological benefits, making the recipient feel comforted and cared for, and produces a unique sense of well-being.[12] However, when the general benefits of massage are combined with the effect of specific essential oils being rubbed into the skin, the healing dynamics already at work can take on a completely new dimension.

The actual techniques of aromatherapy massage are adapted mainly from the Swedish massage style, combined with a more individualistic approach to body work, adopted from the intuitive massage style initiated in the early 1960s. The theory behind the preparation of the essential oils themselves is based largely on the ideas of the French dermatologist, Marguerite Maury. Her concept of the individual prescription is still utilized by most professional aromatherapists working today, and they always prepare an individually chosen blend of essential oils for each client and for each massage session, depending on the needs of the client on each separate occasion.

There are three distinct but overlapping aspects of an aromatherapy massage treatment and this form of therapy can therefore be seen as being beneficial in three quite distinct but interrelated ways:

- ♡ the massage itself and its effects on the body
- ♡ the interraction between therapist and recipient
- ♡ the effect of the essential oils.

Each aspect supports the others in such a way as to provide a multidimensional therapeutic action. During a treatment, the essential oils themselves also interact with the body in two ways:

- ♡ through inhalation (primarily psychological effects)
- ♡ through absorption into the bloodstream via the skin (primarily physiological effects).

JASMINE

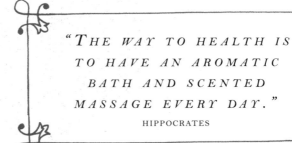

"*THE WAY TO HEALTH IS TO HAVE AN AROMATIC BATH AND SCENTED MASSAGE EVERY DAY.*"

HIPPOCRATES

Touch and smell: a healing synergy

THE SYNERGY OF essential oils and massage has been shown to be a very effective combination in the treatment of stress-related disorders, due to the powerful interaction of touch and smell. During the course of a massage, a certain amount of the essential oils will be absorbed through the skin and into the blood stream to affect the nervous system, as well as other parts of the body directly, by toning, sedating, or stimulating. When this is backed up by a comforting and supportive relationship between patient and therapist, it can provide a vital key to breaking the stress cycle of anxiety, insomnia, and nervous fatigue that underlies so many common physical complaints.

There is increasing evidence to show that stress affects not just the mind, but also the nervous, immune, and endocrine systems, and that it constitutes a factor in physical, as well as mental health.[13]

It is not surprising that stress-related problems are an area in which aromatherapy massage enjoys a great deal of success, because it simultaneously operates on both a physical and psychological level. An aromatic massage, for example, is especially valuable for those who suffer from a number of different responses to stress at the same time. Stress-related illness often presents a wide range of contradictory symptoms. Aromatherapy, rather than dealing separately with individual symptoms such as high blood pressure, indigestion, and back pain, deals with the stress itself. In the words of Dr. Ann Coxon:

"Obviously, the approach of holistic treatment is to help enable people to manage their primary life situation, and the ability of aromatherapy to get at the knot, at the stress reaction itself within the body without using yet more pharmacological treatment is terribly important."[14]

Evidence of the widespread sense of "disease" experienced today in the West is shown in the high consumption of tranquilizers and stimulants, although it is well known that addiction, toxicosis and other side effects can be caused by these products if taken regularly. Any treatment that can help to revitalize and de-stress the organism, without producing detrimental side effects, is therefore of great value. Essential oils, used in the appropriate doses, are safe and harmless, and it is widely agreed that, while they can be highly effective, they "do not cause troubles like those produced by the ordinary psychological drugs."[15]

WARNING

Although aromatherapy massage is effective for both the prevention and treatment of stress-related disorders, it is also very important for the individual to be helped to assess factors such as lifestyle, work patterns, and emotional relationships, and to try to make necessary changes to combat the causes behind the stress reaction directly.

Essential oils to relieve stress

There are many essential oils that are particularly suited to the treatment of stress-related conditions, both on a physical and psychological level. Lavender is possibly the most useful oil employed in this context, because of its regulating effect on the nervous functions, and due to its versatile nature. Other oils which are especially valuable for stress-relief include chamomile, rose, jasmine, neroli, bergamot, geranium, frankincense, and ylang ylang.

JASMINE

CHAMOMILE

LAVENDER

Sources of base oils used in massage

Essential oils used in massage are nearly always diluted in a base or carrier oil. Use good-quality, preferably cold-pressed oils, as they are absorbed more effectively into the skin. Some good carrier oils for general use include sweet almond, sunflower, grapeseed, and coconut oil (see pp. 345–371 for further details on base oils).

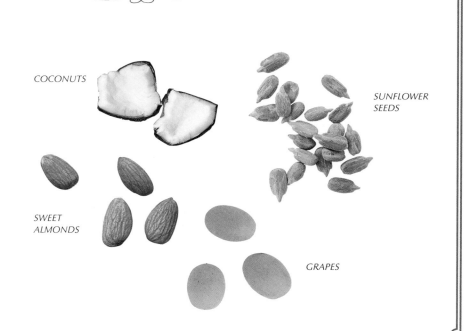

COCONUTS

SUNFLOWER SEEDS

SWEET ALMONDS

GRAPES

Massage techniques

THE FOLLOWING MASSAGE TECHNIQUES should be carried out with a steady, repetitive rhythm. Throughout the massage, try to link the different techniques together into a seamless sequence. If possible, keep at least one hand in contact with the person being massaged at all times, even when moving from one part of the body to another. Before working on the deeper muscles, it is important to warm and relax the superficial ones. While working on a specific part of the body, therefore, the techniques progress from gentle stroking movements to more active rubbing or kneading movements, and eventually to vigorous percussion-type strokes. In general, the more slowly a stroke is performed, the more relaxing it will be. Conversely, the more briskly and rapidly a movement is performed, the more stimulating its effects will be.

BENEFITS OF MASSAGE

♡ Provides a soothing and comforting alternative to verbal therapeutic techniques, such as counseling.

♡ Eases muscular aches and pains and promotes muscle relaxation and tone.

♡ Improves the circulation and lymphatic drainage, and helps to eliminate toxins from the body.

♡ Lowers blood pressure, reduces stress levels, and will help combat insomnia.

♡ Generates confidence and a feeling of well-being by releasing endorphins, the brain's natural opiates.

♡ Stimulates the immune system and strengthens resistance to disease.

♡ Aids digestion, eases constipation, and relieves abdominal spasm.

♡ Imparts a warmth and glow to the skin, and is revitalizing and rejuvenating to the whole body.

♡ Can alleviate tension headaches, and help the recipient to deal with difficult emotions, such as anxiety, depression, grief, or a sense of being unloved.

CYPRESS

MASSAGE CONTRAINDICATIONS

Do not massage in the following cases or conditions:

♡ If you are feeling unwell or drained of energy.

♡ Immediately after a meal.

♡ In cases of infectious disease and/or if you have, or the recipient has, a high temperature.

♡ In cases of serious injury such as torn ligaments or broken bones.

♡ If it causes pain.

♡ Over any areas of skin infection, rashes, cuts, sores, burns, or varicose veins.

♡ Over a recent wound or an operation site that is forming scar tissue.

♡ In cases of acute inflammatory conditions, such as sprains, and some forms of arthritis/rheumatism.

♡ If the recipient has, or has had, thrombosis.

♡ If the recipient has cancer: give hand, foot, or facial treatments only.

♡ If the recipient has, or has had, a serious heart condition or any other serious medical condition.

♡ During the week following a vaccination.

Effleurage: stroking movements

THIS IS THE BASIC STROKING MOVEMENT, and the first technique to be used on any part of the body. Using slow and gentle strokes to cover the surface of the skin ensures that the aromatic oils will be readily absorbed. Effleurage promotes relaxation and draws blood to the area, improving both the assimilation of nutrients and the flow of lymphatic fluids, and aiding the elimination of toxins. It is a soothing and comforting type of movement that can also be used to link other techniques throughout the course of the massage.

STROKING

Using the whole flat area of both palms (not just the fingertips), gently lay your hands side by side on the skin. ♥

1 Slide your hands together rhythmically along the skin, to cover a large or small area.

2 At the end of each stroke always return to your starting position by skimming lightly over the surface.

3 This movement is best employed on the back.

GLIDING

This is a variation of the basic stroking movement, performed with the hands gliding together, side by side and pointing in opposite directions, as shown in steps 1 and 2. The hands may also be placed one on top of the other when extra pressure is needed. As with stroking movements, at the end of each stroke you should always return to your starting position by skimming lightly back over the surface of the skin (as shown in step 3). This movement is a particularly useful stroke for massaging the recipient's arms and legs. ♥

STEP 1   *STEP 2*   *STEP 3*

PULLING

Like stroking, this is a firm, but gentle, rhythmic movement, but here the emphasis is on pulling rather than pushing. Using alternate hands, methodically work your way along a specific area and back again, with a slight lifting and pulling stroke. This is especially useful for the sides of the torso or the limbs. ♥

STEP 1

STEP 2

STEP 3

Petrissage: kneading movements

THESE TECHNIQUES INVOLVE picking up and slightly squeezing or twisting the muscles and are used on all muscular and fatty regions of the body. Using the whole hand, or just the fingertips, the muscle is first squeezed and then released in a rhythmic fashion. As it is released, the muscle relaxes. The overall effect is to pump the vessels of the muscles, so that circulation is improved and lymphatic activity increased. It is an effective technique for easing muscular tension and bringing warmth to an area. Always relax a muscle with effleurage before attempting petrissage.

KNEADING

The hands are placed on either side of a muscle, with the palms slightly facing each other. The movement is an alternate downward pressure, then a picking up, rolling and squeezing of the muscle. The basic kneading technique is a bit like kneading dough (see illustration on right). It is applied on muscular areas, such as the shoulders, back, and limbs. Picking up, which involves lifting up the muscle and stretching it as far as possible from the bone, and rolling, which involves lifting up a section of muscle and rolling it transversely in both directions, can also be practiced as individual movements. ♥

KNEADING TECHNIQUE

STEP 1

STEP 2

STEP 3

ABOVE Aromatherapy may be an alternative to pills.

WARNING

For people with high blood pressure or epilepsy, or who are pregnant, or receiving medication or medical treatment, or if you intend to massage a baby or young child, see Safety Data, p. 375.

WRINGING

Like kneading, this movement involves squeezing the muscles and the soft underlying tissue adhesions connected to the muscle, in this case with an additional twist. This technique is extremely warming and stimulating, but it is only applicable to the limbs. ❧

WRINGING TECHNIQUE

1 Place the hands side by side on a limb.

2 Grasping firmly with the fingers, start to work the hands in opposite directions as if wringing out a cloth.

3 Work your way up the limb and down again methodically, squeezing the flesh between the hands a little at each stroke.

SQUEEZING

Grasping a portion of flesh, squeezing, and then releasing, is a simple technique which can be applied either to large muscular or fatty areas, or to a small area such as the ear lobes or the pads between the fingers or toes. In the former case, all the fingers and both thumbs are used to exert firm pressure; in the latter, simply the forefinger and thumb are employed (as illustrated).

STEP 1

STEP 2

STEP 3

Friction: rubbing movements

FRICTION TECHNIQUES are carried out using the palms or heels of the hands, the finger pads, the ball of the thumb, the knuckles of a loosely clenched fist, or even the elbow. The movement is usually made in small circles, often stretching the tissue and muscles away from the bone. It helps to increase blood and lymphatic flow, and to break down congestion in the tissues and toxic deposits. Friction can be used to penetrate deeply into the tissues but do not tackle tight or knotted areas without adequate preparation through effleurage and petrissage, or the body will resist and tighten further.

FRICTION TECHNIQUE

RUBBING

Rubbing is the lightest form of friction, using the fingers, palm, or heel of the hand in firm, brisk, circular movements. Some pressure is involved, but it is not specifically localized as is the case with circling and pressing. To exert greater pressure, place one hand over the other (step 3). This movement is stimulating yet comforting, bringing a warm glow to the whole area. It is usually used on the back. ♥

STEP 1   *STEP 2*   *STEP 3*

CIRCLING

Circling is a deeper technique, done with the ball of the thumb, finger pads, or knuckles, in small, circular movements. It works on especially tight areas, and helps eliminate uric acid deposits and other toxins. It can be used around the knee or elbow joint, down each side of the spine, or indeed on any area demanding attention, such as the soles of the feet or the palms of the hands. ♥

STEP 1   *STEP 2*   *STEP 3*

PRESSING

Pressing is a very penetrating technique, which is employed to its greatest effect in shiatsu or pressure point massage. By pressing or stimulating certain points on the skin, it is possible to influence the health of the internal organs and the flow of energy along the meridians of the body. Similar principles also apply in reflexology. To use the pressing technique with confidence, it is necessary to know the main pressure points of the body, how to locate them, and what they may be used for (see shiatsu chart, p. 93, and reflexology chart, p. 92). The point between the eyebrows (step 3) is good for relieving headaches and sinus congestion. Pressing can be carried out with the thumb, the forefingers, or sometimes the elbow. ♡

PRESSING TECHNIQUE

STEP 1

STEP 2

STEP 3

WARNING

Pressure should not be applied directly to any area causing pain, and should penetrate only as deeply as the body is willing to receive it.

Tapotement: percussion-like movements

THESE ARE ALL VIGOROUS, brisk movements that can be incorporated into an aromatherapy massage to give the sequence a more stimulating and toning effect. Tapotement consists of a series of light blows made in quick succession, with the movement springing from loosely held wrists. It is a good movement for breaking down fat, eliminating toxins, toning the muscles, and generally stimulating the circulation.

PUMMELING

Using loose fists, and keeping the wrists close together, gently pummel the skin with the padded side of the fists. This technique can be used on fleshy parts of the body (as illustrated) and also over muscular areas, such as the shoulders. ♥

STEP 1

STEP 2

STEP 3

WARNING

Tapotement should never be used on paralyzed muscles, on pregnant women, or on delicate areas of the body, such as the neck or abdomen.

Hacking should never be performed on or over bones.

LEFT Essential oils used in massage are almost always diluted in a base oil.

HACKING

This is performed with the outer sides of the hands, keeping the wrists close together. Use brisk alternate chopping strokes with the hands, but do not let them rise too high above the body. This movement feels very good when it is carried out on fleshy parts of the body, such as the buttocks. ♡

STEP 1

STEP 2

STEP 3

CUPPING

This movement should be performed with the fingers slightly extended and the palms cupped to form a hollow. It should not sound like a slap. Cupping is a very effective technique for use on the areas of the thighs and buttocks, but it can also be used on the upper back, where it offers surface and capillary stimulation. It is generally used on fleshy areas. Cupping is a bouncy, brisk massage movement. ♡

STEP 1

STEP 2

STEP 3

Other useful techniques

ALTHOUGH THESE ADDITIONAL techniques are not specific to aromatherapy massage, they can all be useful movements to incorporate into a full aromatherapy body massage when required for particular problems.

DRAINING

This technique is used specifically when performing a manual lymphatic drainage massage (MLD). Draining improves the circulation of lymphatic fluids, aiding the elimination of toxins via some of the main lymph nodes of the body, especially those on each side of the groin and beneath the armpits (others are in the neck). The direction of the stroke is always toward these nodes, using a firm sliding pressure. Making a V-shape between the fingers and thumbs (steps 1 and 2) is a good way of draining the limbs. ♥

DRAINAGE TECHNIQUE

STEP 1

STEP 2

STEP 3

WARNING

Check with your medical practitioner before undergoing drainage massage if you suffer from a serious illness or inflamed lymph glands, or if receiving medication.

STRETCHING

Like pressing (p. 87), stretching has more in common with shiatsu than with the usual aromatherapy massage routine. However, it is a useful technique for easing muscular tension—especially beneficial as part of an aromatic sports massage or as a pre-exercise warm-up. Stretches should always be gentle and firm, with a brief pause at the end—never jerky. Always ask permission and check for contraindications such as a stiff neck or slipped disk, which require gentle treatment only, before performing any stretch. ♥

STEP 1

STEP 2

STEP 3

FEATHERING

This term refers to touching the skin very lightly and gently—or even moving the hands just above the surface of the skin in a stroking fashion. Feathering may be performed either at the beginning, or, more commonly, right at the end of a whole sequence or series of strokes, to give a feeling of completion. Used right at the end of the massage sequence, feathering allows the contact between the masseur and the recipient to be gradually diminished, and ensures that the massage does not end too abruptly. It can also be employed (as shown, below) as a kind of "auric" massage to cleanse the subtle envelope surrounding the body, and remove any residues of tension from the recipient on this level. ♥

STEP 1

STEP 2

STEP 3

Reflexology points

Reflexology is a specialized form of massage based on the theory that the body is divided into zones that run the length of the body. The soles of the feet reflect these zones and can enable the experienced reflexologist to detect "imbalances" in the body. The application of pressure on the correct "reflex points" can help to correct these.

ANGELICA ROOT

Shiatsu points and meridians

The Japanese massage technique of shiatsu or "finger pressure" is based on the same principles as acupuncture. Combining acupressure, massage, elements of physiotherapy, and osteopathy, it aims to restore a balanced flow of energy within the meridians, enhancing well-being and vitality, through the application of pressure on specific points along the meridians.

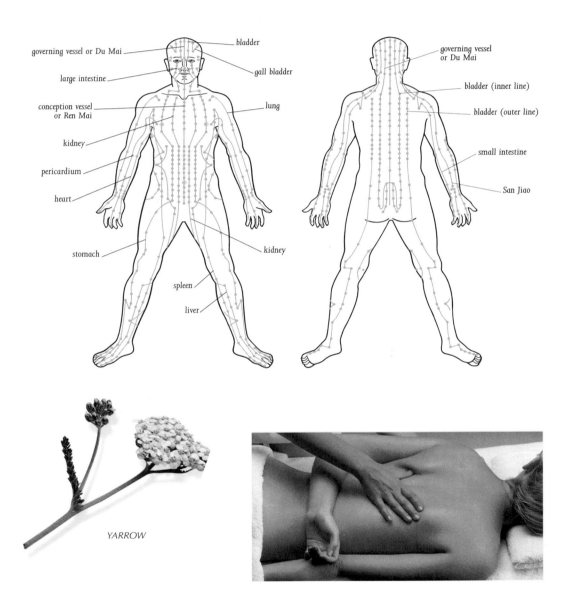

YARROW

Giving a massage

BEFORE GIVING A MASSAGE, it is important to ensure that both you and the recipient are comfortable with the atmosphere in which it is to take place. Massage is best undertaken in a quiet room, and the only language needed is the language of touch.

Massage should be a nonverbal type of therapy. Silence and touch are two of the most important elements or principles at work during a massage and become a language of their own. In general, keep words to a minimum during a massage, and if you need to speak, do so in a quiet tone. If the recipient wants to speak, remain receptive and responsive to what he or she has to say without engaging in or encouraging conversation.

During the course of the massage, it is not unusual for the recipient to experience a release of emotion, such as laughing or crying. Again, do not block or suppress this expression, but just let it come and go naturally without passing judgment.

THE ENVIRONMENT

The easiest place to do a massage is on a massage table or a massage couch. This needs to be adjusted to the right height so that you can get enough leverage for deeper tissue work but do not need to stoop, or bend your back too much. Alternatively, a futon or a piece of foam padding 1–2 inches (2.5–5cm) thick, placed on the floor, also works well. This can be covered with a clean cotton sheet and/or a towel. The most important thing is to feel comfortable while you are performing the massage and to be able to move freely around the person, and to change your position with ease. Make sure you are not strained or uncomfortable during the massage.

The room in which you give the massage (or the environment) should be warm enough—a person with massage oil on their skin becomes easily chilled. Always cover areas of the body which are not being worked on with a towel. The place should be secluded and quiet enough for there to be a minimum of disturbance— interruptions or loud noises can be disconcerting. Quiet background music is optional depending on the situation and preferences of the recipient. Do not use direct overhead lighting: the light source should be as natural as possible and slightly dimmed.

ABOVE Before a massage, ensure that you ask the recipient about his or her personal health record and choose your oils accordingly.

Before you begin

Before beginning a massage, it is important to ask the recipient about his or her personal health record and check for any contraindications, such as a skin infection, inflammation, or illness (see Contraindications panel, p. 81). For a guide to preparing massage oils, see p. 36, and for base oils for blending, see pp. 345–371.

Allow at least an hour for a full-body massage, and plan to give extra time for a prior consultation.

♡ Check your nails are short enough beforehand.

♡ Wash your hands and remove any rings.

♡ If you have long hair, make sure that it is tied back.

♡ Wear loose clothes, and check that your clothing will not impede the massage.

♡ Prepare the massage oil in a bowl, and keep it warm and accessible.

♡ Ask the recipient to remove jewelry, glasses, or contact lenses.

♡ While you withdraw, ask the recipient to take off all his or her clothing apart from underpants and to wrap him or herself in a large towel. (If he or she feels uncomfortable about removing items of clothing, adapt your routine to suit these particular requirements.)

♡ Ask the recipient to lie down comfortably, face down, arms by his or her sides.

♡ Adjust one towel to cover the recipient's back and buttocks, and cover the legs and feet with another large towel.

♡ Ask the recipient to relax and let the body go as limp as possible, and to let you move or lift his or her limbs as required.

♡ Ask if he or she needs a pillow for support, and for him or her to move the head from one side to another if the neck is getting stiff—unless the massage table has a special "face hole."

♡ Quietly take a few deep breaths to center yourself, and to tune in to the needs of the person you are about to massage.

The complete massage sequence

Having ensured that the environment is suitable and that there are no specific contraindications, you can start the full-body massage sequence. First of all, check that the recipient of the massage is lying comfortably, positioned face down, and that he or she is warmly covered with one or two towels. The arms should be lying alongside the body and the head resting to one side—a cushion may be required. Before beginning the massage or removing any portion of the covering, gently lay both your hands on the recipient's back, one at the base and one at the top of the spine. Breathe deeply a few times while allowing your hands to remain in place. This helps to attune the recipient of the massage to your touch.

A FULL BACK MASSAGE DOES MUCH TO ALLEVIATE THE EFFECTS OF STRESS FELT THROUGHOUT THE WHOLE BODY, AND BRINGS RELIEF TO ACHING AND KNOTTED MUSCLES.

Massaging the back

GENTLY PEEL BACK the towel to expose the whole of the recipient's back. Make sure that your hands are warm by rubbing them briskly together if necessary, before pouring a little of the prepared massage oil into the palm of just one hand.

1 Stroking: Rub your hands together, then place both hands at the base of the recipient's spine, with your fingers pointing toward his or her head. Slowly slide your hands up the back, one on each side of the spine, until you reach the neck. Fan your hands out over the shoulders and slide them down the sides of the torso and back into the starting position. Repeat several times, using smooth, rhythmic strokes so that the whole of the back is coated with a thin layer of oil.

2 Pulling: Without losing contact with the recipient's skin, move both your hands to one side of his or her torso, just above the hips. Then, using alternate hands with a firm and rhythmic pulling motion, work your way slowly up the side of the body to beneath the arm and back down again. Repeat a few times before performing the same movement on the other side.

3 Rubbing: Before working on the back's muscular areas with deeper pressure, loosen the whole area around the neck and shoulders with a brisk, circular rubbing movement, using the flat of your hands. One hand can be placed on top of the other to make the movement more vigorous and bring greater warmth.

4 Kneading: Using a firm but gentle kneading movement, gradually start to work your way around all the fleshy, muscular parts of the back, paying particular attention to any possible areas of tension around the neck, shoulders, and upper buttocks.

5 Circling: Having released some of the muscular tension in the back, it is now possible to work more deeply on any particularly tight or knotted areas, using small, circular movements with the thumbs or fingertips. It may be helpful to lift the recipient's arm across his/her back (as illustrated) in order to penetrate more deeply into the area beneath the shoulder blades. Support the shoulder with one hand, and lift it slightly while working with the other hand. Then repeat on the other side.

6 Pressing: Positioning yourself at the recipient's head, run your thumbs firmly down the channels on either side of the spine with a smooth, slow, pressing movement. Glide the hands up each side of the torso and repeat this movement several times.

7 Stroking/Feathering: To complete the sequence use slow, stroking movements over the entire area. Standing at the recipient's head, start with your hands at the top of the back, fanning the hands out over the buttocks and up the sides of the torso. Gradually make the strokes slower and lighter, until your hands barely touch the skin. Cover the back with a towel before moving on to the legs.

Massaging the back of the legs

PEEL BACK THE towel to expose one or both legs, depending on the warmth in the room. It is important that the recipient stays warm and relaxed. Apply more oil to your hands if necessary.

1 Gliding: Place the hands, one above the other, on the ankle of the recipient. Slowly glide your hands together to the top of the leg, then run them down each side of the limb until they are back to their original position. Repeat several times, ensuring that the whole of the back of the leg is oiled.

2 Wringing: Start with the hands next to each other, grasping the ankle lightly. Then using a firm wringing movement, start to work your way rhythmically up the leg and down again, squeezing the flesh between your hands with each change of position. Avoid the delicate area behind the knee, focusing rather on the muscles of the calf and upper thigh.

3 Kneading: Knead the calf muscles and then the thigh and buttocks, with rhythmic strokes. Pay special attention to any especially tight or knotted areas, and again avoid the delicate area at the back of the knee.

4 Hacking: Use a rhythmic hacking motion on the fleshy parts of the upper thigh and buttocks— and, more gently, on the calf if it is sufficiently developed. This movement, like the following one, is quite a vigorous technique which may not apply if you are performing a very soothing or relaxing type of massage. It is, however, extremely beneficial for releasing deep-seated muscular tension, and helping to break down fatty deposits.

5 Pummeling: To further stimulate the circulation and release tension in the fleshy area of the thighs and buttocks, use a rhythmic pummeling motion with gently clenched fists. (Cupping, using lightly cupped hands, is also best employed in this area.)

6 Draining: To encourage lymphatic drainage, make a V-shape between the thumb and forefinger of each hand and lay one hand above the other on the recipient's ankle. Using the V-shape to press in an upward motion, start to run your hands alternately up the back of the leg in a firm, rhythmic movement. Continue up to the thigh, then lift and replace each hand in turn at the ankle, before repeating.

7 Gliding: Finish the sequence of movements on the leg by repeating the initial gliding movement, allowing the strokes to get gradually lighter. Cover the leg with a towel and go on to the other leg. Finally, when both legs have been massaged, you may place one hand on each leg and glide them up both legs together, before covering the legs with a towel.

To proceed to the front of the legs, quietly ask the recipient to turn over, help him or her to reposition the towels, and ensure that he or she is comfortable.

A GOOD MASSAGE ON THE BACK OF THE LEGS CAN STIMULATE THE LYMPHATIC SYSTEM AND IMPROVE CIRCULATION.

HYSSOP

Massaging the front of the legs

CAREFULLY REMOVE the toweling from one or both legs. Make sure your hands are sufficiently oiled (adding more if necessary) before laying them gently, one above the other, on the ankle of the recipient to begin.

1 Gliding: Slowly glide both hands together up toward the thigh, then down each side of the leg and back into the starting position. Repeat several times.

2 Squeezing: Place your hands side by side on the thigh, and grasp the fleshy part between your thumbs and fingers. Then begin to squeeze the muscles along the top of the upper leg using firm, rhythmic pressure. Move your hands up and down the upper leg, between the knee and the thigh several times in this manner.

3 Kneading: Having warmed up the muscles, start to work more deeply into any areas of tension in the upper leg and thigh using a rhythmic kneading movement. In order to knead the calf muscles with greater ease, raise the recipient's knee and use your body to prevent the foot from slipping forward. Support the recipient's raised knee with one hand while using your other hand to work on the muscles of the calf. Gently lower the raised leg.

PEPPERMINT

4 Circling: Starting with your thumbs beneath the recipient's kneecap, circle the thumbs in alternate directions around the knee until they cross above the kneecap. Then circle them back again and repeat. Now begin to work all around the knee and upper leg with small circular movements of the thumb or fingertips. Avoid pressing on the shinbone while working at all times, as this can be painful.

5 Gliding: Return to the initial gliding movement (or insert a draining movement here) to complete the leg massage. Cover the leg with the towel and repeat the sequence on the other leg. Having completed both legs, you may place one hand on each ankle and glide the hands up both legs together as shown, allowing the strokes to become slower and lighter. At the end of these movements, cover both legs with a towel.

TIRED AND HEAVY LEGS CAN BE HELPED WITH A VARIETY OF MASSAGE TECHNIQUES, TO GIVE THE RECIPIENT A FEELING OF RENEWED ENERGY AND LIGHTNESS.

Massaging the feet

UNCOVER ONE OR BOTH FEET. Check that your hands are only lightly oiled, and that you are comfortably positioned. It is important to bear in mind the sensitivity of this area. For more detail on the significance of various areas of the foot, see the reflexology chart on page 92.

1 Stroking: Using both hands, gently stroke the recipient's foot, from the toes toward the ankles. Repeat several times in a rhythmic manner.

2 Rubbing: Carefully supporting the foot with one hand, gently cup the fingers of your other hand around the heel of the foot. Using a firm, circular rubbing movement, massage the whole of this area. This position can also be used to flex and loosen the ankle.

3 Circling: While continuing to support the foot firmly with one hand, use the thumb (or knuckles) of your other hand to make small circular movements all over the sole of the foot. Be aware of the sensitivity of this area, and the fact that some spots may be particularly tender or congested. (A reflexology chart may be used to identify the significance of these different areas, see p. 92.)

THERE ARE THOUSANDS OF NERVE ENDINGS IN THE FOOT, AND A RELAXING MASSAGE TO THE FEET WILL HELP ALLEVIATE NERVOUS TENSION AND RESTORE VITALITY.

4 Pressing: Having covered the entire sole, continue to support the foot with one hand while working on the top of the foot with your other hand. Using the thumb or fingertips, press gently but firmly down the channels running between the bones of the foot. Starting with the channel between the big toe and the next toe, slowly work your way down each channel at a time, until you reach the little toe.

5 Squeezing: Still supporting the foot, grasp the fleshy pads between the big toe and the next toe, using the thumb and forefinger of one hand. Squeeze gently, then slowly pull your hand away. Repeat between each of the toes in turn.

6 Stretching: While still supporting the foot with one hand, grasp the sides of the big toe between the thumb and forefinger of your other hand. Squeeze and pull the toe, with a stretching movement, until your fingers slide off at the end. Repeat with each of the toes in turn.

7 Stroking/Feathering: Complete the sequence on the foot by stroking it all over, moving the hands rhythmically from the heel toward the toes. Finally, using a light feathering movement, stroke the foot in the direction of the toes, until your hands are hardly touching the skin. Cover the foot with a towel before repeating the sequence on the other foot. You may finish by stroking/feathering both feet together, before covering them both.

Massaging the hands and arms

UNCOVER ONE ARM at a time from beneath the toweling. Check that your hands are sufficiently oiled, then place them, one above the other, on the wrist of the recipient.

1 Gliding: Keeping the hands together, glide them firmly up the arm to the shoulder, returning down the sides of the arm and back to the wrist. Repeat this movement several times.

2 Rubbing: Supporting and lifting the arm a little with one of your hands, use the fingers of the other hand to cup the elbow. Rub the area gently, using slow circular movements. Replace the arm gently beside the body.

3 Kneading: Using both hands together, start to knead the muscles of the forearm and upper arm in a rhythmic motion. Pay special attention to any tight or knotted areas, before moving on to the hand.

4 Stroking: Check that your hands are lightly oiled before beginning on the hands—although the hands (like the feet) require very little oil for general massage purposes. Using both hands, cover the entire surface of the recipient's hand with smooth stroking movements.

5 Circling: With the recipient's palm facing upward, use small, gentle circular movements with your thumbs (or knuckles) to massage all over his/her palm. Hold the back of the hand with your fingers while pressing firmly with the thumbs. For a more elaborate, but very effective, technique, use the following hold:

Place the little finger of your left hand between the recipient's (right) forefinger and middle finger, with the fourth and middle finger of your left hand between his or her forefinger and thumb. At the same time, place the little finger of your right hand between his or her middle and fourth fingers, the fourth finger of your right hand between his or her fourth and little finger, and the middle finger and forefinger of your right hand on the other side of his or her little finger. Push all your fingers back hard against the back of his or her hand so that the palm is stretched and taut. Making small circular movements with your thumbs, work over the whole surface of the palm.

6 Pressing: With the recipient's palm facing down, and using one of your hands as a support, use the other hand to press firmly down the channels between the bones on the top of the hand. Press and slide your thumb evenly down the hand to between the thumb and forefinger, then take each channel in turn until you reach the little finger.

7 Squeezing: Gently squeeze the fleshy pads between each of the recipient's fingers, using your thumb and forefinger. Pay particular attention to the muscular area between the thumb and forefinger.

8 Stretching: Supporting the recipient's hand with the palm down, use your other hand to massage the joints of each finger in turn. Then squeeze the outer edge of each finger and give it a firm pull or stretch, until your fingers slide off at the end. To give an additional stretch, while still supporting the wrist with one hand use the other hand to push all the recipient's fingers back together in an arc.

9 Stroking/Feathering: Finish this sequence by stroking the hand from the wrist toward the fingers several times. Hold the hand firmly in yours for a few seconds, before sliding your hands lightly off at the fingertips. Repeat this last movement several times, allowing your touch to become progressively lighter. Cover the hand and arm with a towel, then repeat the same sequence on the other side.

TENSION OFTEN CREEPS INTO THE HANDS AND ARMS; MASSAGING THEM HELPS RELEASE PENT-UP ANXIETIES AND PROMOTES A SENSE OF WELL-BEING.

SANDALWOOD

Massaging the abdomen and chest

FOLD THE TOWEL carefully back from the abdomen and chest. Make sure your hands are warm and well oiled before placing them on each side of the recipient's navel with your fingers toward his or her head. Do not lose skin contact as you work.

1 Stroking: Gently stroke your hands up the center of the recipient's chest, over the shoulders, and down each side of the torso. Repeat several times. If the recipient is a woman and is uncertain about having her chest massaged, this area can remain covered and the movement restricted to her abdominal region only.

2 Pulling: Place your hands together on the side of the torso, next to the hips, then, using a firm, rhythmic pulling motion with alternate hands, work your way up toward the armpits and down again. Repeat on the other side.

3 Circling: Rest your hands lightly on the abdomen, then slowly begin to move the hands one after the other in a large, gentle circular motion, always moving in a clockwise direction. As one hand completes the circle, you will have to lift off the other hand repeatedly to let the first hand pass, then replace it again and continue with the circling movement.

MASSAGING THE ABDOMEN STIMULATES THE DIGESTIVE SYSTEM AND IMPROVES THE ELIMINATION OF WASTE PRODUCTS. A CHEST MASSAGE HELPS PREVENT STIFFNESS AND INFLEXIBILITY IN THE NECK AND SHOULDERS.

4 Stroking: Standing at the head of the recipient, place both your hands gently on his or her upper chest. With a smooth stroking movement, fan your hands out over the top of the chest, continue toward the shoulders, back along the shoulder blades and up to the base of the neck. Without losing skin contact, resume the starting position and repeat several times.

FRANKINCENSE

5 Rubbing: Start by cupping your hands over the recipient's shoulders, then, with a gentle circular movement, use your palms to rub his or her upper arms, chest and shoulders all the way up to the base of the neck. Cover the chest and abdominal region with a towel. Alternatively, this sequence can be completed with stroking movements to the whole of the upper torso before covering it over.

Massaging the neck

STAND BEHIND THE recipient's head. Oil your hands and place them side by side on each side of the neck. The shoulders and neck can hold a great deal of tension, so allow ample time for this area.

1 Pressing: Start by pressing your thumbs firmly into the hollow between the base of the neck and the shoulder blades, on each side. Use your weight to increase the pressure, hold for a few seconds, then release. Move your thumbs along the shoulders a fraction and press. Repeat until you have covered the whole length of the top of the shoulders.

2 Pulling: Ask the recipient of the massage to lift his or her shoulders and back up a little, to let you slide your hands beneath the upper back, with the palms up. Place one hand on each side of the spine, with your fingers curved slightly upward. Ask the recipient to relax back as you slowly pull your hands toward you, giving the muscles on either side of the spine a good stretch. Remove your hands from beneath his or her neck, and repeat twice more.

ANISEED

3 Stretching: Place both your hands firmly beneath the neck at the base of the skull, clasping your fingers together at the back of the recipient's head. Very gently, lift and stretch his or her neck toward you, keeping the movement even and straight. Hold for a few seconds, then release.

4 Stroking: Gently move the head to the right, supporting it with your right hand, then place your left hand on the recipient's shoulder. With a slow and gentle stroking movement, slide your left hand along the shoulder and up the neck, to just behind the ear. Repeat the movement several times. Then gently massage the area at the base of the skull with the fingers to release any tension.

5 Circling: With the recipient's head still to one side, place your fingers at the base of the neck. Using the tips of the fingers, make small circling movements all the way up the neck, then along the base of the skull toward the ears. A great deal of tension can become trapped in this particular area, so repeat this sequence several times very slowly. Slowly move the head to the left and repeat the last two movements, then return the head to an upright position.

MANY OF THE TENSIONS THAT WE FEEL MANIFEST THEMSELVES IN THE NECK. A GOOD NECK MASSAGE HELPS GET RID OF STIFFNESS.

Massaging the face and scalp

STAND AT THE END of the table behind the recipient's head. Make sure that your hands are sufficiently oiled, then begin with step 1. This is the last stage of the full-body massage.

1 Stroking: Start by placing your hands very gently on the recipient's forehead at the hairline in order to establish contact, perhaps stroking his or her hair a little. Then oil your hands lightly, and positioning yourself behind his or her head, place the palms of your hands on either side of the chin. With a gentle sweeping movement, slide your hands from the throat, across the cheeks, and up to the forehead, avoiding the delicate area immediately around the eyes. Let the strokes get gradually firmer, until you are pressing slightly upward against the jawbone. Repeat several times, slowly, until the face is lightly lubricated all over.

2 Stroking: Now place your thumbs together in the center of the recipient's forehead. Slowly start to stroke his or her forehead from the center down toward the temples, using your thumbs. Begin with the panel next to the hairline and progress gradually in strips, moving toward the eyebrows, until the whole of the forehead has been covered.

A FACIAL MASSAGE IMPROVES CIRCULATION AND BRINGS A HEALTHY GLOW TO THE SKIN. HEADACHES AND TENSION DISAPPEAR, AND THE RECIPIENT EXPERIENCES A DEEP SERENITY.

3 Circling: Using small movements, circle the temples lightly with the fingers. This is extremely soothing and can help to calm mental tension and provide relief from headaches or anxiety.

4 Pressing: Place both your thumbs on the bony ridge above the eyes, in the center, next to the nose. Press down quite firmly, hold for an instant, then release. Move each of your thumbs out a few inches/centimeters and repeat the pressure. Repeat this movement until you reach the outer corners of the eye. Then continue, using slightly less pressure, along the bony ridge beneath the eye, again starting on the inner side of the socket.

5 Circling: Again using small circular movements, this time with the forefingers, begin to massage the area on each side of the nose, starting near the bridge and working downward. Repeat on the cheeks on either side of the nostrils, across the upper lip area, and over the chin.

6 Squeezing: Now gently grasp the recipient's ear lobes between your thumbs and forefingers and give them a squeeze. Pinch the edges of the ear all the way around from bottom to top and then back again. Finally, pull the ear lobe downward two or three times—this is good for headaches.

7 Circling: Slide your hands around to the back of the neck. Starting behind the ears, begin to work your fingers all along the underside of the ridge at the base of the skull. Without letting the hair get too oily, continue to massage all over the recipient's scalp, using your fingers and thumbs.

8 Stroking: Finish by stroking the recipient's forehead and brushing the hair gently back from the forehead (as you began), using progressively lighter and lighter strokes.

9 Feathering: To complete the entire massage sequence, move the hands over the recipient's face (and the rest of the body if you wish), using a light sweeping movement and without touching the skin's surface at all. On a subtle level, this helps to disperse any residue of physical or psychological tension that may have been released during the massage.

When the massage is over, encourage the recipient to relax peacefully for a few minutes at least, in order that the full benefits of the massage can be assimilated. Any surplus oil can be removed using paper tissues or, if the situation allows, with a warm, moist towel. Withdraw discreetly to wash your hands, while the recipient "comes round" and gets dressed.

Massage for specific areas

APART FROM PERFORMING the full-body massage detailed on pp. 96–111, it is also possible to concentrate on one part of the body, such as the back, feet, hands, or face, or to use massage for purposes other than relaxation or stress-relief. For example, massage can be used specifically to stimulate the body, and may be enjoyed as a sensual experience between lovers or developed as a bonding link between parent and child. Curative and diagnostic massage techniques, such as shiatsu and reflexology, focus on specific parts of the body—the meridian lines in the body, and the feet, and various forms of massage are used in the treatment of illnesses.

BACK

A back massage can be an extremely relaxing experience in itself, if time is too limited to carry out a complete body sequence. A great deal of tension is often trapped in the muscles of the back, neck, and shoulders—the back is also the part of the body which allows for the greatest absorption of aromatic oils. Simply refer to the section on the back in the full-body sequence (see pp. 96–97), but allow more time for each set of strokes, and adapt your technique specifically to the needs of the recipient.

HANDS AND FEET

Massaging the feet and hands can be a valuable form of treatment, especially in situations where the recipient is ill, or feels uncertain about receiving a more intimate type of contact. It is also useful in hospitals, for example, where it may not be possible to move the patient, or as a complementary form of therapy alongside other types of medication or treatment. The soles of the feet contain nerve endings that connect to all the organs, glands, and systems of the body. This is the principle behind reflexology (see p. 92). It is therefore possible to treat the whole body simply by massaging the feet—refer to the relevant section in the full-body massage sequence (pp. 102–103) as a guide.

FACE

Performing a facial massage requires the most refined and sensitive type of touch. The facial massage sequence, detailed in the complete massage (see pp. 110–111), clearly lends itself to application as part of a beauty treatment or as a general boost to the complexion. It stimulates the circulation, nourishes the deep dermal tissues, and imparts a healthy glow to the surface of the skin. However, a face and scalp massage should not be regarded solely as a cosmetic aid, since it is also very effective in relieving stress-related complaints, especially the more psychological conditions such as insomnia, headaches, or depression. Always make sure the face is cleansed of any makeup before commencing.

Self-massage treatments

ALTHOUGH SELF-MASSAGE MAY never be as relaxing as receiving a massage, it still has many benefits. One of the main advantages is that it can be done where and when it is required, without another person's assistance. Self-massage can benefit the whole body.

THE SHOULDERS AND NECK

Ease the shoulders up and down a few times, using a circular movement, and gently move the head from side to side. Then rub the neck, shoulders, and scalp firmly with both hands, using the fingertips to massage the whole area with small circling movements (illustrated right). Tilt the head to one side and stroke the opposite shoulder, and down the arm to the elbow. Repeat on the opposite side. This can be done while sitting in a traffic jam, or at a desk.

Self-massage can be performed in the bathtub, in a car, on the bed, or while sitting at a desk—whenever you most need it. The areas most easily worked on are neck, shoulders, arms, hands, and feet.

EASING TENSION

HEADACHES AND EYE STRAIN

To relieve headaches or the strain of VDU work, cup your hands over the eyes and look into the darkness. Then circle the temples with the middle fingers, and sweep the fingers from the center of the forehead out toward the sides (as illustrated right).

PROMOTE WELL-BEING

This can be carried out in the bathtub, on a bed, or on the floor. The best part of the body to massage in this case is the soles of the feet—this way we can give ourselves a complete self-treatment (see reflexology diagram, p. 92).

RELIEVING HEADACHES

Massage during pregnancy

MASSAGE DURING PREGNANCY can be extremely helpful, especially in the last few months, when the body can begin to feel strained, and very heavy. Since a pregnant woman is unable to lie on her stomach, some types of massage need to be performed while she is lying on her side or seated in a chair. A good alternative position for performing a massage treatment to the back during pregnancy is for the woman to sit astride a chair, with the front of her body supported by a cushion. Massage to the neck and shoulders can help to alleviate muscular tension and anxiety.

Lower back pain is a common problem, as are feelings of physical tiredness and nervous exhaustion, especially toward the end of pregnancy. Massage to the back can help to ease aches and pains, and help revitalize the whole body.

Local massage to the hands, feet, neck, and face are also very beneficial. For example, gentle massage to the feet and ankles can help to overcome edema (swelling) when performed regularly. A massage to the neck and face can give a boost to self-confidence and promote a sense of well-being.

WARNING

Special care and precautions should always be taken when performing any kind of massage during pregnancy because of the sensitivity of the growing child. All essential oils should be used in a very diluted form. For specific contraindications during pregnancy see Safety Data, p. 375.

NECK MASSAGE

BACK MASSAGE

LEFT Toward the end of pregnancy neck and shoulder massage can release tension.

Baby massage

MANY DOCTORS NOW accept the power of massage to ease anxiety in sick babies and children. New studies indicate its ability to help healthy infants, too. Research has shown that babies who are massaged are more alert, gain weight faster, sleep more soundly, and suffer less anxiety than nonmassaged infants.

Massage can also reduce stress levels in parents, help them to be more responsive to their child's needs, and aid in the natural bonding process. Conditions such as hyperactivity, insomnia, colic, and stomach ache respond well to massage. With a few exceptions, babies over the age of six weeks, and young children, can safely be massaged on the legs, arms, back, and stomach. This can be done three or four times a week, or even every day. A pre-bath massage lasting for 20 minutes will often make a restless child go straight to sleep at bed-time.

WARNING

Babies should not be massaged during the six-week period after their birth, for at least a week after a vaccination, or if they have joint problems. Essential oils should be used in the correct dilution according to age. See Safety Data, p. 375.

1 General massage to the feet, legs, arms, and torso is very soothing and relaxing and is good for insomnia and restlessness.

2 Rubbing the back or stomach gently, using a diluted aromatic oil, with a circular clockwise movement can ease colic, stomach ache, or other complaints.

3 Performing a simple local massage, to the hands or feet, for example, helps to establish a caring contact. This can be a very valuable aid to establishing trust, intimacy, and a loving bond between parent and child.

Sports and detoxifying massage

MASSAGE CAN BE beneficial both before and after exercise, and also as an aid to the body's natural process of eliminating toxins, as an anti-cellulite treatment, and for people recovering from illness.

SPORTS MASSAGE

A stimulating or sports massage tends to use deeper pressure and more vigorous movements than a massage aimed primarily at relaxation. Deep-tissue massage employs techniques such as kneading, rubbing, hacking, and pummeling traditionally associated with masseurs in Turkish baths. Exercise is the most important way of stimulating the circulation and increasing vitality.

WARNING

Some forms of exercise, such as jogging or aerobics, can have negative side effects in the long term. Studies show that yoga, fast walking, and swimming are more gentle, but effective, ways of staying fit.

RIGHT Warming up before sport prevents injury. Pre-and post-sports massage can prevent and treat problems.

DETOXIFYING MASSAGE

A detoxifying or manual lymph drainage (MLD) massage gently pumps toxins and foreign material such as bacteria and lymph fluids through the body's network of lymph canals. It can help clear acne and eczema, and can be used to treat edema (swelling due to water retention). In some hospitals, it is used to help reduce painful swellings following breast cancer treatment. A detoxifying massage may also help to shift cellulite and break down fatty deposits. Cupping, squeezing, and draining (see pp. 85–90) are especially valuable in this context. In MLD massage, the stroke should always be in the direction of the nearest lymph node.

WORKING ON THE CALF

MASSAGING THE THIGH MUSCLES

SQUEEZING THE MUSCLES

Sensual massage

MASSAGE CAN ALSO be a very sensual experience, and massage between partners can help to bring a new depth to the relationship, as well as to enhance sexual enjoyment. Make sure the room is warm and comfortable beforehand, and select the aromatic oils you wish to use. Some oils have a reputation for having aphrodisiac qualities, but it is best to choose oils with scents that appeal to both partners.

1 An aromatic massage is a relaxing and enjoyable experience in itself, promoting new levels of intimacy. It also provides an opportunity to explore different experiences and sensations.

2 A sensual or sexual massage need not focus entirely on the erotic regions of the body, but on the sensitivity of the body as a whole.

3 Like love-making, sensual massage between partners should be a two-way communication in which each person has the opportunity to touch and be touched.

PATCHOULI

PART THREE

♡

Aromatic Remedies

Medical aromatherapy

Essential oils have been used by specialist French doctors and surgeons for many years to treat a wide range of complaints. Depending on the practitioner and on the particular case, aromatherapy may be used exclusively, in conjunction with conventional treatment, or with other forms of alternative medicine. Professional practitioners may also prescribe essential oils for internal use as well as using them in the ways described so far in this book.

The treatment of serious medical complaints, and internal use, are the sphere of qualified medical practitioners, but many forms of aromatherapy can safely be used at home to treat minor illnesses or to act as a backup to conventional medical treatment. A large section of this part of the book (pp.133–237) covers the home use of essential oils for specific complaints. Ailments are grouped into body systems, and as a quick way of finding a particular ailment the appropriate treatment, there is an index of ailments, beginning on page 399.

"WHILST BEING THE OLDEST OF ALL SYSTEMS, PHYTOTHERAPY AND AROMATHERAPY ARE ALSO THOSE WHICH HAVE MOST EFFECTIVELY PROVED THEMSELVES."

DR. JEAN VALNET

TAGETES

CELERY SEED

Clinical aromatherapy

IN FRANCE TODAY, many medical doctors and hospitals prescribe essential oils as an alternative to antibiotic treatment, whereas in most other countries the idea of using natural aromatics as a form of medical treatment is still very radical.

Until recently the very concept of clinical aromatherapy has been ignored or treated sceptically by scientists, and by many in orthodox medical circles. However, such attitudes are beginning to change and plant medicines are being revaluated using modern research techniques. It is now accepted that many modern medications can have harmful side effects and that growing numbers of bacteria are becoming resistant to once successful synthetic medications.

The use of essential oils to fight infectious disease by oral prescription does, however, require great care and a high degree of medical expertise. In France, doctors have the opportunity to incorporate a more naturopathic approach (using herbs and essential oils) into their treatment program only after they have undertaken the full orthodox medical training. In sharp contrast, qualified aromatherapy masseurs and those working in the field of beauty therapy in the UK are only permitted to use the oils externally, and professional bodies such as the International Federation of Aromatherapists clearly indicate that employing aromatic oils for internal use is outside their jurisdiction.

Essential oils can indeed be extremely dangerous if they are taken by mouth without qualified supervision.

This is because, although natural products, they are highly concentrated, and, in an undiluted form, can damage the delicate mucous membranes of the digestive system. Some essential oils, for example pennyroyal, can also be highly toxic when ingested, even in small amounts, and can even cause death.[16] The safety aspects of using essential oils for aromatherapy purposes have therefore been justly highlighted by the media over the last 20 years, with the result that such potentially dangerous oils as pennyroyal have been withdrawn from sale. Regulations covering usage, contraindications, and general safety data have also made the purchase of essential oils by the general public much more strictly controlled and have ensured a much higher degree of safety. Legally, all essential oils should now carry precise safety data on the label, including the warning "Do not take internally" and "Keep out of reach of children." Considering the potential dangers of misusing oils, it is indisputable that the practice of clinical aromatherapy should be the preserve of highly qualified professionals. It is beyond the scope of the majority of people, including most aromatherapists working in the field of alternative health care.

RIGHT Pennyroyal is extremely toxic when ingested and should never be taken internally.

BELOW No essential oil should be taken internally unless recommended by a highly qualified practitioner.

WARNING

Taking essential oils internally can cause adverse reactions, and, in extreme cases, may even be fatal.

SCIENTIFIC STUDIES

The device known as the aromatogram promises to open the way for the use of natural aromatic medicine in the clinical field, and to help make the therapeutic use of essential oils accepted within the established medical arena. As a surgeon during World War II, Dr. Jean Valnet used essential oils for the treatment of both physical and psychiatric disorders, sometimes administering them by oral means, with outstanding success. His method, which involved testing specific oils on cultured bacteria taken from the site of the infection, was used not only to ascertain the minimum dosage levels required for various essential oils, but also to find which oils were best suited to treating a particular infection.

The results often showed that several oils had similar effects on the same infection. This is thought to be because they help to create a healthy environment in which pathogens are unable to survive. According to Valnet: "… one can select them [the oils] according to their primary healing powers, such as those oils which act in the region of the lungs: niaouli, eucalyptus and pine, or on the urinary system: juniper and sandalwood … determined by the aromatogram."[17] Most importantly, Valnet also discovered that bacteria treated with essential oils do not develop resistance as they do with antibiotics.

A demonstration of the aromatogram at a meeting of the Royal Society of Medicine in London in 1995 caused widespread interest. Of particular value to many who were present was the ability of certain essential oils to clear up infections caused by MRSA (methicillin-resistant *Staphylococcus aureus*). Essential oils could prove to be very useful allies in the fight against these new strains of "superbug."

This is thought to be true because antibiotics are, chemically, relatively simple substances; "they may only involve a single molecule, and that is why bacteria are constantly able to develop resistance to them. Aromatic oils, on the other hand, are very complex, containing an array of molecules in different proportions which reinforce each other."[18] It has been found that if the most active anti-infection ingredient in an essential oil is extracted and used on its own, it is less effective.

One enthusiastic British physician has initiated the use of essential oils in his general practice. He does not advocate abandoning modern antibiotics, but believes that they should be used, by those trained in both systems, in harmony with essential oils. "For instance, an inner ear infection (caused by pseudomonas) needs to be brought under control very quickly with antibiotics or there is a danger of the eardrum bursting … But it makes far more sense to treat [a fungal infection of the toenail] locally with an oil which can actually penetrate the nail, rather than handing out a powerful drug that has known effects on the liver and will probably knock out some of the bacteria in your guts as well."[19]

The delicate balance of benign bacteria naturally found in the gut and the vagina is upset not only by antibiotics but also by other common medications such as the contraceptive pill, anti-inflammatory drugs, and antacids. Rosalind Blackwell, a medical herbalist who trained in France, regularly prescribes aromatic oils internally for specific conditions, especially to rebalance intestinal flora and clear up all sorts of chronic infections, such as thrush or cystitis. Fully aware of the dangers of using essential oils internally, she carefully monitors dosage levels and systematically checks her patients for any signs of adverse effects. Although many common conventional drugs are far more toxic than natural aromatic materials, Blackwell stresses the fact that aromatic oils should only be used internally by specifically trained practitioners.

Other fully qualified medical herbalists have also started to use essential oils as part of their treatment program. One British medical herbalist, Colin Nicholls, uses the aromatogram regularly to diagnose and treat his patients using essential oil and herbs. In one case history, a woman came to him suffering from chronic cystitis. Clary sage, an essential oil with an estrogen-like quality, was indicated by the aromatogram, even though it does not have outstanding bactericidal properties. Yet, when the woman took the oil in the form of a vaginal pessary, clary sage got rid of the infection. Putting the estrogen balance right meant that the body could take care of the infection itself. This shows the high degree of accuracy and unique value of individually tailored aromatic remedies when the aromatogram is used as a diagnostic technique.

RIGHT Many bacterial infections have developed a resistance to antibiotics. Alternative methods of treatment may provide the key to dealing with such illnesses.

ABOVE AND ABOVE RIGHT The bacterium Staphylococcus aureus *(above) can be successfully treated with essential oils (above, right).*

Diagnosis and prescription

THE AROMATOGRAM is clearly a very sensitive and highly refined diagnostic tool when applied to the field of clinical aromatherapy. However, Jean Valnet, like other doctors, also made use of other more traditional diagnostic measures, including examining the presenting symptoms of the patient and making an assessment of their overall disposition.

When faced with any kind of illness it is always beneficial to build up an overall picture of the individual concerned and to highlight any contraindications that may be relevant. In the context of clinical aromatherapy, for example, a person who is using high levels of paracetamol should not be given oils containing certain phenols, because both these chemicals have similar elimination pathways and this can lead to an overdose. Before performing an aromatic massage, it is important to make an overall assessment to ensure that there are no contraindications, as in the case of thrombosis, where massage itself is inadvisable. Certain essential oils are also contraindicated in conditions such as epilepsy, high blood pressure, and pregnancy

.

OTHER DIAGNOSTIC TECHNIQUES

Other diagnostic techniques that are of particular value for the practice of aromatherapy, apart from the conventional examination tests, are those associated with reflexology. This is used as a form of treatment in its own right, but it is also a useful diagnostic tool. It consists of an examination of the feet by a trained practitioner. Problematic areas show up as points of congestion or pain in particular points on the soles of the feet, which are linked to specific areas of the body. Iridology may also sometimes be used. Here, areas of discoloration within the iris of the eyes are interpreted as an indication of areas of the body in which there may be problems. Even within the context of clinical aromatherapy, it is valuable to assess the overall temperament and disposition of the individual concerned rather than simply focus on the presenting symptoms.

EUCALYPTUS BARK

LEFT An experienced practitioner will know the character and therapeutic value of an individual oil, such as eucalyptus, before mixing it with others.

PRESCRIBING SPECIFIC BLENDS

In medical herbalism, when preparing a prescription, it is common to mix a number of herbs together to make an individual remedy—usually given in the form of a tincture (an alcohol-based preparation) or an infusion/decoction (a tea made by infusing the herbs in boiling/cold water). The reason for combining herbs in this way is that they can have a synergistic effect upon one another. This means that the therapeutic potential of a single herb is enhanced by the chemical combination with other plant materials; in other words, the end product is greater than the sum of its parts. In medical herbalism, it is also valuable to mix herbs together in order to target different aspects of a particular complaint.

In aromatherapy, likewise, essential oils are usually mixed together to create a synergistic blend or personalized remedy. In this way, each blend develops a unique chemical structure and therapeutic action determined by the combined constituents of all the essential oils used. Unlike herbs, however, essential oils cannot be prepared as aqua-based (water-based) solutions, because they do not mix with water. They are too concentrated to be taken or used on the skin in any way in an undiluted form, but they do mix readily with alcohol and with vegetable oils and fats. When essential oils are prescribed for internal use, they are therefore mixed with an alcoholic base beforehand (much like a tincture) or made into pessaries using a fatty base (e.g. cocoa butter), for insertion into the anus or vagina. This method of medication is not generally used in Britain or the US except as a form of local treatment, but in Europe as a whole it is widely used as a way of introducing therapeutic substances into the system through absorption.

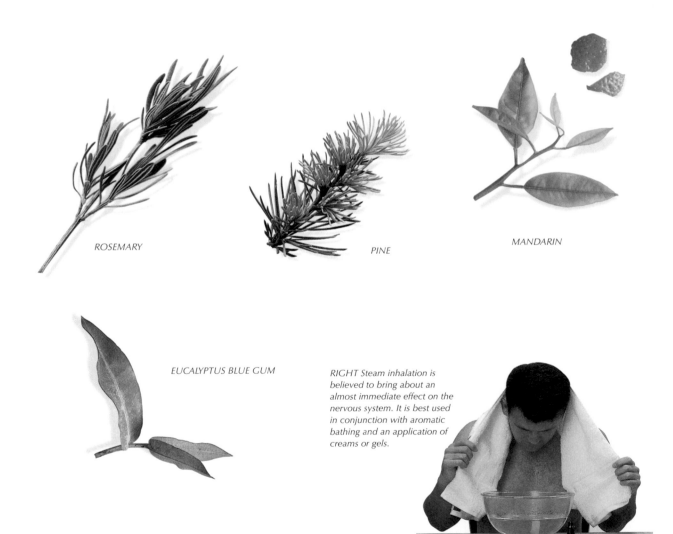

ROSEMARY

PINE

MANDARIN

EUCALYPTUS BLUE GUM

RIGHT Steam inhalation is believed to bring about an almost immediate effect on the nervous system. It is best used in conjunction with aromatic bathing and an application of creams or gels.

PRESCRIBING FORMS OF TREATMENT

Research has shown that oral prescription is not always the most effective form of aromatherapeutic treatment. Even within the context of clinical aromatherapy, both Gattefossé and Valnet advocated a wide range of treatment methods, to be used simultaneously. These included steam inhalations and aromatic bathing, as well as application to the skin using a suitable oil or cream base. This method of treatment means that a multiplicity of substances—specifically combined to treat the illness as it manifests in the particular patient—is absorbed into the body in a variety of ways. Gattefossé found, for example, that the inhalation method brought about an almost immediate effect on the nervous system, in contrast to the slow absorption rate via the digestive system when essential oils were administered orally.

The experienced practitioner can take advantage of all these nuances in the behavior of essential oils to formulate a unique prescription and form of treatment that is tailored to the patient, and makes optimum use of the oils' qualities. For most practitioners, perhaps the most important ingredients in preparing any kind of aromatic remedy are knowledge and experience. Initially, it is imperative to get to know the character and therapeutic potential of each essential oil in its own right before mixing it with others. In considering a blend of oils to treat coughs and congestion, take eucalyptus blue gum (*E. globulus*), for example: it has a camphoraceous, sharp, slightly herbaceous scent; its principal areas of action are as an expectorant, bactericidal, antiseptic, and febrifuge agent; its main chemical constituent is cineole; it is specifically indicated for infectious disease and respiratory illness—especially congested coughs and bronchitis; it is contraindicated for very young children (due to toxicity levels) and will cause the skin to tingle if more than about 3 to 5 drops are added to the bath water.

Having got to know an individual oil, with all its strengths and weaknesses, it is possible to move onto its immediate family. There are various other types of eucalyptus oil, apart from *E. globulus*, but only a few are used therapeutically—notably *E. citriodora* and *E. radiata*. Related family members, in this case of the Myrtaceae family, include tea tree, cajeput, niaouli, West Indian bay, allspice, clove, and myrtle.

Other oils to combine in the case described on p. 127 might include lavender (*L. officinalis*), an effective sedative and tonic to the nerves; and benzoin (well known as an ingredient of friar's balsam, used for chesty conditions), with a mild warming, drying,

and soothing effect on the whole respiratory system. The synergistic combination of myrtle, lavender, and benzoin also represents a balance of top, middle, and base notes or an accord—as described in the section on perfume blending (see p. 70). Mixed in equal proportions, these blended essences could then be used for vaporization, in baths, or for local massage. If the infection persisted, a little tea tree oil could be included for its powerful antimicrobial properties, but it has to be admitted that many children dislike its strong medicinal smell.

There are no magic rules for creating a good aromatic blend or "synergy": it is just a matter of using a combination of common sense, knowledge, and intuition. Whether preparing a blend for massage or for other simple aromatherapy uses, try to match the remedy to the person being treated as precisely as possible, and avoid discordant or unpleasant combinations of aromas. Always consult the safety data for each individual oil (see pp. 239–343) and check for any contraindications before using an aromatic remedy.

PEPPERMINT

MYRTLE

CHAMOMILE

LEFT Some oils, such as myrtle and chamomile, are particularly useful for treating children, as they are mild and not too stimulating.

Case study: treating a child with a cough

The subtlety of the way in which aromatherapy treatment can be tailored by a clinical practitioner to suit an individual case is illustrated in the following case study of a child who is suffering from a chesty cough. In this case there is also insomnia (due to coughing at night) and it is thought that there may be an underlying nervous component in the disposition of the child. In such a case, it is vital to use remedies that will simultaneously combat and support the different aspects of the overall condition, on both a physical and emotional level. Here, the following types of action are required: expectorant (to expel mucus or phlegm); bactericide (to fight infection); balsamic (to soothe irritation); sedative (to induce sleep); nervine (to strengthen and calm the nerves). A herbal tea or syrup using a combination of remedies including chamomile (relaxant), coltsfoot (expectorant), echinacea (antimicrobial), and peppermint (decongestant) would be indicated in this case. For each aspect of the illness there is a choice of oils to be used. In this example, myrtle would be a good oil to include in the prescription as a general aid for the child suffering from a chesty cough and insomnia. This is because although myrtle shares many of the properties of eucalyptus oil (widely used in the treatment of coughs and colds), it is much milder (thus it is more suitable for children), and is not so stimulating (thus it would not interfere with sleep patterns).

The chemistry of essential oils

AN IMPORTANT ASPECT to consider when combining essential oils for therapeutic effect is their chemistry. Essential oils are very complex chemical compounds—a single oil can be composed of hundreds of chemical constituents. The majority of these constituents, however, can be grouped into eleven main chemical families, as shown in the panel below.

A knowledge of the chemical components of essential oils is important for several reasons. Essential oils which share a high proportion of common constituents generally blend well together. For example, clary sage and bergamot combine well because they both contain a high proportion of linalyl acetate (an ester), although they belong to different botanical families and odor groups. The chemical makeup of an individual oil, or a blend of oils, can also provide a very useful key to its potential properties and bioactivities, on both a physiological and psychological level.

The book *L'Aromathérapie Exactement* shows an analysis of the eleven basic chemical families, each of which has an overall stimulating, sedating, or balancing effect. To make the analysis, a grid or scale was produced by spraying essential oils between two electric plates, then noting down their properties. It was found that chemical components with a negative charge, which were attracted to the positive pole, exhibited stimulating, tonic, and warming properties, whereas those components attracted to the negative pole exhibited relaxing, cooling, and anti-inflammatory properties. The effect of individual essential oils and their blends could therefore theoretically be predicted according to their major constituents and their polarity. The different chemical families are graded and coded in detail, and placed in order of their stimulating and relaxing properties.

Esters are generally the most relaxing of the chemical families whereas phenols are the most stimulating. Certain other activities or properties have also been found to be generally associated with

Constituents

The main families of chemical constituents are:

- ⚶ ESTERS: relaxing
- ⚶ ALDEHYDES (aliphatic): relaxing
- ⚶ KEYTONES: relaxing
- ⚶ SESQUITERPENES: balancing
- ⚶ LACTONES AND COUMARINS: balancing
- ⚶ OXIDES: mildly stimulating
- ⚶ ACIDS: mildly stimulating
- ⚶ ALDEHYDES (aromatic): mildly stimulating
- ⚶ MONOTERPENES: stimulating
- ⚶ ALCOHOLS: stimulating
- ⚶ PHENOLS: stimulating

BELOW Oils, which should be stored in dark bottles, are largely stimulating, balancing, or relaxing (sedating) in their effects, as determined by their major ingredients. Red is used to represent oils that are stimulating, purple is used to show that an oil is balancing, and blue is used to show that it has sedating effects.

RED—STIMULATING

PURPLE—BALANCING

BLUE—SEDATING

particular chemical groups. For example, esters are generally considered to have good anti-inflammatory, fungicidal, and cicatrizant (wound-healing) properties. Phenols, on the other hand, display excellent antiseptic and bactericidal properties, although they can also cause skin irritation. For details of the main chemical families found in the oils referred to in this book, see pp. 377–379.

Nevertheless, as Dr. Lis-Balchin points out in her book *Aromascience: The Chemistry and Bioactivity of Essential Oils*, it would be wrong to group together essential oil components of similar chemistry, and assume that certain biological properties can be allocated to these groups with complete predictability. She points out that similar components can influence the action of different essential oils in different ways.[20]

Therefore, although it is interesting to keep the chemical constituents and related potential biological effects in mind, and to use this as a guide to the expected action of individual essential oils, it remains, at best, an estimation. Of greater value in this field are the clinical research studies that have been carried out on the specific effects of botanically classified essential oils. Many such studies have been published, providing precise information on the bioactivity and pharmacology of individual essences.

Among such studies is the systematic research into the possible stimulating or sedating effects of specific essential oils on the nervous system undertaken by

Gattefossé, Valnet, and Rovesti earlier this century. Using the inhalation method, they found that certain essential oils stimulated the nervous functions on a purely physiological level, while others helped induce relaxation.

Further research aimed at distinguishing between those oils which have a sedative effect and those which have a stimulating effect was then taken up in Japan by recording brain wave patterns. During each experiment, the subjects had electrodes attached to their scalp which showed their normal electroencephalogram (EEG) trace, while the measuring device used was the contingent negative variation (CNV) curve, an electrical brain wave pattern created by anticipation. True to expectation, initial studies showed that lavender suppressed the CNV trace, while jasmine increased it—in other words, lavender had a sedative effect and jasmine a stimulating one.

However, some of the CNV traces on individual oils were contrary to expectation. Notably, neroli and rose, which had previously been classified as sedative oils, were shown to have a stimulating effect on brain wave activity, while lemon and sandalwood, which were thought to be stimulating, both showed a marked sedative effect. Subsequent research has shown that some oils can simultaneously stimulate brain activity and sedate other parts of the nervous system, or vice versa. While neroli and rose essence do indeed stimulate the brain and uplift the spirits, at the same time they

EFFECTS OF OILS MEASURED BY CNV CURVE

BASIL
BERGAMOT
ROSEWOOD
CHAMOMILE
CLOVE
GERANIUM
LEMON
LEMONGRASS
MARJORAM
NEROLI
PATCHOULI
PEPPERMINT
ROSE
SAGE
SANDALWOOD
VALERIAN
YLANG YLANG

LEFT Brain wave patterns recorded in the contingent negative variation (CNV) curve, reveal whether a particular essential oil is sedative (left) or stimulating (right).

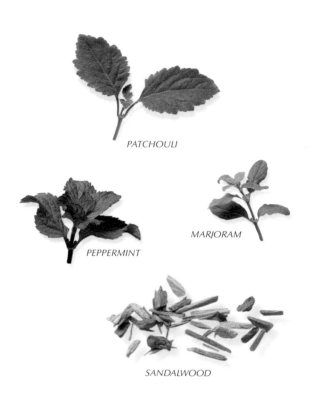

PATCHOULI

PEPPERMINT

MARJORAM

SANDALWOOD

reduce the heartbeat and blood pressure, and soothe the nerves. Many oils, such as bergamot and geranium, also have this dual-action capacity, and have been found to have special value in stress-related disorders through helping to establish a state of calm vitality. Certain oils, such as lavender, can also produce a stimulating or sedative effect depending on the state of the individual concerned—such oils are known as "adaptogens." In the polarity test, lavender shows an almost equal balance of stimulating and sedative components, which may help to account for its regulating effect. On the other hand, clove oil, well known to be a stimulant in treatment and containing approximately 70 percent phenols, shows an overall stimulating quality in polarity tests and the well-known relaxing and calming oil of Roman chamomile, with over 70 percent esters, was proved to be an overall relaxant.

On a purely psychological level, results show that the response can also vary or change according to concentration levels. Gattefossé had noted earlier that some essences were stimulating in small doses, but sedative in larger amounts—much like wine. For example, "angelica essence at low doses stimulates the brain, but at high doses it becomes a narcotic."[21]

BASIL

LEMON

YLANG YLANG

LEMONGRASS

NEROLI

The effects of inhaled essential oils on the nervous system

The sedative or stimulating effects of some of the essential oils tested by Gattefossé, Valnet, and Rovesti are shown below. Geranium proved to be an adaptogen, able to be both sedative and stimulating, depending on the circumstances.

SEDATIVE
aniseed
bergamot
carrot seed
chamomile
clary sage
cypress
geranium
lavender
lemongrass
marjoram
melissa
neroli

STIMULATING
angelica
basil
borneol (camphor)
cardamom
cinnamon
clove
fennel
geranium
jasmine
lemon
pine
rosemary
sage
sandalwood
sweet orange
ylang ylang

APHRODISIAC
borneol (camphor)
cinnamon
clove
myrtle
rose
sage
ylang ylang

ANAPHRODISIAC
borneol (camphor)

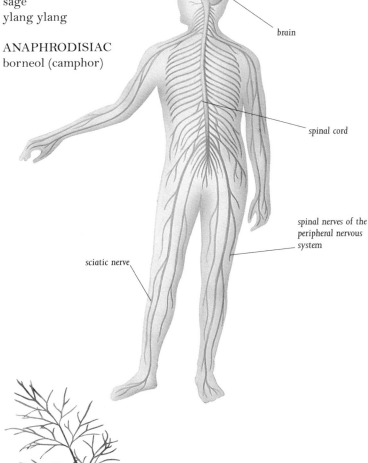

brain

spinal cord

spinal nerves of the peripheral nervous system

sciatic nerve

LEFT The oil obtained from fennel is generally stimulating to the nervous system.

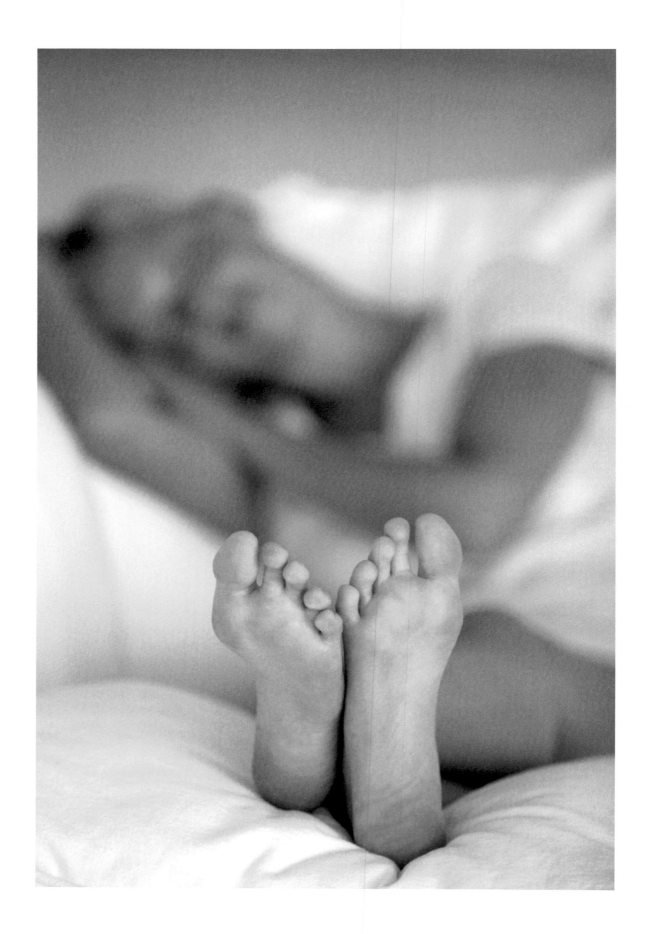

Aromatic remedies

MEDICAL AROMATHERAPY has many useful home applications. The simple treatments, such as aromatic bathing and steam inhalation, described in the first part of the book (pp. 37–40) can all be varied and used for medicinal remedies, and the massage and facial oils, moisturizers, toner-cleansers, and simple creams and gels described throughout the book can be used in treating medical complaints or common skin problems. From the facing page to page 217, a range of frequently occurring medical problems and suitable aromatherapeutic remedies is described.

This section begins with advice on home first-aid remedies, and then covers common medical problems and methods of treatment and prevention. Aromatherapy oils that may be useful are highlighted in each case, and methods of using them described, but advice on dietary and other factors, and on complementary methods of treatment, is also given. Instead of being listed alphabetically, the complaints covered on these pages are divided into the following body systems: the skin, first aid (p. 135); skin disorders (p. 140); the skin, beauty care (p. 158); hair and scalp care (p. 166); bones, muscles, and joints (p. 171); circulatory system and heart (p. 177); respiratory system (p. 185); mouth, teeth, and gums (p. 194); digestive system (p. 198); genitourinary/endocrine systems (p. 205); immune system, infectious diseases (p. 220); nervous system (p. 228). For a complete list of entries see the index on p. 399. Always note any Warning boxes or notes on Safety data for remedies described, and consult the profiles of the oils used in treatments on pp. 239–343 for further information on each particular oil. Do not treat serious or long-term medical problems without the advice of a fully qualified physician.

RIGHT Many forms of aromatherapy can be used safely at home. Herbal tea with chamomile can help with troublesome digestion, as well as relaxation.

THE SKIN: FIRST AID

Bruises

INITIAL PAIN AND swelling are followed by blue, purple, or blackish discoloration of the skin, fading to yellow or brown. This indicates that the underlying tissue is damaged as a result of a knock or pressure. The skin becomes especially prone to bruising when the diet is lacking in vitamin C. Obese and anemic people are most susceptible to bruising. Frequent bruising of the skin may also indicate a kidney complaint.

DIETARY FACTORS

Eat foods high in Vitamin C or take a course of Vitamin C tablets—recommended daily intake is 60mg.

OTHER MEASURES

The Bach Flower Rescue Remedy is recommended if there is shock. Raise and support the injured part if necessary.

CLINICAL NOTES Case

study notes show tea tree to be an effective bruise remedy: "Suppurating bruise checked in 24 hours using solution diluted 1:40 as a compress. Condition cured in one week by continuing this treatment." SEE J. LAWLESS, *TEA TREE OIL*, P. 48.

Methods of use

♡ For minor bruises, an application of neat lavender or tea tree oil reduces inflammation, and speeds up the healing process.

♡ If the swelling is severe, apply an ice compress to ease inflammation. Then gently apply witch hazel lotion to which have been added a few drops of chamomile (Roman or German) or lavender oil. Apply this treatment two to three times a day until the condition clears.

♡ Arnica ointment is one of the most effective bruise remedies.

WARNING

Severe bruising can cause considerable internal bleeding—if worried, seek medical help.

Arnica must not be applied to broken skin.

ABOVE Yarrow oil can also be used in dilution to treat bruises.

Aromatherapy oils

Lavender, tea tree, chamomile (Roman and German), fennel, hyssop, geranium, cypress, yarrow.

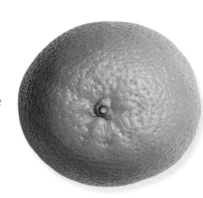

RIGHT A high intake of Vitamin C may help prevent frequent bruising. Oranges are a good source.

Burns

BURNS ARE classified into three degrees of severity: superficial (redness and swelling); intermediate (swelling and blistering); and deep (numbness and charring). They can be caused by dry heat, or moist heat (scalds), and are among the most common household injuries. Burns can also be caused by contact with chemicals, radiation, or electricity.

DIETARY FACTORS
Eat plenty of garlic to help build up the immune system and combat any infection. Alternatively, take a course of garlic capsules.

OTHER MEASURES
The Bach Flower Rescue Remedy is recommended if there is shock. See also Sunburn (p. 138).

WARNING
Severe burns, especially if accompanied by shock, require immediate medical attention.

Avoid fatty oils or ointments when treating burns during the initial stages, as they can cause the skin to "fry."

CLINICAL NOTES
Minor burns respond extremely well to treatment with essential oils, which reduces pain, prevents blistering or infection, and promotes healing without scarring. Both lavender and tea tree oil are being increasingly employed for treating burns in hospitals. SEE LAWLESS, *TEA TREE OIL*, P. 49, *LAVENDER*, P. 55.

Natural bisabolol, found in German chamomile, has been shown to be: "More effective than synthetic racemic bisabolol in healing burns." *POTTER'S NEW CYCLOPAEDIA OF BOTANICAL DRUGS AND PREPARATIONS*

BELOW A gauze dressing with a few drops of essential oil is placed on the burn.

Methods of use

♡ Immediately hold the affected area under the cold tap for ten minutes, then apply neat lavender or tea tree oil to the burn. Reapply at least three times a day until the skin has healed.

♡ For larger areas, especially if there is inflammation, apply an ice compress. Then gently apply a lotion made from 8 to 10 drops each of lavender and German chamomile oil in a 2fl oz (50ml) bottle of distilled water, lavender water, or rose water, shaken well. Shake the bottle before each application.

♡ Cover with a sterile gauze treated with a few drops of lavender, tea tree, or German chamomile. Replace the dressing every few hours. Do not use adhesive plasters.

♡ Calendula cream or oil helps the skin to heal in the latter stages and prevents scarring.

Aromatherapy oils
Lavender, tea tree, German chamomile, eucalyptus blue gum, geranium, yarrow.

Cuts/wounds

SMALL CUTS, grazes, and scratches are some of the most common injuries. Where glass, rust, splinters, or dirt are concerned, special care should be taken to avoid secondary infection.

DIETARY FACTORS

Slow healing may be due to lack of Vitamin C, which also leaves the body more open to infection, especially when the skin is broken. Eat foods rich in Vitamin C or take Vitamin C tablets. Garlic is indicated for infection.

OTHER MEASURES

The Bach Flower Rescue Remedy is recommended if there is shock.

WARNING

Seek immediate medical help in cases of severe bleeding or very deep wounds, which may require stitching.

Do not apply fatty oils or ointments to broken skin during the initial stages of healing, as these can delay the formation of scar tissue.

LEFT Garlic capsules may be taken to guard against infection.

RIGHT Lavender has excellent healing properties and is often used to treat cuts and wounds.

CLINICAL NOTES

Tea tree and lavender are excellent first-aid remedies for all skin abrasions and wounds, due to their excellent antiseptic and wound-healing properties. They do not sting the exposed raw skin, even applied neat, while encouraging a rich flow of blood to the damaged area. They also prevent scarring. Clinical research has shown tea tree to be especially effective for septic conditions, pus-filled infections, and dirty wounds: "… it dissolved pus and left the surfaces of infected wounds clean, so that its germicidal action became more effective without any apparent damage to the tissues … most effective germicides destroy tissue as well as bacteria."

SEE J. LAWLESS, *TEA TREE OIL*, P. 9.

Aromatherapy oils

Tea tree, lavender, chamomile (both Roman and German), yarrow, myrrh, patchouli, benzoin, palmarosa, eucalyptus blue gum, clove.

Methods of use

♡ Cleanse with water, to which a few drops of any of the above essential oils have been added, removing any dirt or fragments.

♡ Apply a few drops of neat lavender or tea tree oil. Cover with a plaster if required—but let the skin breathe whenever possible. Reapply several times a day until the skin has healed.

♡ For splinters, clean the area gently, then apply neat lavender or tea tree oil. Cover with a warm clay poultice and leave for two hours.

♡ Remove the splinter with tweezers, then apply a few drops of lavender or tea tree oil and cover with a plaster.

♡ For swelling, apply a cold compress of witch hazel lotion to which have been added a few drops of chamomile or lavender oil. Apply two or three times a day.

♡ Cover larger injuries with a sterile gauze semi-saturated with lavender or tea tree oil. If the wound is weepy or slow to heal, include a few drops of myrrh or yarrow. Myrrh can also be applied neat to weepy wounds.

♡ Calendula cream or oil helps the skin to heal in the latter stages, and prevents scarring.

Sunburn

THE SKIN is red, itching, and tender, eventually becoming hot and swollen. In severe cases it can turn lobster red, with acute pain, blistering, and peeling. Sunburn is a type of radiation burn due to overexposure to the sun. Radiation burns can also be caused by direct ultraviolet light (e.g. sunbeds) or reflected light (e.g. mountain snow). People with fair skin (and children) are more susceptible to burning than people with dark skin, until their pigmentation increases.

DIETARY FACTORS
Drink plenty of water, or other liquids, to avoid dehydration. People who are especially prone to sunburn can increase their tolerance levels by taking para amino benzoic acid (PABA), a member of the B-vitamin family.

OTHER MEASURES
Sunbathe for short periods only, using effective sunscreens (jojoba oil is equivalent to a factor 6 sunscreen) and avoid the midday sun (12–3pm). Keep vulnerable areas covered by wearing loose clothes and a hat. See also Burns, Heat rash.

CLINICAL NOTES
Clinical evidence has shown that lavender and tea tree can provide great relief from the effects of burns.
SEE J. LAWLESS, *TEA TREE OIL*, P. 49 AND *LAVENDER OIL*, PP. 50, 55.

Chamomile (Roman and German), and rose oil have also both been used clinically in the treatment of radiodermatitis (burned, red, and sore skin caused by radiotherapy).
SEE J. LAWLESS, *ROSE OIL*, P. 20, DATA BASE, VOL. I. P. 7.

WARNING
Overexposure to the sun can cause skin cancer. Excessive sunbathing also causes the skin to wrinkle and turn leathery.

Avoid fatty oils or ointments when treating sunburn during the initial stages as they can cause the skin to "fry."

Methods of use

♥ For patches of sunburn, apply lavender or tea tree oil neat.

♥ For large areas, make up a lotion using 3 to 4 drops of lavender, chamomile (Roman or German) or tea tree oil (or a blend) in 1 tbsp (15ml) of distilled water (or chamomile or rose or lavender water) and dab the area gently.

♥ Soak in a lukewarm bath containing 8 to 10 drops of chamomile (Roman or German), lavender, or tea tree oil; afterwards gently apply a light moisturizing lotion to the skin.

♥ Calendula cream or (infused) oil containing a few drops of rose, chamomile (Roman or German), or neroli oil, helps the skin to heal in the later stages, and prevents scarring.

Aromatherapy oils
Lavender, tea tree, rose, chamomile (Roman and German), yarrow, geranium, neroli.

Stings/bites

STINGS AND BITES vary from minor to severe, and there may be swelling or a gash. Poisoning or an allergic reaction can cause further inflammation and pain, fever, or headaches. Among the more common bites and stings are those of jellyfish, dogs, bees, wasps, ticks, bedbugs, fleas, horseflies, gnats, sandflies, hornets, and mosquitoes. It is important to try to identify the exact cause, since the different types require individual antidotes.

DIETARY FACTORS
Vitamin C helps the skin to heal more quickly. Garlic is indicated for infection.

OTHER MEASURES
The Bach Flower Rescue Remedy is recommended if there is shock. Prevention is always better than cure in the case of all bites or stings.

CLINICAL NOTES
Tea tree oil is traditionally used in Australia for bite and stings, including those of mosquitoes, sandflies, fleas, horseflies, wasps, and bees, and some types of spider and jellyfish.
SEE J. LAWLESS, *TEA TREE OIL*, P. 79.

In France, lavender oil has been traditionally used. Lavender has also successfully treated adder bites.
SEE J. VALNET, *PRACTICE OF AROMATHERAPY*, P. 81.

WARNING
Bee stings can cause an allergic reaction, with severe swelling—seek medical help immediately if this happens.

Snake bites can be extremely dangerous, especially in tropical countries. Get help immediately.

Bites from rabies-infected animals or poisonous snakes, and severe insect stings inside the mouth or throat, require immediate medical attention.

Methods of use

♡ Bee stings: Remove the sting with tweezers (avoid squeezing the venom sac). Apply an ice-cold compress saturated in a solution containing 1 tsp (5ml) bicarbonate of soda, and 1 tbsp (15ml) chamomile or lavender water (or distilled water mixed with a few drops of chamomile or lavender oil). Reapply frequently until the swelling subsides.

♡ Ant bites and hornet sting: Treat with a compress as described for bee stings (above).

♡ Jellyfish/sea urchin stings: Remove any spikes or tentacles carefully, then apply neat tea tree or lavender oil. Repeat at intervals.

♡ Mosquito and other insect bites: Apply neat lavender or tea tree oil (or a blend of the two). Repeat every hour, or as required. If there is inflammation, apply an ice-cold compress with a few drops of chamomile, lavender, or melissa oil. To soothe irritation and prevent infection, add 8 to 10 drops of the above oils to the bathwater daily.

♡ Ticks and leeches: Apply neat tea tree oil to the live tick or leech and surrounding skin and leave. After 20 minutes, remove by hand those ticks or leeches that have not already fallen off. Apply the neat oil to the bite three times a day for a week to soothe any irritation and prevent possible infection.

♡ Snake bites: Call for medical help. Do not move the bitten area, and tie a bandage around the limb to slow down the circulation. For adder bites, apply copious lavender oil.

♡ Spider bites: Mix 2 to 3 drops each of tea tree and lavender oil in 1 tsp (5ml) alcohol or cider vinegar and apply three times a day.

♡ Wasp stings: Apply a cold compress saturated with cider vinegar and 2 drops of lavender or tea tree oil. Reapply fresh compresses frequently until the swelling subsides.

Aromatherapy oils
Lavender, tea tree, chamomile (Roman and German), melissa, basil, bergamot.

THE SKIN: SKIN DISORDERS

Eczema

ECZEMA AND dermatitis are terms for a variety of inflamed or irritated skin conditions with redness, flaky skin rashes, and itching, leading to blisters, weepy sores, and scabs. In hives there is burning and itching, and white bumps, red blotches, or small boils. Sometimes large red weals may appear. Cradle cap affects very young babies. A thick, yellowish crust develops on the scalp, and there is often scaling behind the ears. Atopic (chronic) eczema is associated with inherited allergic tendencies, especially to dairy, or wheat products. Contact dermatitis is the result of hypersensitivity to an irritant such as detergents or cosmetics, dust or wool. The reaction may appear some time after the initial contact, or the skin may suddenly react to a familiar substance.

Aromatherapy oils

Chamomile, tea tree, yarrow, rose, melissa, lavender, myrrh, patchouli, benzoin, carrot seed, cedarwood, Virginian juniper berry, neroli, bergamot, geranium.

DIETARY FACTORS

Lack of fatty acids in the diet has been associated with atopic eczema, and too little pantothenic acid (Vitamin B5) has been connected with allergic tendencies. Vitamin C and the B vitamins are indicated. Evening primrose oil is also beneficial. It may be necessary to consult an allergy specialist.

OTHER MEASURES

In contact dermatitis, try to isolate the allergen by a process of elimination. In both atopic eczema and contact dermatitis, aim to reduce stress levels and emotional anxiety.

CLINICAL NOTES

Clinical studies and case histories have shown tea tree oil, chamomile oil, and rose oil to be effective in various forms of dermatitis and eczema.

References

BOILS see ABSCESSES page 144

CRADLE CAP see ECZEMA page 140

ONYXIS see NAIL INFECTIONS page 148

PARONYCHIA see NAIL INFECTIONS page 148

WHITLOWS see NAIL INFECTIONS page 148

WARNING

Even mild essential oils, such as chamomile, can cause an allergic reaction in some individuals, especially children. Always carry out a patch test (see p. 375) before applying any oil for treatment. It may be necessary to experiment with different essential oils and types of treatment, due to the individual nature of the problem.

Methods of use

♡ For patches of sunburn, apply lavender or tea tree oil neat.

♡ Although pure lavender or tea tree oil can be effective, very low dilutions (1 percent or less) are better suited to conditions involving allergies.

♡ Apply a soothing cold compress, dipped in rose or chamomile or lavender water to which 1 to 2 drops of the following oils have been added: weepy eczema—patchouli or myrrh; scaly eczema—rose or melissa; inflamed eczema—chamomile or yarrow; infected eczema—tea tree or lavender. Repeat as required.

♡ If the skin will tolerate light creams or oils, make up the following mild blend: 5 tsp/25ml calendula cream/oil or evening primrose oil with 5 to 6 drops of blended chamomile, lavender, and rose (or melissa).

♡ Apply to the affected area twice daily.

♡ Add a few drops of a recommended oil to the bathwater as a general measure. A handful of baking soda in the water can reduce itching.

♡ Treat eczema of the scalp, and cradle cap with 2 to 6 drops (according to age) of lavender or tea tree oil blended with 1 tbsp (15ml) of slightly warmed olive oil. Rub gently into the scalp, leave for 5–10 minutes, then wash out. Avoid the eyes while rinsing. Repeat daily initially, then use lavender or tea tree shampoo regularly to prevent recurrence.

Barber's rash

BARBER'S RASH, *tinea barbae*, or shaving rash, is characterized by a mass of small red pimples on the face and neck—the skin is also often flaky and sore. The rash is a fungal infection. The condition is aggravated by shaving, and can be compounded by acne.

DIETARY FACTORS
Eat plenty of garlic, or take a course of garlic capsules, to help build up the immune system and combat infection.

OTHER MEASURES
Avoid using after-shaves containing alcohol, and harsh chemical products, including scented soaps, which aggravate the skin. See also Acne (p. 145).

CLINICAL NOTES
Clinical studies in California (1991) showed tea tree oil to be effective against various types of tinea, including *tinea barbae*.

SEE J. LAWLESS, *TEA TREE OIL*, P. 16.

Aromatherapy oils

Tea tree, lavender, myrrh, lemongrass, patchouli, peppermint, lemon eucalyptus, geranium.

Methods of use

♡ Add 10 to 12 drops of tea tree oil to a 2fl oz (50ml) bottle of lavender water and shake well. Apply to the affected area using absorbent cotton. Shake the bottle well before each application.

♡ Make up a soothing, nourishing cream or oil using 3 to 4 drops each of tea tree, lavender, and myrrh in 5 tsp (25ml) of calendula cream or (infused) oil. Apply sparingly, morning and night.

♡ Put a few drops of tea tree oil (or any of the above oils) in a basin of warm water for washing.

PEPPERMINT

LEFT Tea tree oil can be applied neat or diluted.

Athlete's foot

THIS IS CHARACTERIZED by red, soggy, or flaky skin, and itching between the toes. The soles and heels may become white and scaly. Fingers or nails may also be affected. The skin may become cracked and painful. Athlete's foot is a highly contagious fungal infection. Excessive perspiration and poorly ventilated footwear are often contributory factors to the condition.

DIETARY FACTORS
Eat garlic or take garlic capsules to help build up the immune system and combat infection. Vitamin A is necessary for the health of the skin. If you are very run down, take a course of multivitamin and mineral supplements.

OTHER MEASURES
Do not wear hosiery or footwear made from synthetic materials, and go barefoot to air the feet when possible. Meticulous hygiene is vital.

CLINICAL NOTES
Pure tea tree oil was used successfully to treat athlete's foot in research trials carried out by Dr. M. Walker in 1972.

Aromatherapy oils
Tea tree, lavender, myrrh, lemongrass, peppermint, patchouli, lemon eucalyptus, geranium.

Methods of use

♥ Wash and dry the feet thoroughly, then apply neat tea tree oil—repeat two or three times daily. If the skin is soggy, dissolve the tea tree oil in a little alcohol for the first few days.

♥ Soak the feet for 5–10 minutes daily in a tea tree oil foot bath. Use 5 to 10 drops in a bowl of warm water; a little added cider vinegar is also helpful.

♥ Make a foot powder for daily use by mixing 3 tbsp (45ml) unperfumed talc or cornflour with 5 to 6 drops each of tea tree, lemon eucalyptus (or lemongrass), and lavender. Allow the base to absorb the oils for 24 hours before applying.

♥ If the skin is cracked and painful, apply 3 to 4 drops each of tea tree, lavender, and myrrh in 5 tsp (25ml) of calendula (infused) oil or cream.

NEAT TEA TREE OIL

RIGHT A foot powder or soak made from lavender, talc, tea tree, and eucalyptus can help treat athlete's foot.

Abscesses/boils

AN ABSCESS or boil is a localized painful swelling containing pus and/or serum (tissue fluid), which can occur on any part of the body. The cause appears to be an invasion by bacteria such as staphylococci or streptococci, usually occurring when the body is run down or stressed, at times of hormonal upheaval, or due to a blood disorder. Poor diet and acne are often found to be contributory factors.

DIETARY FACTORS

To purify the system, avoid stimulants, eat lots of fresh fruit and vegetables, and drink plenty of water or herb teas. Include garlic in the diet, or take a course of garlic capsules, to stimulate the immune system.

OTHER MEASURES

Never burst a boil or abscess. Immaculate hygiene is vital to stop the infection spreading. See also Acne (p. 145), Toothache/tooth abscess (p. 194), Stress (p. 236).

CLINICAL NOTES

Medical research has confirmed that tea tree oil is especially effective against boils and abscesses because it penetrates the skin to combat the infection and disperses the pus without making it necessary to break the skin. In a series of clinical trials, it was also shown that tea tree oil: "encouraged more rapid healing without scarring than conservative treatment."

SEE J. LAWLESS, *TEA TREE OIL*, P. 13.

Methods of use

♡ Never wait for the boil or abscess to burst—treat it as soon as it begins to appear by dabbing with neat tea tree oil. Repeat two or three times a day.

♡ If the boil/abscess has already formed, apply a warm poultice of clay containing 3 to 4 drops of tea tree oil. Leave for 30 minutes to draw the liquid or pus, then bathe with water.

♡ Apply a hot compress dipped in a solution of boiled water, a little cider vinegar, and a few drops of any of the recommended oils. Then dab with neat tea tree oil. Repeat the treatment two or three times daily.

♡ If the boil/abscess is severe, apply a gauze pad that has been saturated with tea tree oil for 12 hours. Cover with a plaster. Add 8 to 10 drops of tea tree, bergamot, or lavender oil (or one of the other recommended aromatherapy oils) to the bathwater as a general disinfectant measure.

Aromatherapy oils

Tea tree, lavender, bergamot (bergapten-free), myrrh, chamomile (Roman and German), lemon, galbanum, grapefruit, eucalyptus blue gum, lemon eucalyptus.

LEFT Staphylococci bacteria cause skin infections, such as acne or boils.

LEFT Citrus oils such as mandarin and grapefruit can be useful in treating abscesses and boils.

Acne vulgaris

THIS CONDITION is characterized by a blemished complexion, enlarged pores, spots, pimples, and blackheads—sometimes boils or abscesses can develop. The face, neck, upper chest, and back are affected. The pores become congested due to overactivity of the sebaceous glands. This is especially common during adolescence, the menopause, and before or during menstruation. Acne can be exacerbated by poor diet (especially an excess of fat, oil, and sugar), too little exercise, lack of hygiene, stress, and other emotional factors.

DIETARY FACTORS

A good diet is important. Drink plenty of water and herb teas, such as chamomile, peppermint, echinacea, and lemon balm, and reduce tea, coffee, and alcohol to a minimum. Vitamin A (retinol) deficiency can cause the pores to become blocked, causing whiteheads (goosepimply skin) and blackheads. Recommended nutritional supplements include evening primrose oil, garlic capsules, zinc, and Vitamins A and B.

OTHER MEASURES

Take regular exercise and make time for relaxation. Moderate exposure to sunlight is also beneficial. Wash gently with an unscented pH-balanced soap, and avoid heavy makeup, especially face powders. See also Abscesses/boils (p. 144), Oily skin (p. 160), PMS/PMT (p. 209), Stress (p. 236).

CLINICAL NOTES

Tea tree oil has been highlighted for use against acne in several scientifically controlled blind trials. In Australia (1990), it compared favorably with benzol peroxide, a widely used chemical acne treatment, and had fewer side effects.

SEE J. LAWLESS, *TEA TREE OIL*, P. 15.

Methods of use

♡ Apply neat tea tree oil night and morning using a cotton bud.

♡ To stimulate the lymphatic system, aid elimination, and reduce stress, have a massage once a week, using 7 to 8 drops each of rosemary, geranium, and fennel in 2fl oz (50ml) of a light base oil.

♡ To make a cleansing lotion, mix together 5 tsp (25ml) witch hazel, 3fl oz (75ml) lavender water, 1 tbsp (15ml) glycerine, 7 drops each of lavender and bergamot (bergapten-free), and 3 drops each of tea tree and chamomile oil. Shake well before using.

♡ Make up a healing/nourishing moisturizing oil or cream by mixing 3 drops of lavender and 1 to 2 drops each of patchouli and geranium in 5 tsp (25ml) of apricot kernel oil or a bland cream.

♡ Once or twice a week, apply a deep-cleansing mask containing 5 tsp (25ml) of wet clay paste and 2 to 3 drops each of tea tree, bergamot, and lavender oil.

♡ Steam the face for 10 minutes, two or three times a week, using a few drops of tea tree, bergamot (bergapten-free), and lavender oil in a bowl of steaming hot water. Then apply cold water to which have been added 1 tbsp (15ml) of cider vinegar and a few drops of geranium or cypress oil.

♡ Add 8 to 10 drops of any of the recommended oils to the bathwater, as a disinfectant measure. When washing the face, add a few drops of tea tree oil to the water in the basin.

Aromatherapy oils

Tea tree, bergamot, geranium, lavender, rosemary, cypress, sandalwood, lemongrass, juniper, palmarosa, petitgrain, chamomile, patchouli, lemon eucalyptus.

Warts/verrucae

WARTS ARE BENIGN growths commonly occurring on hands, fingers, face, elbows, or knees. Plantar warts or verrucae usually occur on the soles of the feet, often at the base of the toes. Small black dots are visible at the center of the verruca. Both types are notoriously difficult to get rid of. Both are caused by a papilloma virus. Warts usually disappear of their own accord eventually, but because they are unsightly, most people resort to a cure.

DIETARY FACTORS
Vitamin E has been found to inhibit the formation of warts. Garlic builds up the immune system.

OTHER MEASURES
Verrucae are contagious. Wear rubber socks when swimming to prevent spreading infection.

WARNING

Anal and genital warts, and those on the larynx, require medical attention.

TAGETES

ABOVE *Lemon is a traditional cure for warts, which are caused by a virus.*

CINNAMON LEAF

Methods of use

♡ Treat warts with neat tree tea oil three times a day. This may take a month or more to be effective.

♡ Verrucae should be covered daily with an equal-parts mixture of tea tree and lemon eucalyptus oil, then covered with a plaster. After a few days, the black roots of the verruca should be dug out with a needle. Treatment should be continued for about six weeks until the skin has healed over.

♡ Add a few drops of any of the recommended oils to the bathtub or a footbath to speed up the process, and as a disinfectant measure.

♡ Once the wart or verruca has gone, apply wheat germ or calendula cream or oil, with a few drops of myrrh added, to encourage healing and prevent reinfection.

Aromatherapy oils

Tea tree, clove, cinnamon leaf, lemon eucalyptus, Virginian cedarwood, lemon, tagetes.

Corns/calluses

CORNS AND CALLUSES are areas of hard, thickened skin, generally found on the toes. A corn can form an inverted pyramid that presses into the deeper layers of skin, causing pain. Distorted nails and nail-bed infections often develop. Rheumatism or arthritic conditions, but especially poorly fitting footwear, can contribute to the problem.

DIETARY FACTORS
Lack of Vitamin A in the diet can cause a buildup of dead skin cells, making the skin dry and thickened. Vitamin A is vital for the healthy functioning of the skin.

OTHER MEASURES
Correctly fitting footwear is essential for the prevention and treatment of corns and calluses. See also Nail infections (p. 148), Warts (p. 146).

Aromatherapy oils

Tea tree, tagetes, carrot seed, lavender.

Methods of use

♡ Soak the feet daily in a bowl of warm water containing 1 tbsp (15ml) cider vinegar, a handful of sea salt and a few drops of tea tree oil. Dry thoroughly, then rub the dead skin away gently with a pumice stone or metal nailfile.

♡ After bathing, apply pure tea tree or tagetes oil to the area, then cover with a plaster. Repeat daily—it may take several weeks to see any result, but the treatment is effective in the long run.

♡ As the condition improves, to maintain and promote healthy skin, apply an ointment or oil made from 3 to 4 drops each of lavender, carrot seed and tea tree oil in 5 tsp (25ml) of calendula cream or oil.

LEFT Wearing well-fitting shoes and walking barefoot whenever possible help to prevent corns and calluses.

Nail infections

IN INFECTED NAILS the cuticle becomes inflamed, red, and painful and there can be a slight pus discharge. The skin beneath the nail becomes discolored, and the nail itself furrowed and distorted. The most common infection, *Paronychia* (whitlows), is often caused by contact with detergents. Onyxis is a fungal infection caused by a strain of *Candida albicans*.

DIETARY FACTORS
Adequate protein and Vitamins A and E are important for healthy nails.

OTHER MEASURES
Do not wear nail varnish. Use rubber gloves for washing up or using chemical cleaners to protect the hands.

CLINICAL NOTES
Tree tree oil is very effective because of its penetrating, fungicidal, and antiseptic properties.
See J. LAWLESS, *TEA TREE OIL*, P. 14.

Methods of use

♡ Rub the infected nails three times daily with pure tea tree oil for two or three minutes, massaging the oil into the nailbed.

♡ Mix 1 tsp (5ml) wheat germ oil, 4 tsp (20ml) borage or carrot (base) oil, and 5 to 6 drops each of lavender, rosemary, and carrot seed oil. Massage into nails and cuticles at least once a week as a preventive measure.

Aromatherapy oils

Tea tree, petitgrain, eucalyptus blue gum, lavender, tagetes, rosemary, carrot seed.

LEFT An oil made with carrot seed and wheat germ can be massaged into the nails to treat infection.

ABOVE Nail infections can result from frequent wearing of nail varnish or from washing clothes and dishes without wearing rubber gloves.

Dhobi itch

INFLAMED PIMPLES appear on the inside of the upper thigh, and merge to form a scaly, red, and itchy patch with a clearly marked edge. The condition is properly called tinea cruris. This fungal infection usually affects men, especially in hot weather.

DIETARY FACTORS
Eat garlic or take garlic capsules to help build up the immune system.

OTHER MEASURES
Avoid wearing tight trousers, and let the skin breathe as much as possible. Wash towels and clothing thoroughly.

CLINICAL NOTES
Scientific studies have shown both tea tree oil and lemongrass oil to be effective against tinea infections.
SEE M. LIS-BALCHIN, *AROMASCIENCE*, PP. 68, 100.

Aromatherapy oils

Tea tree, myrrh, lavender, lemongrass, peppermint, patchouli, lemon eucalyptus, geranium.

Methods of use

♡ Add 8 to 10 drops of tea tree and lemon eucalyptus or lemongrass oil to the bath water as a disinfectant measure on a regular basis.

♡ Wash and dry thoroughly, and apply neat tea tree oil to the inflamed area twice a day.

♡ As a preventive measure, apply an ointment or lotion made from 3 to 4 drops each of lavender, myrrh, and tea tree oils in 5 tsp (25ml) calendula cream or (infused) oil.

RIGHT Eating garlic regularly helps to keep the immune system functioning well and so ward off many infections.

MYRRH

LEMONGRASS

Heat rash

THIS RASH OF TINY red blisters can affect any part of the body, and is very itchy. It is the result of sweat glands being blocked through heat or humidity. An allergic reaction may also be implicated.

DIETARY FACTORS
Drink plenty of cold water to cool the body and prevent dehydration. If you are especially prone to heat rash, increase tolerance levels by taking para amino benzoic acid (PABA), a member of the B-vitamin family.

OTHER MEASURES
Keep in the shade; expose the affected area to air; wear a hat, and cover up with light cotton clothing when going out in the sun. See also Eczema (p. 140).

CLINICAL NOTES
Clinical research has demonstrated that rose oil or water can help to alleviate heat rash.
SEE J. LAWLESS, *ROSE OIL*, P. 70.

Methods of use

♥ Add 5 to 6 drops of blended rose (or tea tree), chamomile, and lavender oil to 5 tsp (25ml) rose water, shake well, and gently dab the affected areas, using a saturated cotton pad.

♥ Mix 4 to 5 drops of lavender with a handful (one cup) of baking powder, and add this to a lukewarm bath. Immerse the whole body in the water, and soak for at least 10 minutes.

Aromatherapy oils
Lavender, chamomile (Roman and German), tea tree, rose.

RIGHT Anyone who spends time in the sun should wear a hat or some other form of protective head covering.

Impetigo

TINY RED SPOTS, initially, turning into inflamed patches or pus-filled sores, which blister and then crust over. It usually affects the face, scalp, and neck, but sometimes the hands and knees. This highly infectious skin disease, which mainly affects children, is usually caused by an invasion of streptococcus or staphylococcus bacteria, often as a result of an infected scratch or insect bite.

DIETARY FACTORS
Eat plenty of garlic, or take a course of garlic capsules, to build up the immune system.

OTHER MEASURES
Immaculate hygiene is vital to prevent the infection spreading. See also Alopecia (p. 167), Abscesses/boils (p. 144).

CLINICAL NOTES
Scientific studies have shown that tea tree oil is very effective in treating both the infection and the irritation of this contagious skin condition.
SEE J. LAWLESS, *TEA TREE OIL*, P. 15.

Aromatherapy oils

Tea tree, lavender, myrrh, patchouli, chamomile (Roman and German), benzoin.

Methods of use

♥ Apply pure tea tree oil to the affected area using the tip of the finger or a cotton bud. Repeat the treatment twice a day.

♥ If an open sore has developed, clean the area thoroughly with distilled water to which a few drops of tea tree oil have been added. Then cover with a lint or gauze compress or a dressing that has been saturated in a solution containing 5 tsp (25ml) lavender water and 5 to 6 drops of tea tree oil. Fix this in place for an hour using adhesive tape (around the edge), then remove the dressing, allowing the sore exposure to air. Repeat as required.

♥ Add 5 to 10 drops of lavender or tea tree oil and a cup of cider vinegar to the bathwater or washing water as a disinfectant measure.

RIGHT This highly infectious skin disease mainly affects children, often as a result of an infected insect bite or scratch.

Ulceration

WITH VARICOSE ULCERS, the skin initially takes on a papery-thin appearance, due to lack of blood and oxygen to the area. This fragile tissue can quickly develop into open, often painless, sores—usually on the lower legs or feet. Varicose ulcers can often form on the lower legs as a result of varicose veins. Elderly people are particularly prone to this condition, especially if they suffer from poor circulation—some merely have to scratch the skin on their lower legs and it develops into a sore which can be very slow to heal. Tropical ulcers, or naga sores, also start with papery-thin skin. These ulcers usually occur in hot, humid climates. Again, a large, painless sore develops, often on the feet or legs, due to a bacterial infection, poor nutrition, or environmental factors.

DIETARY FACTORS
Eat plenty of fresh foods—especially those rich in fiber and Vitamins E, C, D, and A. Cut down on dairy products, and avoid tea, coffee, and alcohol. Take zinc as a nutritional supplement, and a course of multivitamin tablets.

OTHER MEASURES
Keep the affected area raised as much as possible: bed rest is recommended. Avoid very hot baths. When sufficiently recovered, take gentle exercise as a preventive measure. See also Low blood pressure (p. 179), Varicose veins (p. 183).

CLINICAL NOTES
Gattefossé and Valnet used lavender successfully for the treatment of long-standing varicose ulcers.
SEE J. LAWLESS, *LAVENDER OIL,* P. 10.

Medical cases illustrate that lavender and tea tree oil are very effective. "Many cases of extreme ulcerations of the legs, with considerable suppurations, which have not responded to treatment by any other means, have been quickly cured with Ti-trol (tea tree oil)."
SEE J. LAWLESS, *TEA TREE OIL,* P. 104.

Aromatherapy oils
Tea tree, lavender, German chamomile, myrrh, bergamot (bergapten-free), geranium, yarrow.

Methods of use

♥ Bathe the sore gently with a warm, diluted solution of lavender, bergamot, and/or tea tree oil by adding a few drops to a bowl of distilled or boiled water.

♥ Apply neat lavender or tea tree oil to the sore. If the skin is very fragile, spray with distilled water to which have been added 3 to 4 drops each of bergamot, tea tree, and lavender oil per 5 tsp (25ml) water (a new indoor plant spray is suitable). Shake well before use and reapply every hour. Keep the sore open to the air as much as possible.

♥ Cover the ulcer with a clean melamine dressing, only when necessary (e.g. for sleeping).

♥ To improve the circulation, and as a preventive measure, massage the feet regularly, using a blend of 3 to 4 drops each of rosemary, cypress, and geranium in 5 tsp (25ml) carrot base oil or sweet almond oil.

♥ As the condition improves, gently apply the following ointment, with upward strokes, once daily: 5 tsp (25ml) calendula cream or oil, with 3 to 4 drops each of lavender (or bergamot), tea tree, and myrrh.

Psoriasis

PSORIASIS is a noncontagious skin disease that varies enormously in severity. Symptoms include chronic scaling, plaques, ringed lesions, smooth red areas, and acute pustules. It is believed to be caused by a dysfunction of skin enzymes, with increased turnover of epidermal cells and a dilation of dermal capillaries. Psoriasis can be precipitated by allergies, environmental factors, and stress.

DIETARY FACTORS
Assess diet for possible allergens. Take 6 x 500mg evening primrose oil daily.

OTHER MEASURES
Sunlight and sea water often give temporary relief. However, psoriasis is a difficult condition to treat, and may involve a variety of approaches. Psychotherapy, hypnotherapy, nutritional, and allergy advice are particularly recommended. See also Alopecia (p. 167), Stress (p. 236).

CLINICAL NOTES
In clinical studies 60 percent of sufferers benefited from taking evening primrose oil.

Methods of use

♡ Make up a thick lotion by blending 5 tsp/25ml avocado oil and 5tsp (25ml) borage seed or evening primrose oil with a little wheat germ oil, and adding 15 drops of tea tree, and 5 drops each of cajeput and myrrh oils. Apply at least twice daily to the affected area.

♡ Mix together 5 tsp (25ml) cider vinegar, 3fl oz (75ml) lavender water, 10 drops each of lavender, cajeput, and tea tree oil. Shake well, and rub into the scalp several times a week.

♡ Add a handful of Dead Sea salt and a few drops of the above essential oils to the bath as a general measure.

Aromatherapy oils
Tea tree oil, cajeput, myrrh, lavender, Virginian cedarwood, angelica.

DEAD SEA SALT

ABOVE Use avocado oil on the skin.

Ringworm

RINGWORM (*tinea capitis*) usually affects the scalp, causing scaly skin and itching—temporary bald patches may also appear. It can also be found on elbows, knees, and other areas in the form of a characteristic, scaly ring. A number of different fungal organisms may be responsible, including *Trichophyton mentagrophytes* and *Microsporum audounii*. It can be picked up from pets and farm animals.

DIETARY FACTORS
Garlic builds up the immune system and combats infection.

OTHER MEASURES
Avoid wearing synthetic fibers. Expose the affected area to fresh air and sunlight as much as possible. Strict hygiene is essential to avoid reinfection. Combs, towels, clothes, and bedding should be disinfected by adding a few drops of tea tree oil to the wash. See also Alopecia (p. 167).

CLINICAL NOTES
Studies show that tea tree, lemongrass, lemon eucalyptus, and grapefruit oils are all effective.

Methods of use

♡ Apply neat tea tree oil to the affected areas. Repeat three or four times a day.

♡ For ringworm of the scalp, apply neat tea tree oil in the same manner, then wash the hair daily with a tea tree oil shampoo.

♡ Add 8 to 10 drops of tea tree oil, or any of the other recommended oils, to the bathwater regularly as a general disinfectant measure.

♡ As the condition improves, make a healing and nourishing cream or oil using 3 to 4 drops each of tea tree, lavender, and myrrh oil in 5 tsp (25ml) of calendula cream or infused oil. Apply morning and night.

Aromatherapy oils
Tea tree, lemongrass, lavender, myrrh, peppermint, lemon eucalyptus, patchouli.

ABOVE Ringworm can be carried by sheep.

LEMONGRASS

Scabies

SMALL, RED, ITCHY PIMPLES which can become infected. Common areas affected are the groin, penis, nipples, and skin between the fingers. This highly contagious skin disease is caused by the itch mite, *Sarcoptes scabiei*. In sheep-farming areas, it is commonly transmitted from the wool of the sheep to farm workers. It does not require close contact to pass from one person to another. The female mites lay eggs under the skin, and when hatched the mites burrow their way out, causing severe irritation and itching.

DIETARY FACTORS
Garlic builds up the immune system to combat infection.

OTHER MEASURES
Frequently wash linen and clothes using a few drops of tea tree oil in the washing water. Sponge the mattress down, using a 10 percent solution in alcohol.

CLINICAL NOTES
Dr. Valnet cites Helmerich's Ointment as efficacious. This contains gum tragacanth, lemon, peppermint, lavender, clove, and cinnamon essential oils.
SEE J. VALNET, *THE PRACTICE OF AROMATHERAPY*, P. 147.

Methods of use

♡ Add 8 to 10 drops of lavender or tea tree oil to bathing and washing water, as a disinfectant measure.

♡ Wash the skin gently, then treat the affected area with a lotion made from 2fl oz (50ml) glycerine, and 5 drops each of tea tree, lavender, lemon eucalyptus, clove, and peppermint oils— apply two or three times a day.

Aromatherapy oils

Tea tree, lavender, bergamot (bergapten-free), peppermint, clove, rosemary, lemon eucalyptus, eucalyptus blue gum, pine, thyme, lemongrass, cinnamon leaf, lemon.

ABOVE *The scabies mite lays its eggs under the skin. When they hatch, the mites tunnel their way out, causing violent itching and blisters.*

PEPPERMINT

CINNAMON LEAF

Chilblains

SMALL, PAINFUL, or itchy, reddish-blue swellings, mostly on the toes, fingertips, nose, or ears. In extreme cases these can cause ulceration. They result from poor circulation, or extreme cold. The condition is aggravated by rubbing.

DIETARY FACTORS

Since vitamin and mineral deficiency (notably of calcium and silicon) can contribute to the problem of chilblains, it may be beneficial to take a multimineral and vitamin supplement daily. Rutin, a bioflavonoid, has also been used successfully in the treatment of circulatory disorders, and dietary supplements may help.

OTHER MEASURES

Exercise and warm clothing are important preventive measures. See also Low blood pressure (p. 179).

CLINICAL NOTES

The British Herbal Pharmacopoeia (1983) cites capsicum or cayenne pepper as specifics for chilblains, applied as an ointment. The essential oil of black pepper shares similar qualities.

Aromatherapy oils

Black pepper, tea tree, lemon, lavender, rosemary, geranium, ginger, pine.

Methods of use

♡ For unbroken chilblains only, add 2 to 3 drops of black pepper oil to 1 tsp (5ml) calendula or arnica cream and massage the area gently.

♡ If the toes are affected, prepare a warm footbath to which a few drops of any of the recommended oils have been added. Soak the feet for 10 minutes at least once a day.

♡ A regular massage treatment to improve the circulation is beneficial, using the following concentrated blend: 10 drops each of rosemary and pine, and 5 drops each of black pepper and ginger in 2fl oz (50ml) of sweet almond oil. Add a little wheat germ oil as a preservative. Local blood supply can also be improved by massaging the feet or affected area with the above blend.

LEFT Poor circulation may cause chilblains and can be improved with dietary ginger, as illustrated, or ginger oil massage.

Cold sores

THESE PAINFUL blister-like sores are usually found on the lips or face. They are infectious and can be spread to other parts of the body or to other people quite readily. The cause is the virus Herpes simplex I, which can lie dormant in the body, only to flare up when the system is under stress. Some people are particularly prone to cold sores, especially when run-down or after exposure to cold winds, excessive heat, or illness.

DIETARY FACTORS
Take Vitamin C and B in the diet or as supplements. Allergies can also be involved, so it is beneficial to assess any dietary indications.

OTHER MEASURES
Strict hygiene is vital to stop the infection spreading to other parts of the body or to other people. See also Stress (p. 236).

CLINICAL NOTES
Clinical studies have shown that pure tea tree oil is a very effective remedy for cold sores, especially if they are treated early on.
SEE J. LAWLESS, *TEA TREE OIL*, P. 16.

Genuine melissa oil is used clinically for treating cold sores in Germany by aromatherapy doctors.

Aromatherapy oils

Tea tree, melissa, lavender, bergamot (bergapten-free), myrrh, geranium, lemon eucalyptus, chamomile (Roman and German).

Methods of use

♡ Use neat tea tree oil to dab the sore spot as soon as it begins to develop—this can stop the cold sore from developing altogether. Repeat frequently until the condition has cleared.

♡ Add 3 drops of tea tree oil (or a blend of lavender, melissa, and tea tree) to 1 tsp (5ml) alcohol or cider vinegar. This astringent lotion may be used in place of pure tea tree oil during the initial stages of treatment, but only if the skin is unbroken.

♡ In the later stages of healing, apply 3 to 4 drops each of tea tree, bergamot (bergapten-free) and lavender or myrrh in 5 tsp (25ml) hypericum or calendula (infused) cream or oil.

MELISSA

RIGHT Myrrh will ease painful cold sores and boost the immune system.

RIGHT Early treatment with tea tree oil or a homemade blend of oils in cider vinegar can sometimes prevent cold sores from developing.

THE SKIN: BEAUTY CARE

Aging skin

CELL DIVISION slows down with age, and the epidermis (outer layer of the skin) becomes thinner, losing tone, and suppleness. Wrinkles develop, and age spots and thread veins are also common. Smoking, drugs, poor diet, too much sun, central heating, and stress can all speed up the aging process.

DIETARY FACTORS

Overeating and overindulgence generally are implicated in hastening aging. A diet rich in fiber and fresh produce, with a minimum of additives, helps promote healthy skin. It is important to drink plenty of liquids daily, although alcohol, tea, and coffee should be drunk in moderation only. Recent research has shown that age degeneration largely results from oxidation caused by the highly reactive chemical compounds known as free-radicals. Antioxidants, notably Vitamins A (beta-carotene), C, selenium, and E, can protect the body from this damage.

OTHER MEASURES

Aging is inevitable, but a healthy lifestyle with adequate exercise and relaxation, and a balanced disposition can certainly help to keep the signs of aging at bay. Despite our youth-oriented culture, age itself should not be rejected. See also Scarred skin (p. 163), Sensitive skin (p. 164).

CLINICAL NOTES

Marguerite Maury demonstrated that essential oils can do much to slow down the effects of aging by encouraging the skin cells to regenerate, as documented in *Guide to Aromatherapy: The Secret of Life and Youth.*

References

CHAPPED SKIN see CRACKED SKIN page 162

GREASY SKIN see OILY SKIN page 160

MATURE SKIN see AGING SKIN page 158

THREAD VEINS see SENSITIVE SKIN page 164

WRINKLES see AGING SKIN page 158

Aromatherapy oils

Rose, frankincense, sandalwood, neroli, geranium, lavender, carrot seed, elemi, galbanum, myrrh, palmarosa, patchouli.

LEFT Eating plenty of fresh fruit and vegetables gives vitality and helps to keep the face and body looking young.

Methods of use

♥ Instead of soaps and alcohol-based products, use a natural toner/cleanser twice daily. In a dark, well-stoppered bottle mix 7 drops each of geranium and lavender oils and 3 drops each of frankincense and neroli (or petitgrain) oils in 3fl oz (75ml) of rose water. After one month, filter into a similar container (use a coffee filter-paper). Add 5 tsp (25ml) glycerine and shake well.

♥ Regular use on face and neck of an oil or cream containing cytophylactic oils (stimulating new cell growth) is vital. A good basic blend for face and neck is as follows: to 5 tsp (25ml) jojoba, almond or grapeseed oil (or a bland cream base), add 1 tbsp (15ml) wheat germ oil, 1tbsp (15ml) rosehip seed oil (or another rich vegetable oil, such as apricot kernel, avocado, hazelnut, borage, evening primrose, or peach kernel), and 10 to 15 drops (in total) of lavender, rose, neroli, or petitgrain, and frankincense essential oils.

♥ To treat and help prevent wrinkles around the eyes, apply a little wheat germ oil or rosehip seed oil, gently to the area before retiring.

♥ Gentle facial massage, avoiding the delicate area around the eyes, helps to improve the circulation and muscle tone. Use any of the recommended oils in a light base oil.

♥ Use a face mask once a week. A basic mask can be made by mixing 2 tbsp (30ml) clay, 2 tsp (10ml) runny honey, 1 tsp (5ml) water, 4 to 5 drops (in total) of carrot seed, frankincense, and lavender oils.

Oily skin

OILY OR GREASY skin is especially common during adolescence, when hormonal changes promote the overproduction of sebum (the natural skin oil). Oily skin is more prone to developing large pores, blackheads, whiteheads, and pimples.

DIETARY FACTORS
Eating saturated fats contributes to the problem. Oily skin on the nose, forehead, and chin (combination skin) is associated with a lack of Vitamin B2 (riboflavin)—found in lamb's liver, yeast, and wheat germ. Eat lots of fresh fruit and vegetables and drink plenty of water, fruit juices, and herb teas.

OTHER MEASURES
Wash gently with an unscented pH-balanced soap. Adopt a suitable skin-care routine, and avoid heavy makeup. Moderate exposure to sunlight is also beneficial. See also Acne (p. 145).

CLINICAL NOTES
Antiseborrheic oils are tea tree, geranium, bergamot, juniper, cedarwood, and lavender. Regulating oils are geranium, lavender, and palmarosa.

CHAMOMILE

Methods of use

♡ To make a cleansing lotion mix together 5 tsp (25ml) witch hazel, 3fl oz (75ml) lavender water, 1 tbsp (15ml) glycerine, 7 drops each of lavender and geranium, 3 drops each of bergamot and sandalwood oil.

♡ Make a moisturizing oil or cream by mixing 2 to 3 drops each of lavender, geranium, and patchouli or palmarosa oil, 1 tbsp (15ml) wheat germ oil, and 5 tsp (25ml) apricot kernel oil or a bland cream. Use in moderation twice daily. Wipe away any excess after 15–20 minutes.

♡ For a reviving cosmetic vinegar mix 4 tsp (20ml) cider vinegar with 5 drops lavender oil, and add 4 tbsp (60ml) rose water and 4 tsp (20ml) witch hazel.

♡ Once or twice a week apply a mask made from 5 tsp (25ml) wet clay paste with 6 to 7 drops (in total) of tea tree, bergamot, and lavender oils.

Aromatherapy oils

Tea tree, bergamot (bergapten-free), geranium, lavender, rosemary, cypress, sandalwood, lemongrass, clary sage, juniper, palmarosa, petitgrain, chamomile (Roman and German), patchouli, lemon eucalyptus, cedarwood.

Dry skin

THIS TYPE of complexion is fine and close-textured, but it is also the most brittle, often having a fragile appearance. It becomes wrinkled more easily than greasy skin, and is also prone to flaking, and conditions such as eczema or psoriasis. In severe cases, thread veins or cracks can develop. Dry skin is aggravated by exposure to central heating and too much sun.

DIETARY APPROACH

Take a supplement of brewer's yeast, which is rich in biotin; assess the diet to check Vitamin A content; if required, take a course of Vitamin A supplements; use cold-pressed vegetable oils in food preparation: walnut, borage, and evening primrose oil especially.

OTHER MEASURES

Moisturize the skin regularly, and protect from extremes of cold and heat. See also Aging skin (p. 158), Cracked skin (p. 162).

CLINICAL NOTES

Rose oil, in the form of an ointment, is beneficial even for extremely dry skin, and has been used in clinical practice for the treatment of skin damaged by radiotherapy.
SEE J. LAWLESS, *ROSE OIL*, P. 20.

Methods of use

♡ Blend 2 to 3 drops each of rose, geranium or palmarosa and lavender, 5 tsp (25ml) of apricot kernel oil, and 1 tbsp (15ml) of a rich oil such as avocado, borage, evening primrose, wheat germ, or rose-hip seed oil. Use as a moisturizer.

♡ A good toner or cleanser for dry skin is made by mixing 7 to 8 drops each of chamomile, lavender, and sandalwood with 3fl oz (75ml) of rose water in a dark, well-stoppered container. After one month, filter, using coffee filter-paper, then add 5 tsp (25ml) glycerine and shake well. Use twice daily.

♡ A mask for dry skin can be made by mixing 2 tbsp (30ml) clay, 2 tsp (10ml) honey, 2 tsp (10ml) cornstarch, 1 egg yolk, 1 tsp (5ml) evening primrose oil or rosehip seed oil, and a few drops of rose, lavender, or sandalwood oil. Leave on the skin for 15 minutes, then rinse off with cool water.

Aromatherapy oils

Rose, sandalwood, neroli, lavender, chamomile, palmarosa, rosewood, geranium, benzoin, myrrh.

ABOVE Create your own moisturizer out of the oils listed above and use regularly to counteract the effects of central heating and the sun.

Cracked skin

CRACKED OR CHAPPED skin is a common problem on the feet and hands, but it can occur on the face, especially around the mouth, or on other parts of the body. The cracks can be painful. Exposure to cold, or skin complaints such as psoriasis or eczema can cause or aggravate the condition. Lack of Vitamin B (especially B2, B6, and biotin), and of fatty acids may be associated with cracked skin.

DIETARY FACTORS
Include cold-pressed vegetable oils (especially walnut and borage oil), and natural sources of Vitamin B, such as brewer's yeast, liver, and wheat germ.

OTHER MEASURES
Protect the skin from extreme cold, and treat exposed and affected skin with rich, moisturizing oils, such as unrefined avocado oil and wheat germ oil. See also Dry skin (p. 161).

CLINICAL NOTES
German chamomile ointment is used medicinally for the treatment of cracked skin.

Methods of use

♡ Mix 3 to 4 drops each of myrrh, German chamomile, and patchouli/benzoin oils with 5 tsp (25ml) calendula cream. Massage the cream into the skin night and morning.

♡ To nourish and moisturize very dry skin, add a few drops of rose oil to 5 tsp (25ml) wheat germ, borage, walnut, avocado, or rosehip seed oil (or a blend of these) and apply daily.

BORAGE

AVOCADO

Aromatherapy oils

Myrrh, patchouli, lavender, German chamomile, benzoin, tea tree, rose, sandalwood.

RIGHT For very dry skin, mix rose oil, wheat germ, borage, walnut, avocado, or rosehip oil and apply daily.

Scarred skin

SOME SCARS ARE pigmented—a common feature of birth marks—although most are flesh-colored. Most are caused by burns or deep wounds. However, a severe case of chicken pox can leave permanent pock marks, as can infected boils, spots, or abscesses. Stretch mark scars, following pregnancy or sudden weight loss, are also common.

DIETARY FACTORS

Lack of folic acid is associated with the slow healing of sores, and with a grayish-brown skin pigmentation. Vitamins C, E, and F or essential fatty acids (such as linoleic acid) are vital for the speedy healing of skin tissue.

OTHER MEASURES

To prevent scars and stretch marks, lubricate the skin, and treat wounds or boils with cicatrizant (healing, cell regenerating) oils immediately. See also Aging skin (p. 158), Chicken pox (p. 223), Pregnancy (p. 216).

CLINICAL NOTES

Vegetable oils rich in Vitamin E (such as borage and wheat germ) are especially good for repairing scarred skin. Rose oil, especially in combination with rosehip seed oil, is also very beneficial for the treatment of all types of scars, including pigmented scars, stretch marks, old injuries, and surgical scars.

Methods of use

♡ Add 1 tsp (5ml) of rosehip seed, wheat germ, or borage oil to 1 tsp/5ml of a hypo-allergenic cream base, with 1 drop of rose, lavender, or neroli oil. Apply at least twice daily.

♡ To prevent stretch marks, mix 1 tbsp (15ml) each of wheat germ, borage and rosehip seed oil in 5 tsp (25ml) jojoba, grapeseed or sweet almond oil. Up to 6 drops of rose, neroli, frankincense, or lavender (or a combination of these) may also be added. After the fourth month, use this twice daily for light massage to the belly and breasts. This blend can also help to get rid of existing stretch marks.

♡ Add 1 to 2 drops each of neroli, rose and lavender to 5 tsp (25ml) of jojoba, apricot or peach kernel oil, or to an anti-allergenic cream or lotion. Use as a daily moisturizer.

Aromatherapy oils

Rose, frankincense, neroli, lavender, elemi, galbanum, sandalwood, palmarosa.

LAVENDER

LEFT Vitamin C, found in oranges and other citrus fruit, is essential for skin regeneration.

Sensitive skin and thread veins

SENSITIVE SKIN can be of any skin type, although it is usually fine-textured and delicate (like a baby's). It is easily irritated or sensitized by substances such as cosmetics, perfumes, or detergents. Thread veins mainly affect those with fair or sensitive complexions, though they can also be a sign of aging. They appear as very fine red lines on the cheeks, giving the face a ruddy appearance. Sensitive skin is commonly a hereditary condition, and may be associated with allergic tendencies. Thread veins are caused by a circulatory problem, which causes the capillary walls to dilate or stretch—like varicose veins.

DIETARY FACTORS
Sensitive skin will often react adversely to chemical food additives; alcohol, coffee, and tea should also be cut to a minimum.

OTHER MEASURES
Avoid exposure to harsh sunlight and extremes of heat or cold. For sensitive skin, it is important to avoid all possible irritants, such as lanolin or alcohol-based toiletries and perfumes, and to use only the most gentle essences. See also Aging skin (p. 158), Varicose veins (p. 183).

CLINICAL NOTES
Rose is a remarkable ally in the fight against thread veins, due to its tonic and astringent effect—but it does require perseverance.

Methods of use

♥ Avoid harsh soaps and products that dehydrate the skin. Instead make a natural cleanser by adding 5 to 6 drops each of chamomile and lavender, and 2 to 3 drops of rose to 3fl oz (75ml) of rose water in a well-stoppered, dark container. Filter, using coffee filter paper, after one month, add 5 tsp (25ml) glycerine and shake well. Apply with a cotton pad, morning and night, before moisturizing the skin.

♥ For thread veins and sensitive skin, blend 2 to 3 drops each of rose, neroli, or petitgrain, and lavender oils with 5 tsp (25ml) witch hazel and 3fl oz (75ml) orange flower water and apply to the cheeks twice a day.

♥ For moisturizing the skin, add 5 to 6 drops (in total) of rose or chamomile or lavender oil to 5 tsp (25ml) jojoba, apricot, or peach kernel oil or an antiallergenic cream or lotion. Use daily. For thread veins, mix 1 tbsp (15ml) of rose-hip seed oil or a hypoallergenic cream with 3 drops of rose oil and gently massage into the affected area twice daily.

♥ For inflamed thread veins, apply soothing compresses of rose water to the cheeks.

♥ Avoid clay masks, and instead use face packs containing honey, which is soothing and moisturizing, and suitable for thread veins, sensitive, and dehydrated skin.

ABOVE Rose oil makes an excellent treatment for sensitive skin.

Aromatherapy oils

Rose, chamomile, lavender, jasmine, neroli, carrot seed, yarrow.

Perspiration

THE PRODUCTION OF perspiration or sweat is the body's natural cooling device. Vigorous exercise and heat cause an increase in perspiration rate. Stress, anxiety, or fear can cause the body to break out in a "cold sweat." Perspiration only becomes a problem when bacteria on the skin's surface cause it to break down, producing lactic acid—which has an offensive odor.

DIETARY FACTORS

Drinking plenty of water ensures that the body is constantly flushed out and cleansed. In hot climates, it is particulary important to drink plenty of water and to take extra salt to replace that which is lost in sweat.

OTHER MEASURES

Wash regularly, using bactericidal tea tree soaps; avoid wearing clothes made from synthetic fibers (nylon, polyester, lycra); wear footwear made from leather or other materials that allow the skin to breathe.

WARNING

Using chemical deodorants to prevent perspiration altogether is not healthy since it blocks the pores. Aluminum-based deodorants can cause dermal irritation.

CLINICAL NOTES

The classic eau-de-Cologne/ deodorant oils are bergamot, neroli, lavender, and rosemary (sometimes with thyme, orange, lemon, and petitgrain added). This aromatic blend from Cologne rapidly became well known for its cooling, refreshing, deodorant, and antiseptic properties.

SEE P. DAVIS, *AROMATHERAPY: AN A–Z.*

ABOVE *Rosemary is used in many soaps, cosmetics, and perfumes to refresh and invigorate the body.*

Methods of use

♡ Add 5 to 6 drops (in total) of lavender, tea tree, and/or rosemary oil, and 1 tbsp (15ml) of cider vinegar to a bowl of warm water, and soak the feet nightly for 5 minutes. Add 8 to 10 drops of any of the recommended oils to the bathwater.

♡ A few drops of tea tree oil can be mixed with a little witch hazel and rubbed into the soles of the feet or beneath the arms in the morning.

♡ A classic eau-de-Cologne can be made as follows: 100 drops (5ml) bergamot, 50 drops (2.5ml) lemon, 50 drops (2.5ml) lavender, 30 drops (1.5ml) neroli or petitgrain, 10 drops (0.5ml) rosemary oils. Add to 5fl oz (150ml) vodka and leave in a cool, dark place to mature for at least a month.

♡ Add 10 drops bergamot, 5 drops lemon, 5 drops lavender, 3 drops neroli or petitgrain, and 1 drop rosemary oil to 2fl oz (50ml) of a base oil such as sweet almond or grapeseed to make a cooling, refreshing body oil.

Aromatherapy oils

Tea tree, petitgrain, cypress, rosemary, bergamot, grapefruit, myrtle, neroli, thyme, lemon, orange, lime, mandarin, lavender.

HAIR AND SCALP CARE
Greasy hair

THE CONDITION of the hair reveals a great deal about an individual's overall health and can affect a person's whole appearance. Greasy, lank hair not only looks unattractive, it is also difficult to style or control. Greasy hair, like oily skin, is caused by overactivity of the sebaceous glands in the scalp. Frequent washing with harsh detergent shampoo strips the hair of its natural oils, and induces an ever greater production of sebum.

DIETARY FACTORS
Eating too many junk or fast foods such as potato chips, or fried foods, and especially saturated fats, can contribute to overproduction of sebum (oil) in the hair follicles and scalp. A nutritious diet, rich in minerals and vitamins (especially Vitamins B, C, and F or essential fatty acids) is vital for the growth of healthy hair and for regulating seborrhea.

MANDARIN

OTHER MEASURES
Use a mild pH-balanced shampoo that will not strip the hair of its protective acid mantle, and a natural bristle brush for brushing the hair. See also Dandruff (p. 168), Alopecia (p. 167).

References
DAMAGED HAIR see DRY/DAMAGED HAIR page 169

HAIR LOSS see ALOPECIA page 167

PEDICULOSIS see HEAD LICE page 170

SEBORRHEIC DERMATITIS see DANDRUFF page 168

CLINICAL NOTES
Tea tree and West Indian bay oil are used in commercial shampoos for greasy hair, while rosemary oil is used in pharmaceutically prepared lotions and liniments. Lavender oil also makes an excellent conditioning treatment for oily hair.
SEE J. LAWLESS, *LAVENDER OIL*, P. 72.

Methods of use

♡ Choose a mild or pH-balanced shampoo that will not strip the hair of its protective acid mantle, and add 20 to 30 drops of rosemary, bay, and bergamot or sandalwood oil per 3½fl oz (100ml) shampoo (or 2 to 3 drops to 1tsp (5ml) of shampoo). Try to leave at least three days between shampoos.

♡ As a conditioner for oily hair, mix 10 to 12 drops (in total) of rosemary, sandalwood, and lavender with 5 tsp (25ml) of slightly warmed jojoba oil (or sunflower seed oil) and massage thoroughly into the scalp. Wrap in warm towels and leave for an hour if possible. Wash out—applying the shampoo before the water, or the hair will remain oily. Repeat once a week.

♡ Mix 2fl oz (50ml) lavender water (rose water or orange flower water), 2fl oz (50ml) witch hazel, 1 tbsp (15ml) cider vinegar, and 3 drops each of grapefruit, West Indian bay or rosemary, and lavender. Massage into the scalp between shampoos as required. Add 3 drops of lavender, rosemary, or bay and 1 tbsp (15ml) of cider vinegar to the final rinse water. This will help to remove detergent residue and restore the acid equilibrium of the scalp.

Aromatherapy oils

Bergamot, cedarwood♡, cypress♡, sandalwood, lemon♡, lime♡, grapefruit, rosemary, West Indian bay, juniper♡, lavender, mandarin♡, pine♡, tea tree, patchouli, petitgrain, clary sage, Spanish sage, yarrow.

Note: The oils marked ♡ are unstable in shampoo or detergent.

Alopecia

ALOPECIA—hair loss—can be patchy, or it can result in total baldness. It mainly affects men, but some women are also prone, especially after middle age. In men, the condition is generally inherited. Poor nutrition, hormonal upheaval, and stress are also contributing factors. In women, the most common cause of hair loss is the overuse of hair dyes, permanents, and bleaches. Illness, and the side effects of chemotherapy and radiotherapy, can cause dramatic hair loss.

DIETARY FACTORS

Cut down on tea, coffee, and alcohol and eat foods that are rich in vitamins and minerals. Vitamins B, C, and F (essential fatty acids) are especially good for the hair, as is inositol, found in liver, wheat germ, oatmeal, molasses, and yeast. A course of yeast tablets and a lecithin supplement are recommended.

OTHER MEASURES

Avoid chemical treatments and wash the hair once a week only, using a mild pH-balanced shampoo.

CLINICAL NOTES

Essential oils help combat hair loss by stimulating the hair follicles (roots), and, especially in combination with massage, by promoting the circulation: Studies have shown that...
"pure lavender essence used as a scalp massage reduces hair loss and encourages regrowth."
SEE C. MEUNIER, *LAVENDER AND LAVENDINS*, P. 198.

Aromatherapy oils

West Indian bay, rosemary, lavender, German chamomile, clary sage, juniper, Spanish sage, yarrow.

Methods of use

♡ Local massage is effective if carried out regularly. Make a scalp massage oil by mixing 3 tbsp (45ml) coconut oil, 3 tbsp (45ml) wheat germ oil, and 7 to 8 drops each of West Indian bay, rosemary, and lavender oils.

♡ To encourage hair growth and to treat baldness (alopecia), mix 10 to 12 drops of rosemary or lavender with 5 tsp (25ml) of slightly warmed jojoba oil, castor oil, or extra virgin olive oil and massage thoroughly into scalp. Wrap in warm towels and leave for an hour. Wash out—but apply shampoo before the water, or the hair will remain oily. Repeat once a week.

♡ Mix 1 tbsp (15ml) cider vinegar with 3 drops each of West Indian bay, rosemary, and lavender oils, and add to 3½fl oz (100ml) of lavender or rose or orange flower water. Shake well and massage the mixture into the scalp.

♡ Alternatively, rub a few drops of neat lavender oil into the scalp.

♡ Add a few drops of any of the above oils to the shampoo at each wash, or to the final rinse water.

LEFT As a herbal remedy, try rinsing with nettle infusion.

Dandruff

DANDRUFF CAN BE mild or severe. In pityriasis, and simple dandruff, small, dry flakes of dead skin are released into the hair from the scalp, spoiling its appearance. In seborrheic dermatitis, however, the greasy patches of skin may become infected, causing scabbing and inflammation. Seborrheic dermatitis is aggravated by overactive sebaceous glands. Chemical hair preparations, poor diet, and stress can contribute.

DIETARY FACTORS
Faulty diet and food allergies are often a major cause, especially when combined with greasy hair. Evening primrose oil capsules and Vitamin E will help most cases of dandruff.

OTHER MEASURES
Use a natural bristle hair brush, and avoid brushing the hair when it is wet. If the condition persists, have a food allergy test.

CLINICAL NOTES
Scientific research has demonstrated that lemongrass oil is effective specifically against *P. ovale*, a fungus or yeast infection that causes dermatitis.
SEE M. LIS-BALCHIN, *AROMASCIENCE*, P. 68.

Aromatherapy oils

Tea tree, chamomile, citronella, clary sage, lavender, lemongrass, lemon eucalyptus, rosemary.

Methods of use

♡ Mix 25 drops of tea tree oil (5 drops of lemongrass oil may also be added) with 2fl oz (50ml) of slightly warmed jojoba or coconut oil.

♡ Massage thoroughly into scalp. Wrap in warm towels and leave for an hour. Wash out, using about 5 drops of tea tree oil to 1 tsp (5ml) of a mild shampoo. Apply the shampoo before the water, to prevent the hair remaining oily. Repeat once a week.

♡ Use up to 5 drops of tea tree oil to 1 tsp (5ml) mild shampoo on a daily or regular basis.

♡ Between washes, if required, rub a few drops of pure tea tree oil into the scalp using the fingertips.

♡ Add a few drops of any of the recommended oils to the final rinsing water when washing the hair.

BELOW Chamomile is especially indicated for dry, irritated, or sensitive scalp conditions.

Dry/damaged hair

DRY, STRESSED, OR overtreated hair tends to become dull, frizzy, and difficult to manage. The hair becomes brittle, and the ends split more easily. It is often the result of frequently subjecting the hair to chemical treatments, such as permanents, bleaching, or artificial coloring. Exposure to the sun and heat treatments also dry out the hair.

DIETARY FACTORS

Protein deficiency results in brittle hair and nails, while a lack of essential fatty acids (found in cold-pressed vegetable oils) causes dry hair and a scaly scalp. A nutritious diet is vital for the growth of healthy hair.

OTHER MEASURES

Use a mild pH-balanced shampoo, which will not strip the hair of its protective acid mantle, and a natural-bristle brush. See also Alopecia (p. 167), Dandruff (p. 168).

Aromatherapy oils

Sandalwood, ylang ylang, lavender, chamomile (Roman and German), rose, geranium, petitgrain, neroli, clary sage, Spanish sage, yarrow, rosemary, tea tree.

Note: Ylang ylang is not stable in shampoo or detergent.

Methods of use

♥ Choose a mild or pH-balanced shampoo and add 20 to 30 drops (in total) of chamomile, lavender, and geranium per 3½fl oz (100ml) of shampoo (or 2 to 3 drops of essential oil to 1 tsp (5ml) of shampoo).

♥ Mix 10 to 12 drops (in total) of chamomile, petitgrain, and lavender with 5 tsp (25ml) of slightly warmed jojoba oil, castor oil, or extra virgin olive oil. Massage thoroughly into the scalp. Wrap in warm towels and leave for an hour. Wash out—but apply the shampoo before the water, or the hair will remain oily. Repeat once a week.

♥ As a final rinse for dry hair, add 3 drops of lavender, petitgrain, geranium, or chamomile oil, and 1 tbsp (15ml) cider vinegar to the rinsing water. This will help to remove detergent residue and restore the acid equilibrium of the scalp.

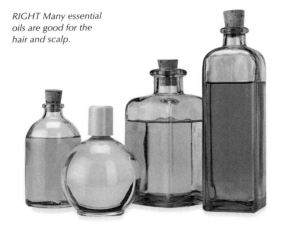

RIGHT Many essential oils are good for the hair and scalp.

YARROW

Head lice

LICE ARE SMALL, grayish, bloodsucking insects that live in the hair. They keep very close to the scalp and can be difficult to see because they are no bigger than a pinhead. Lice can pass very quickly from one head of hair to the next. The first sign of their presence is often that the scalp starts to itch. This occurs after the lice have multiplied enough to cover the scalp with thousands of tiny bites. The lice also lay tiny, grayish-white eggs—the nits—which attach themselves firmly to the hair, usually near the scalp. The eggs are hard to see, and can also be quite difficult to remove.

DIETARY FACTORS
To prevent lice, eat plenty of garlic regularly.

OTHER MEASURES
Regular combing can usually keep lice infestations at bay. If any member of the family does get lice, it is vital that all family members check their hair and carry out preventive treatments. Brushes, combs, towels, and pillowcases should be thoroughly washed and disinfected, using a few drops of tea tree oil in the washing water.

CLINICAL NOTES
Several essential oils can kill lice, but do not prevent their eggs from hatching. Therefore, they must be used regularly (at three-day intervals) until all the eggs have hatched or been removed. These remedies are less toxic than commercial treatments, and actually improve the quality of the hair rather than damaging it.

LEFT Lice multiply rapidly in the hair, by laying tiny eggs. Their bites cause an uncomfortable itching sensation in the scalp.

RIGHT A scalp rub of a recommended oil and a special fine-toothed comb, available from pharmacies, can be used as part of the treatment.

Methods of use

♡ During an outbreak, use a lavender or tea tree oil shampoo daily to prevent contamination. Add 1 to 3 percent of lavender or tea tree oil to a mild or pH-balanced shampoo (use 20 to 60 drops per 3½fl oz (100ml) of shampoo, or 2 to 3 drops to 1 tsp (5ml) of shampoo). Leave for 10 minutes before rinsing. Also add a little lavender oil to the conditioner or final rinse water.

♡ To counteract lice or eggs, make up an alcohol-based scalp rub by adding 1 tsp (5ml) of lavender and tea tree oils to 5 tsp (25ml) vodka, and 3fl oz (75ml) water. Leave for at least an hour (overnight if possible), then wash out. Finally comb the hair carefully with a fine-toothed comb. Repeat every three days from the start of an infestation until the condition has cleared up.

♡ If the scalp is too irritated or sensitive to use alcohol, replace the alcohol and water in the scalp rub with a vegetable oil.

Aromatherapy oils

Eucalyptus blue gum, lavender, tea tree, cinnamon leaf, rosemary, geranium, clove, thyme.

BONES, MUSCLES, AND JOINTS

Rheumatism

GENERALLY, RHEUMATISM (like fibrositis) refers specifically to muscular pain, whereas arthritis is associated with pain located within the joints. The onset of rheumatic tendencies is often gradual, and the exact cause can be difficult to define—however, the condition nearly always signifies long-term friction, either of a purely physical, or of a more subtle, psychological nature. A slight, though progressive, aching in the muscles can suddenly flare up, usually in association with stress, or environmental factors, such as exposure to cold or damp, or a change in diet.

DIETARY FACTORS
Since rheumatism, like arthritis, is aggravated by an accumulation of toxins in the system, the diet should be adjusted in a similar manner (see Arthritis, p. 174).

OTHER MEASURES
It is most important to assess the overall lifestyle: "It is essential to treat the whole being, (for) when the unique picture of the individual is taken into account, it is possible to open the gates for quite a miraculous healing to occur."
SEE HOFFMAN, *THE HOLISTIC HERBAL*, P. 83.
See also Muscular pain (p. 173).

References
ACHES AND PAINS see MUSCULAR PAIN page 173
GOUT see ARTHRITIS page 174
HOUSEMAID'S KNEE see BURSITIS page 176
MUSCULAR SPASM see CRAMP page 175
OSTEOARTHRITIS see ARTHRITIS page 174
RHEUMATOID ARTHRITIS see ARTHRITIS page 174
SPORTS INJURIES see SPRAINS/ STRAINS page 172
TENNIS ELBOW see BURSITIS page 176

CLINICAL NOTES
Spike lavender and juniper oil are current in the *The British Herbal Pharmacopoeia* for the treatment of rheumatic pain, applied topically.

Methods of use

♡ Massage is helpful for rheumatic pains because it stimulates the circulation and helps remove toxins. For a concentrated massage oil mix 3 to 4 drops each of lavender, juniper, rosemary, and black pepper or ginger oil in 5 tsp (25ml) St. John's wort oil. Apply by massage to the area twice daily.

♡ Add 8 to 10 drops of any of the recommended oils to the bathwater whenever required for pain relief, and to increase mobility.

♡ Alternate hot and cold compresses, using a few drops of lavender or chamomile oil, can help relieve pain and swelling. Leave each compress in place for 10 minutes before changing.

Aromatherapy oils

For detoxifying—fennel, juniper, carrot seed, celery seed, lemon, tea tree, angelica, grapefruit.
For inflammation—chamomile, lavender, yarrow.
Analgesic (pain killers) for stimulating greater mobility—pine, spike lavender, marjoram, rosemary, ginger, black pepper, eucalyptus blue gum, cardamom, peppermint, clove.

RIGHT Fennel can be very helpful for rheumatic aches and pains, both as part of the diet, and as fennel seed oil rub, mixed with a base oil.

Sprains/strains

SPRAINS CAUSE PAIN and tenderness around the joint, made worse by movement, with swelling and bruising. A strain is characterized by a sudden, sharp pain at the site of the injury. There can be swelling, stiffness, and cramp. A sprain occurs at a joint where the ligaments and surrounding tissues are wrenched or torn. A strain occurs when a muscle or group of muscles is overstretched by a violent or sudden movement. It is most commonly caused by lifting heavy weights or by taking strenuous exercise.

DIETARY FACTORS
Adequate Vitamin C in the diet is vital for the rapid healing of tissues and bones.

OTHER MEASURES
Rest and support the affected area. Elevate an injured limb, using cushions.

CLINICAL NOTES
The traditional remedy for application to slow-healing sprains, *Oleum spicae*, was made by combining spike lavender oil and turpentine (pine oil).

WARNING
Severe sprains or strains are difficult to distinguish from fractures: in all doubtful cases, seek medical help immediately.

Methods of use

♥ Apply a cold compress (with ice) to which a few drops of chamomile oil have been added. Repeat as often as possible to reduce the swelling. Do not massage. Wrap in a bandage moistened with witch hazel lotion and rest as much as possible.

♥ As the swelling subsides, gently apply the following cream or oil: 3 to 4 drops each of pine, lavender, and rosemary oil in 5 tsp (25ml) calendula cream or oil. Alternatively, use a liniment moistened with a few drops of any of the recommended oils (or a blend).

♥ Apply arnica ointment to the skin locally for bruising—unless the skin is broken.

♥ To encourage healing, soak in a warm bath containing 8 to 10 drops of one of the recommended oils and 3 tbsp (45ml) sea salt.

LEFT Pine is used in many ointments to treat sprains and strains.

Aromatherapy oils

Spike lavender, lavender, chamomile, pine, rosemary, eucalyptus blue gum, thyme, marjoram.

Muscular pain

MUSCULAR ACHES AND PAINS can affect any part of the body. Many people carry tension in their necks and shoulders, which causes the muscles to become tight and painful. Muscular pain can be caused by overexertion, poor posture, cold or damp, injury, stress, and tension. It can also be related to other complaints, such as rheumatism, arthritis, lumbago (lower back pain), or a "slipped disk."

DIETARY FACTORS

Muscular aches and pains can indicate lack of biotin (this can be destroyed by taking antibiotics). The best natural source of biotin is yeast. Lack of Vitamin E can also lead to muscular degeneration, causing stiffness and pain: supplements of evening primrose or borage oil are indicated.

OTHER MEASURES

Take gentle exercise (yoga, swimming); assess stress levels; avoid sudden, strenuous exercise without sufficient training. Alexander Technique can help improve habitual poor posture; osteopathy is indicated if there is a slipped disk or structural problem.

CLINICAL NOTES

It is well known among keen sports players that the combination of essential oils and massage is very effective for muscular aches and pains, as well as a valuable preventive treatment: "Rosemary is ... a very good oil to use for tired, stiff, and overworked muscles. I have used it very successfully for massage [before and] after training or competing."
SEE P. DAVIS, *AROMATHERAPY: AN A–Z*, P. 293.

Aromatherapy oils

Marjoram, rosemary, black pepper, chamomile, lavender, ginger, pine, juniper, bergamot, grapefruit.

Methods of use

♥ Muscular aches and pains respond well to local massage—make a massage oil by adding about 7 to 10 drops each of lavender, marjoram, and rosemary oil to 2fl oz (50ml) of carrier oil, and rub into the affected area. Best after a warm shower or bath.

♥ Soaking in a hot bathtub is an easy and effective way of relaxing the muscles and bringing instant pain relief. Adding 8 to 10 drops of any of the recommended oils to the water will increase the benefits further.

♥ As a preventive treatment, and to tone the muscles before strenuous exercise, make a massage oil by mixing 10 drops each of rosemary and pine oils with 5 drops each of grapefruit and black pepper oils in 2fl oz (50ml) of a vegetable carrier oil. Rub gently into the whole body, concentrating on the muscles that will have to work the most.

LEFT Rosemary oil is widely used in the treatment of muscular aches and pains.

ABOVE Ginger warms the muscles and the oil is effective in sports massage.

Arthritis

THERE ARE SEVERAL different kinds of arthritis, all forms of joint distress resulting in pain and progressive immobility. The three most common are rheumatoid arthritis, osteoarthritis, and gout. With the former, which can affect all age groups, the connective tissue around the joints (usually the wrists and knuckles) becomes swollen. The skin becomes tight and shiny around the joint, which gradually becomes stiff and sometimes deformed. With osteoarthritis, which usually occurs in the elderly, an aching pain and stiffness develop slowly, usually in the hips, knees, or fingers. Gout is characterized by severe pain and swollen joints, often with a burning sensation. It usually affects the joints of the toes, but also sometimes the fingers. All types signify an inability to eliminate toxic waste efficiently. Heredity, stress, emotional conflict, lack of exercise (or overuse, in the case of osteoarthritis), poor diet (or over-rich food, in the case of gout), or food allergies can all contribute to these conditions.

DIETARY FACTORS
Initially the diet should aim at eliminating toxic waste: drink plenty of water and herb teas; eat salads, fruit, green vegetables, whole wheat bread, pulses, white meat, and fish. Avoid red meat, tea, coffee, alcohol, fried foods, vinegar, spices, refined flour, and sugar products, and all additives and preservatives. Vitamins A, C, D, and E are especially important for healthy bones and muscles. Take 1 tbsp (15ml) cod liver oil, and evening primrose oil supplements daily.

OTHER MEASURES
Take gentle exercise, especially yoga; reassess physical, emotional, and environmental factors—many cases of arthritis are brought on by underlying emotional issues. It is important to identify anything that aggravates the condition, such as stress, cold, and certain foods. It may be valuable to consult a dietary specialist to check for food allergies.

CLINICAL NOTES
Case studies show that aromatherapy is one of the most effective treatments for arthritis through helping to eliminate toxic waste, as well as providing considerable relief from pain and increased mobility.

Methods of use

♥ As an excellent initial detoxifying treatment for all types of arthritis, add 3 drops each of fennel, carrot, or celery seed, and juniper oil (or up to 10 drops of any of the above detoxifying oils) to the bathwater, together with two handfuls of Epsom salt and one of rock salt. Repeat daily for two weeks. Oils (see below) for soothing pain or increasing mobility are also beneficial used in baths.

♥ Make a massage oil to stimulate greater mobility and ease pain by mixing 7 to 10 drops each of lavender, rosemary, and marjoram oil with 2fl oz (50ml) of a vegetable carrier oil. Rub into the area very gently twice daily.

♥ To ease inflammation and pain, apply a cold compress with a few drops of lavender, and chamomile or yarrow oil. To reduce stiffness, a hot compress may be used with oils such as rosemary, marjoram, or black pepper.

Aromatherapy oils

For detoxifying—fennel, juniper, carrot seed, celery seed, lemon, grapefruit. **For inflammation**—chamomile, yarrow, lavender. **For stimulating greater mobility**—pine, marjoram, rosemary, ginger, black pepper, eucalyptus blue gum, cardamom, lavender.

WARNING
Immediately after any kind of heat treatment (baths, massage, compress), the joint should be kept moving to avoid congestion. Never massage directly over a swollen joint.

Cramp

CRAMP OR MUSCULAR spasm causes sudden, intense pain. It can affect both the smooth (involuntary) muscle and the voluntary muscles with which we move our limbs. The calf or foot are most commonly affected (often at night), especially if there is anemia, or during pregnancy. Dysmenorrhea is also a form of cramp, caused by the contraction of the smooth muscles surrounding the uterus wall; stomach cramps often accompany severe indigestion or diarrhea. Poor circulation, exposure to cold, or other factors which cause an insufficient flow of blood to the muscle tissue can all cause spasm. An overworked muscle may also suddenly go into spasm, a common problem for keen sports players.

DIETARY FACTORS

A rich or heavy diet can induce cramps. Avoid swimming immediately after eating a big meal. Lack of pantothenic acid (found in yeast, liver, and wheat germ) may be involved. Cramp can also be caused by a deficiency of salt, sodium, or other elements in the blood. Garlic capsules, calcium, and zinc supplements are recommended. The herb cramp bark, taken as a tea three times a day, is effective.

OTHER MEASURES

Stretch or flex the cramped muscle; then, gently stroke the affected area to warm it up, before applying deeper pressure, finally kneading the knotted muscles. See also Dysmenorrhea (p. 205), Dyspepsia (p. 200), Muscular pain (p. 173), Pregnancy (p. 216).

CLINICAL NOTES

Many case histories bear witness to the fact that essential oils are very valuable for treating and preventing cramp or muscular spasm. "I was troubled by acute pain and spasm in my neck muscles ... I massaged lavender into my neck which greatly reduced the pain and muscle spasm." SEE *INTERNATIONAL JOURNAL OF AROMATHERAPY*, VOL. 3, NO. 1, 1991, P. 24.

Methods of use

♥ To relieve muscular spasm of the limbs, or if a particular area is very tight or painful, massage with a concentrated blend containing 5 drops each of marjoram, rosemary, and lavender oil, and 3 of black pepper or ginger oil in 5 tsp (25ml) base oil or cream.

♥ For stomach cramp, period pains, or muscular spasm brought on by cold, apply a hot compress, using a few drops of clary sage or marjoram oil. Keep it warm with a hot water bottle.

♥ As a preventive treatment after strenuous exercise, make a concentrated massage oil by mixing 7 to 10 drops each of rosemary, marjoram, and lavender oil with 2fl oz (50ml) of a vegetable carrier oil. After a warm shower, rub the oil gently into the whole body, concentrating on the muscles that have worked the most.

♥ Add 8 to 10 drops of any of the above aromatherapy oils to the bathwater after taking strenuous exercise as a preventive measure.

Aromatherapy oils

Rosemary, clary sage, marjoram, black pepper, lavender, ginger, pine, bergamot, juniper, chamomile, coriander.

RIGHT Massage with one of the recommended aromatherapy oils will help relieve cramps which often attack calf muscles.

Bursitis

BURSITIS is characterized by hot, swollen, and tender skin at the elbow joint (tennis elbow), knee joint (housemaid's knee), shoulder, or hips. This is due to inflammation of the bursae—the small, water-filled cushions that enable muscles and tendons to move smoothly at the joint. The condition may be caused by repeated use, friction, or an accident involving a hard knock to the joint. It may also show a degenerative rheumatic or arthritic tendency.

DIETARY FACTORS
Boost the amounts of dietary calcium and magnesium needed to form the synovial fluid that lubricates the joints. Rich sources of calcium include milk, leafy green vegetables, nuts, seeds, and grains. Foods rich in magnesium are whole grains, nuts, and seafood. Vitamin C is also vital for the rapid healing of tissues and bones. Take Vitamin C supplements to aid recovery.

OTHER MEASURES
Rest the joint until the inflammation has subsided. See also Arthritis (p. 174), Edema (p. 184), Rheumatism (p. 171).

CLINICAL NOTES
Clove stem should not be used in aromatherapy treatments due to dermal toxicity. Clove bud oil is officially: "patented for external use in the degeneration of bone, inflammation of joints, bursitis, and the treatment of sinuses."
SEE M. LIS-BALCHIN, *AROMASCIENCE*, P. 45.

> **WARNING**
> Never massage directly over a swollen joint.

Methods of use

♡ Mix 3 to 4 drops each of rosemary, pine, and marjoram or clove oil with 5 tsp (25ml) of calendula cream or oil and apply gently, twice daily, to the affected part of the body.

♡ Initially, if the joint is very swollen, apply a cold compress, using a few drops of lavender or chamomile oil. Repeat as required to reduce inflammation.

Aromatherapy oils
Clove bud, chamomile, spike lavender, yarrow, rosemary, marjoram, pine.

LEFT A cold compress can be held over painful and inflamed areas to reduce pain and swelling.

RIGHT To combat bursitis, boost your intake of magnesium and calcium. Leafy green vegetables are rich in calcium.

THE CIRCULATORY SYSTEM AND HEART

Arteriosclerosis

MANY FORMS OF arteriosclerosis go unnoticed but one of the main symptoms of the most serious form, which affects the coronary arteries, is angina, a severe pain in the chest, and also breathlessness, usually brought on by stress or exercise. The danger of arteriosclerosis is that it can result in a coronary thrombosis (heart attack) or a stroke if the warning signs are not heeded in time. There may also be kidney damage. Arteriosclerosis is caused by a slow buildup of fatty deposits (atheroma) in the lining of the arteries (which carry blood from the heart). This leads to a thickening and hardening of the arterial walls, restricting the flow of blood and oxygen. Atheroma is linked to high blood cholesterol.

DIETARY FACTORS

Eat plenty of fresh, unrefined foods; avoid red meat, animal fats, dairy produce, and refined wheat and sugar products; alcohol, tea, and coffee should be drastically reduced—a glass or two of red wine is permitted. Cut out salt altogether. Raw onions, garlic, and rosemary, Vitamin C and E supplements are all beneficial.

OTHER MEASURES

To reduce stress levels, a more relaxed lifestyle, which includes gentle exercise (yoga or swimming are ideal), should be taken up. Aromatherapy massage can help to reduce stress and anxiety levels. See also High blood pressure (p. 178), Stress (p. 236).

CLINICAL NOTES

Yarrow is current in *The British Herbal Pharmacopoeia* as a specific for thrombotic conditions with hypertension.

References

ANGINA see ARTERIOSCLEROSIS page 177

BLOOD PRESSURE see HIGH BLOOD PRESSURE page 178, LOW BLOOD PRESSURE page 179

FLUID RETENTION see EDEMA page 184

HYPERTENSION see HIGH BLOOD PRESSURE page 178

HYPOTENSION see LOW BLOOD PRESSURE page 179

PILES see HEMORRHOIDS page 182

POOR CIRCULATION see LOW BLOOD PRESSURE page 179

TARCHYCARDIA see PALPITATIONS page 180

Methods of use

♥ Have a massage at least once a week using 7 to 10 drops each of rosemary and lavender oils and 5 drops of valerian oil in 2fl oz (50ml) of vegetable carrier oil.

♥ Rub the above blend of oils into the chest and soles of the feet on a daily basis.

♥ Use relaxing oils such as lavender, marjoram, or chamomile for baths on a daily basis to help to reduce stress levels.

Aromatherapy oils

Rosemary, lemon, yarrow, lavender, valerian, marjoram, juniper, chamomile.

LEFT Valerian, once known as "all heal," has been used as a herbal remedy since medieval times. It is now used to treat angina.

High blood pressure

HIGH BLOOD PRESSURE is a common side effect of the fast pace of 20th-century life. Symptoms may include headaches, palpitations, feelings of anxiety, and restlessness—workaholics are especially prone. The condition, in the long term, may lead to serious kidney disease or heart failure. Prolonged stress, smoking, and arteriosclerosis (the thickening and hardening of the arterial walls); poor diet, especially too much alcohol, salt, animal fats, and caffeine, can all contribute to the problem.

DIETARY FACTORS
Diet should be reassessed: eat plenty of fresh, unrefined foods, especially those containing Vitamin E; avoid red meat, animal fats, salt, and refined wheat and sugar products; stimulants such as alcohol, tea, and coffee should be drastically reduced. Intake of cholin and inositol should be reviewed. Garlic is beneficial.

OTHER MEASURES
General lifestyle, work, and ambitions need to be seriously reassessed for satisfactory long-term results. Other measures may include yoga, meditation, psychotherapy, or counseling. See also Arteriosclerosis (p. 177), Palpitations, (p. 180) Stress (p. 236).

CLINICAL NOTES
Aromatherapy massage has been found to be especially effective in implementing change in this field.

Aromatherapy oils

Lavender, marjoram, ylang ylang, chamomile (Roman and German), clary sage, vetiver, melissa, yarrow, bergamot, valerian, rose, neroli, jasmine.

Methods of use

♡ If possible, put aside some time each week to have a regular professional massage, using a blend of relaxing oils: 7 to 10 drops each of ylang ylang, lavender, and marjoram oil in 2fl oz (50ml) jojoba oil. Self-massage or massage between partners or friends is also valuable.

♡ Take a soothing bath every day, using 8 to 10 drops of relaxing oils such as lavender, ylang ylang, chamomile, or marjoram.

♡ Use relaxing oils, singly or blended, in a vaporizer at home or in the office on a regular basis. Alternatively, put a few drops on a handkerchief for inhalation throughout the day.

GRANARY LOAF

LEFT A good mixed diet, with plenty of fresh fruit and vegetables, fresh fish, cereals, and grains rather than red meat, and vegetable oils rather than animal fats, helps to ensure good health and normal blood pressure.

BELOW Salty foods such as smoked fish should be reduced.

JASMINE

SMOKED MACKEREL

Low blood pressure

ALTHOUGH THIS condition (hypotension) has less potential danger than high blood pressure, it is often accompanied by debilitating symptoms such as dizziness, lightheadedness, constant feelings of tiredness, and sensitivity to the cold (especially the hands and feet). Nervous exhaustion, stress, poor circulation, anemia, and hereditary factors can all contribute.

DIETARY FACTORS

Eat foods rich in Vitamins C and E; also use lots of onions and garlic. Spices such as ginger, coriander, and black pepper can help to stimulate the circulation.

OTHER MEASURES

Fresh air, sufficient exercise, and deep-breathing exercises are beneficial. Brisk massage is particularly useful.

WARNING

Hypotension can be a symptom of a more serious health problem—if worried, seek medical advice.

Methods of use

♥ Make a therapeutic massage oil by mixing 7 to 10 drops each of rosemary, pine, and basil (or 5 of black pepper) oils with 2fl oz (50ml) of a vegetable carrier oil. Apply briskly to the entire body, paying particular attention to the hands and feet.

♥ Add 8 to 10 drops of any of the above aromatherapy oils to the bathwater regularly.

♥ Use stimulating oils in a vaporizer at home or in the office to uplift the mind and invigorate the body.

Aromatherapy oils

Rosemary, pine, basil, fennel, peppermint, West Indian bay, thyme, angelica, Spanish sage, black pepper, caraway, ginger, cinnamon, coriander, clove, camphor.

CORIANDER (CILANTRO)

ABOVE AND RIGHT Fresh garlic and garlic oil in capsule form help regulate blood pressure and protect against heart disease.

Palpitations

THIS IS A GENERAL term used to describe an irregular heartbeat, either "missing a beat" or a rapid fluttering or pounding of the heart. The condition (tachycardia) can be brought on by exercise (which is quite normal), but is also associated with high blood pressure, stress, and panic attacks. It is especially common in women during the menopause.

DIETARY FACTORS

Increase intake of the B vitamins; avoid stimulants, notably nicotine and caffeine; do not eat too much; use garlic in cooking (or take as a supplement); drink relaxing herbal teas, such as chamomile or verbena.

OTHER MEASURES

Training in yoga, meditation, deep breathing, or relaxation exercises can help to reduce stress levels and combat panic attacks.

WARNING

Palpitations may be a sign of an underlying heart disorder—if worried, seek medical advice.

Aromatherapy oils

Ylang ylang, lavender, clary sage, rose, melissa, chamomile, neroli, valerian.

Methods of use

♡ A full-body massage is very effective in reducing stress levels. If possible, have a regular professional massage weekly, using a blend of 7 to 10 drops each of ylang ylang, lavender, and clary sage oils in 2fl oz (50ml) jojoba oil.

♡ For self-massage, use the above blend and rub thoroughly into the soles of the feet. This is very therapeutic and relaxing.

♡ Inhaling ylang ylang (or other relaxing oils) can help calm a rapidly beating heart.

♡ Regular aromatic bathing using ylang ylang, lavender, neroli, rose, or chamomile essential oils helps reduce stress levels and anxiety, which often trigger tachycardia.

ABOVE A full-body massage or self-massage can be effective in reducing stress. Massage the feet using the recommended oils.

BELOW Regular baths using aromatic oils can help reduce stress, which triggers tachycardia.

Cellulite

THIS FATTY, orange peel-like cell tissue commonly found on the thighs, legs, and upper arms, is very stubborn to shift even after considerable weight loss from other parts of the body has been achieved. There is a variety of causes: toxicity is a major factor, whether the cause is environmental or due to diet. Treatment, therefore, should focus on ridding the body of impurities. There is also a hereditary predisposition to developing cellulite.

DIETARY FACTORS

Correct diet is essential in the treatment of cellulite. Eliminate (or reduce) tea, coffee, alcohol, and refined products; use organically produced foods whenever possible; eat lots of raw fruit and vegetables, and drink plenty of spring water or herb teas. Zinc and Vitamins C and B complex are also indicated.

OTHER MEASURES

Even severe cases of cellulite can be reversed if dietary changes are combined with the following measures:

♥ Plan an exercise routine that specifically targets the cellulite (as cellulite often gathers in places that tend to get no exercise).

♥ Give the area a vigorous massage and use a loofah or scrubbing brush briskly while in the bath. This can help to break down congestion within the system, especially when combined with appropriate essential oils.

♥ Take up relaxation and deep breathing exercises to increase the supply of oxygen to the tissues, which is vital in shifting cellulite.

♥ Increase blood circulation with daily dry skin-brushing. Using a brush of real bristle, brush toward the heart, up legs, trunk, and arms, and down from the shoulders, starting with the feet and continuing all over the body.

♥ Have a full-body massage each week, if possible, concentrating on stimulating lymphatic drainage.

CLINICAL NOTES

There are many commercial creams and oils that claim to eliminate cellulite—often with dubious results. Essential oils are only effective if they are used in combination with the other measures stated here.

Methods of use

♥ A full-body massage, using 7 to 8 drops each of rosemary, geranium, and fennel to 2fl oz (50ml) base oil, is very beneficial, helping to increase the circulation generally and improve lymphatic drainage.

♥ Make up a concentrated oil or cream using 3 to 4 drops of carrot seed, grapefruit, and fennel oils in 5 tsp (25ml) of jojoba or carrot carrier oil (or a bland cream) and rub into the affected areas vigorously.

♥ Use 8 to 10 drops of any of the recommended oils (or a combination) in the bathtub. In addition, apply a few drops to a brush or loofah and rub the affected areas briskly in circular movements while bathing.

Aromatherapy oils

Spanish sage, bergamot (bergaptenfree), rosemary, juniper, thyme, grapefruit, celery seed, fennel, geranium, carrot seed, coriander, angelica, mandarin, orange, lime, petitgrain, lemon.

WARNING

Many citrus oils are phototoxic—do not use on the skin before exposing to direct sunlight or using a sunbed.

Hemorrhoids

HEMORRHOIDS OR PILES are swollen veins in the walls of the anus, which can appear on the inside or outside. They may be itchy or painful, and can bleed—surgery may be required in severe cases. Heredity, a sedentary lifestyle, being overweight, sluggish circulation, pregnancy, constipation, and poor diet are all contributing factors.

DIETARY FACTORS

Include plenty of roughage in the diet, such as bran and whole wheat bread; salads and fruit also help to cleanse the digestive system. Drink plenty of liquids daily. Take a course of garlic capsules and Vitamin E supplement.

OTHER MEASURES

Take more exercise, and keep the legs raised as much as possible. Inverted yoga positions are beneficial. See also Varicose veins (p. 183).

CLINICAL NOTES

Ranunculus (pilewort) is specific for this problem, used in topical application. Yarrow oil has well-documented vasoconstrictive properties.

Methods of use

♡ To alleviate symptoms and as a preventive, make up an ointment using 5 to 6 drops each of cypress or yarrow, and geranium oils in 5tsp (25ml) calendula cream (or a gel). Apply topically several times daily, or as required.

♡ Add 8 to 10 drops of any of the above oils to the bathwater, or to a sitz or hip bath daily.

♡ To soothe irritation, use cold witch hazel lotion applied on absorbent cotton.

Aromatherapy oils

Cypress, geranium, yarrow, rose, Virginian cedarwood, clary sage, frankincense, myrrh, myrtle.

BRAN

FRANKINCENSE

GERANIUM

Varicose veins

THESE ARE unsightly and sometimes painful, swollen, or knotted veins, usually in the legs. They are the result of poor circulation and inadequate elasticity in the walls of the veins. Heredity, lack of exercise, standing for long periods, overweight, pregnancy, and poor nutrition all make a contribution to this condition.

DIETARY FACTORS
Have a diet high in fiber; Vitamins E, and C, and rutin (a riboflavonoid found in buckwheat and the pith of citrus fruits) are also indicated; use garlic in cooking (or take as a supplement).

OTHER MEASURES
Take gentle exercise; do not sit with legs crossed; avoid standing for long periods; rest with the legs raised (also when sleeping); inverted yoga postures are beneficial; do not take very hot baths. See also Hemorrhoids (p. 182).

CLINICAL NOTES
Cypress and rose can do much to tone the blood vessels and reduce dilation.

Methods of use

♥ Make up a massage oil or cream containing 7 to 10 drops each of geranium (or 5 of rose), yarrow and cypress oil in 2fl oz (50ml) calendula oil or cream and rub gently into the area around and above the veins. DO NOT press directly on them or below them, and work up the legs toward the heart. The legs should be elevated after massage. Repeat this massage daily.

♥ To help reduce swelling, apply local cold compresses soaked in witch hazel lotion.

♥ Warm (not hot) baths with 8 to 10 drops of a circulatory stimulant such as rosemary or juniper can help improve the condition of the circulatory system as a whole.

Aromatherapy oils

Cypress, geranium, rose, yarrow, Virginian cedarwood, clary sage, frankincense, myrrh.

ROSE

CYPRESS

Edema

IN EDEMA, excess fluid is retained in the body tissues, causing swelling or puffiness. Most commonly found in the ankles, it can also affect the hands, feet, abdomen, around the eyes—or the whole body. Edema or fluid retention is a common complaint, especially during pregnancy and in obesity, and is caused by fluids leaking from the tissues. Allergies, sprains, high blood pressure, PMS, jetlag, and taking oral contraceptives can contribute to this condition.

DIETARY FACTORS

B vitamins are indicated; fennel, celery, parsley, garlic, and onions are beneficial. Drink fennel herb tea.

OTHER MEASURES

If the ankles or feet are affected, keep the legs raised as much as possible, and while sleeping. Massage is one of the best treatments for stimulating the circulation and lymphatic system, and thus eliminating excess fluids. Gentle exercise is a valuable preventive measure. See also Bursitis, Jetlag, PMS.

CLINICAL NOTES

In a venture combining aromatherapy and herbal medicine, a blend of six oils (juniper, lavender, clary sage, chamomile, rosemary, and thyme) was applied by neuromuscular and lymphatic drainage massage to three women suffering from PMS-associated edema twice a month: "It was concluded that the treatment was successful for persistent edema and the synergy between two complementary disciplines was proven."

SEE *DATA BASE*, VOL. I, P. 10.

Methods of use

♥ Add 3 to 4 drops each of rosemary, geranium, and fennel to 5 tsp/25ml of carrier oil or cream. Massage into the affected area using gentle upward strokes (always toward the heart).

♥ If possible, have a full-body lymphatic drainage massage once a week until the condition subsides.

♥ Add 8 to 10 drops of any of the oils listed to a warm (not hot) bath, or to a footbath if the ankles are affected.

Aromatherapy oils

Fennel, geranium, cypress, juniper, rosemary, celery seed, parsley seed, dill, angelica, carrot seed, grapefruit, thyme, lavender, clary sage, chamomile.

WARNING

Generalized edema is often a sign of serious kidney disease or progressive heart failure—seek medical help immediately.

Rosemary and juniper are contraindicated during pregnancy.

RIGHT Celery seed helps eliminate the build-up of toxins in the body.

THE RESPIRATORY SYSTEM

Colds

THE SYMPTOMS of a cold include sore throat, coughing, feverishness, aching limbs, sneezing, fatigue, and catarrh. Secondary infections such as bronchitis, sinusitis, or ear infections may arise. There are at least 30 different strains of the virus that can cause the common cold—or in medical terms, coryza. It is a highly contagious infection affecting the upper respiratory tract, and is picked up by breathing infected air. Exposure to cold, damp conditions, and to stuffy or smoky atmospheres, stress, and being generally run down are all contributory factors.

DIETARY FACTORS

Eating excessive amounts of dairy and wheat products encourages the formation of excess mucus. A cold is the body's attempt to cleanse the system of this congestion. To keep the system clean, eat plenty of fresh fruits and vegetables, particularly those high in Vitamin C (especially lemons, oranges, strawberries) and lots of onions and garlic. Alternatively, if already infected, take a course of garlic capsules and Vitamin C tablets. Cut down on alcohol, tea, and coffee: instead drink herbal teas—especially peppermint, rose-hip, and elderflower—or lemon with honey.

OTHER MEASURES

Rest and keep warm—staying in bed encourages faster recovery and prevents the germs from spreading. See also Coughs (p. 186), Headaches (p. 229), Influenza (p. 226), Throat infections (p. 193).

References

OTITIS see EARACHE/OTITIS page 192
RHINITIS see HAY FEVER page 190
SORE THROATS see THROAT INFECTIONS page 193

Methods of use

♡ For colds with a cough, or chills, make up a warming, concentrated chest rub by mixing 4 to 5 drops each of ginger, thyme, and lavender or hyssop in 5 tsp (25ml) of carrier oil, and apply to the chest and upper back. Repeat at least twice a day.

♡ Use tea tree, thyme, or eucalyptus oil in vaporizers throughout the duration of the illness, but especially at the onset of the cold—this may prevent it from developing at all. Add a few drops of one of these oils to a handkerchief for inhalation throughout the day. Use drops of soothing oils such as myrtle or lavender on the pillow at night.

♡ Add 5 to 6 drops (in total) of tea tree, eucalyptus, or Spanish sage or thyme oil to a bowl of steaming water, cover the head with a towel and breathe deeply for 5–10 minutes, keeping the eyes closed. (Very hot steam is in itself a hostile environment for viruses.) Repeat at least twice a day.

♡ Take a daily hot bath, adding 8 to 10 drops of tea tree, rosemary, or thyme to the water—this combats congestion and fights infection. Lavender, marjoram, or bergamot oil can also be used in baths to soothe aching limbs and encourage restful sleep.

♡ For a sore throat, add 4 to 5 drops of tea tree or Spanish sage or clary sage or thyme to a glass of warm water, mix and gargle at least three times daily.

Aromatherapy oils

Tea tree, eucalyptus blue gum, myrtle, rosemary, marjoram, lavender, cajeput, lemon, pine, thyme, peppermint, bergamot, black pepper, ginger, cinnamon leaf, clove, Spanish sage, hyssop.

Coughs

COUGHING IS A reflex action aimed at clearing the respiratory tract. A cough can be dry and unproductive, or can be accompanied by mucus discharge. Coughs can have several causes, including smoking, and exposure to dust, pollen, or a cold, damp atmosphere. They usually occur in association with an infection such as whooping cough, or with allergies such as hay fever or asthma.

DIETARY FACTORS
Dairy and wheat products encourage the formation of excess mucus. To cleanse the system, eat plenty of fresh fruits and vegetables, especially those high in Vitamin C (including lemons, oranges, and strawberries) and lots of onions and garlic. Cut down on alcohol, tea, and coffee, and instead drink herbal teas—especially peppermint—and lemon with honey. The herb coltsfoot is excellent for persistent coughs, taken as a tea or syrup, three times a day.

OTHER MEASURES
Stop smoking, rest, and keep warm, especially the chest, throat, and neck area. Identify the type of cough (dry, infected, congested) and treat accordingly. See also Bronchitis (p. 188), Colds (p. 185), Fever (p. 227), Headaches (p. 229), Influenza (p. 226), Sinusitis (p. 191), Throat infections (p. 193).

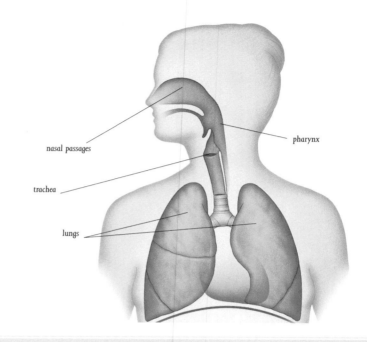

nasal passages

pharynx

trachea

lungs

WARNING
Use no more than 3 drops of the spice oils (eucalyptus, camphor or peppermint) in the bathtub.

Methods of use

♡ To loosen mucus and ease congestion, rub the chest, back, and throat with a blend of warming and expectorant oils: 3 to 4 drops each of lavender, thyme, ginger or hyssop in 5 tsp (25ml) of a light base oil or cream.

♡ Regular steam inhalations will help to soothe a dry cough. Add 2 to 3 drops each of sandalwood, and/or frankincense or benzoin to a bowl of steaming hot water and inhale for 5 to 10 minutes. For congestion, use 2 to 3 drops each of tea tree, lavender, thyme, peppermint, and/or eucalyptus oil. Repeat at least twice a day.

♡ To combat infection, use tea tree, spike lavender, eucalyptus, or thyme (or a combination) in a vaporizer or humidifier in the home, and more soothing oils (sandalwood, benzoin, frankincense, cedarwood, or myrtle) for dry coughs and in the bedroom at night. A few drops of these essential oils may also be put on a handkerchief for inhalation throughout the day.

♡ Hot baths with 8 to 10 drops of any of the recommended oils (or a combination) aid the body's natural response to infection. This also has a similar effect to steam inhalation.

Aromatherapy oils

Warming/tonic (for chills)—angelica, cinnamon, ginger, nutmeg, clove, aniseed. **Soothing/balsamic (for dry coughs)**—benzoin, cedarwood, myrrh, frankincense, galbanum, sandalwood, marjoram.

Expectorant (for excess mucus)—myrtle, peppermint, hyssop, pine, rosemary, lavender. **Antimicrobial/antiviral (for infection)**—eucalyptus blue gum, tea tree, bergamot, thyme, camphor, cajeput, Spanish sage.

Bronchitis

BRONCHITIS indicates an inflammation of the bronchial tubes, and is accompanied by coughing, mucous congestion, chest pain, and aching muscles. Acute bronchitis usually starts with a cold or sore throat, which then develops into a fever that lasts a few days. Chronic bronchitis is a long-term condition, without fever, which is aggravated by smoking, a cold, damp climate, air pollution, and even bad posture, stress, and, sometimes, allergies.

DIETARY FACTORS

Dairy products, white flour products, and junk foods aggravate bronchitis. A wholesome, nutritious diet is essential for building up the body's defenses. Foods rich in Vitamins A and C are especially indicated. Ginger, garlic, onions, and horseradish are good preventive additions to the diet. Take fresh ginger root tea three times a day throughout the winter. The herb coltsfoot, taken as a tea or syrup, is excellent for the treatment of long-term lung weakness.

OTHER MEASURES

Give up smoking. Rest, and keep the whole body warm, especially the chest and neck area. Avoid cold and damp, or very dry, air and open fires. See also Colds (p. 185), Coughs (p. 186), Fever (p. 227), Headaches (p. 229), Sinusitis (p. 191), Throat infections (p. 193).

CLINICAL NOTES

Chronic bronchitis has been successfully treated by inhalations of peppermint, lavender, and sage mixture.

WARNING

Use no more than 3 drops of the spice oils (eucalyptus, camphor, peppermint) in the bathtub.

Acute bronchitis can lead to complications (e.g. pneumonia), especially in the very young and elderly. Professional help should be sought immediately if the condition deteriorates.

Aromatherapy oils

Soothing/balsamic—benzoin, cedarwood, myrrh, frankincense, galbanum, sandalwood, marjoram.

Expectorants—myrtle, peppermint, hyssop, pine, rosemary, lavender. **Antimicrobial/antiviral**—eucalyptus blue gum, tea tree, bergamot, thyme, camphor, cajeput, Spanish sage.

Methods of use

♡ To loosen mucus and ease congestion, rub the chest, back, and throat with a blend of warming and expectorant oils: 4 to 5 drops each of lavender, peppermint, and Spanish sage or clary sage oil in 5 tsp (25ml) of a light base oil or cream. Alternatively, use the same quantities of hyssop, thyme, and angelica oil.

♡ If the cough is dry, regular steam inhalations will help to soothe irritation: add 6 drops (in total) of sandalwood, and/or frankincense or benzoin to a bowl of steaming hot water, and inhale for 5–10 minutes. If there is infection or congestion, use 6 drops of tea tree, thyme, or hyssop, and/or eucalyptus oil. Repeat at least twice a day.

♡ To combat infection, use tea tree, eucalyptus, or thyme in a vaporizer or humidifier in the home, and more soothing oils (marjoram, cedarwood, or myrtle) in the bedroom at night. A few drops of essential oil may also be put on a handkerchief for inhalation throughout the day.

♡ Hot baths with 8 to 10 drops of any of the recommended oils (or a combination), aid the body's natural response to infection. This also has a similar effect to steam inhalation. When feverish, especially if the temperature is high, keep the bath water cool.

Asthma

ASTHMA is characterized by wheezing and shortness of breath, caused by muscle spasm in the bronchi of the lungs. During an attack, the narrowing of the bronchial tubes makes breathing difficult, causing agitation and anxiety. It commonly appears during early childhood, and often ceases at puberty. It usually runs in families, and, as in many allergic conditions, an attack can be brought on by a number of factors, including: diet; contact with allergens such as dust, polish, hairspray, or feathers; cigarette smoke or climatic conditions, such as damp; strenuous exercise; and, especially, by anxiety, fear, or underlying emotional issues.

DIETARY FACTORS

Dairy products, notably cow's milk, are a common trigger for asthma attacks in children. Wheat products, refined sugar, red meat, fizzy drinks, and all types of additives and preservatives are also frequently implicated. The whole diet needs to be assessed carefully on an individual basis. Avoid stimulants (tea, coffee, chocolate), and replace with soothing herbal teas such as chamomile, linden, or lemon balm. Taking a course of Vitamin B complex supplements is recommended.

OTHER MEASURES

Much can be done to alleviate and prevent asthma, if the cause of the attack and the pattern of the illness can be identified. Allergy testing; deep breathing exercises or yoga; psychotherapy, herbal, or homeopathic treatment are all beneficial. Regular massage to the chest, neck, and shoulders, is also helpful. See also Bronchitis (p. 188), Hay fever (p. 190).

CLINICAL NOTES

In one case history, a girl who suffered from frequent asthma attacks and coughs used lavender on a regular basis for massage, baths, and inhalation: "... Despite a two-week camping holiday Jodie did not have to take any Triludan over the summer. Only one asthma attack was experienced." SEE *INTERNATIONAL JOURNAL OF AROMATHERAPY*, VOL. 3 NO. 4, 1991, P. 32, DUST AND DUSTERS.

Methods of use

♥ Mix 3 to 4 drops of lavender, clary sage, frankincense, or benzoin oil with 5 tsp (25ml) sweet almond oil, and use to massage the back in long, sweeping movements, starting at the base of the spine, up over the shoulders, then down the sides of the body.

♥ Use lavender or peppermint (or other recommended oil) in vaporizers at home, and put a few drops on a tissue for inhalation throughout the day, especially at the onset of an attack.

♥ Use 8 to 10 drops of any of the above oils in the bath on a regular basis as a general precautionary and preventive measure.

Aromatherapy oils

Clary sage, cypress, sandalwood, rose, hyssop, melissa, sweet marjoram, benzoin, frankincense, lavender, chamomile, valerian. (With mucous congestion, as in bronchitis: eucalyptus blue gum, peppermint.)

RIGHT This traditional vaporizer uses a night light.

Hay fever

HAY FEVER is an allergic form of rhinitis, an inflammation of the lining of the nose. The symptoms are similar to those of the common cold. The eyes, throat, and mucous membrane lining the nose are generally affected, resulting in sore or streaming eyes, headaches, sneezing, and a blocked or runny nose. Hay fever often starts in childhood but can also suddenly develop in later life. This is generally caused by airborne pollen or spores that are released during the spring and summer months. Different people react to specific allergens. Stress, or feeling run down, may also be a contributing factor.

DIETARY FACTORS

Cut down on milk and other dairy products. A high intake of Vitamin C and garlic can help control the severity of the attack. Eating plenty of local honey also acts as a preventive in some cases. The following tea can be most effective, especially if the treatment starts at least a month before the person's particular hay fever season begins: 2 parts elderflowers, and 1 part each of eyebright, golden seal, and ephedra— take one cupful 2–3 times a day.

OTHER MEASURES

Allergy testing; yoga and other forms of relaxation and deep-breathing exercises may be beneficial measures. See also Coughs (p. 186), Sinusitis (p. 191).

CLINICAL NOTES

The most helpful oils for hay fever are those which combine an antiallergenic or antihistaminic action with balsamic and antiinflammatory properties, notably rose, chamomile, melissa, lemon eucalyptus, lavender, and thyme— especially the milder citrol or linalol types. Thyme is current in *The British Herbal Pharmacopoeia* as specific for respiratory infections, including asthma. Rose is clinically indicated for inflamed mucous membranes and headaches: "... a cream for dry mucous membranes in the nose (Bulgarian rose in eucerit) is very helpful."

SEE D. WABNER, "ROSE OIL: ITS USE IN THERAPY AND COSMETICS," *INTERNATIONAL JOURNAL OF AROMATHERAPY*, VOL. 1, NO. 4, P. 29.

Methods of use

NOTE: Treatment can be a matter of trial and error. Experience has shown that often two or three oils need to be alternated or combined to provide the greatest benefit.

♥ Apply one (or a combination) of the oils listed below left to a tissue to inhale throughout the day— additionally, use in room vaporizers. Use a chosen oil for bathing on a regular basis.

♥ Regular massage to the neck, chest, and back with 4 to 5 drops each of chamomile and lavender, and 3 of rose or melissa oil in 5 tsp (25ml) calendula or a light base oil can be beneficial, and may help to decrease the frequency or severity of an attack.

♥ For sore, red eyes, apply cool compresses of rose water (not the essential oil).

♥ For inflamed mucous membranes in the nose, mix 2 to 3 drops (in total) of rose, chamomile, and/or lavender oil with 1 tsp (5ml) petroleum jelly (such as Vaseline). Apply a small amount to the nostrils 2–3 times a day.

Aromatherapy oils

Chamomile, melissa, rose, lemon eucalyptus, lavender, peppermint, clove, rosemary, lemon, eucalyptus blue gum, hyssop, cajeput, myrtle, basil, marjoram, pine, clary sage, Spanish sage, thyme.

Sinusitis

AN INFECTION or inflammation of the mucous membranes lining the bony cavities behind, above, and on each side of the nose. An acute attack is often accompanied by congested headaches and catarrh, sometimes with fever. The complaint usually follows a cold, hay fever, or prolonged exposure to cold, damp air. Chronic or long-term sinusitis indicates a mild infection that causes the nose to be continually blocked, and a dull pain or feeling of tension to manifest in the area between the eyes. Sinusitis can be aggravated by working or living in overheated or stuffy rooms, and by neck tension.

DIETARY FACTORS

People who suffer from constant or repeated attacks of sinusitis often suffer from allergies, especially to gluten and cow's milk. Cut down or eliminate these mucus-forming foods from the diet and eat plenty of fresh fruits and vegetables, especially those high in Vitamin C (including lemons, oranges, and strawberries), and lots of onions and garlic. Alternatively, take a course of garlic capsules and vitamin C tablets.

OTHER MEASURES

Check for allergies. Fresh air, deep breathing, and gentle exercise can facilitate the easing of nasal congestion. If there is fever, stay in bed. See also Colds (p. 185), Earache (p. 192), Fever (p. 227), Hay fever (p. 191), Headaches (p. 229).

WARNING

Use no more than 3 drops of the spice oils (eucalyptus, camphor, peppermint) in the bathtub.

Sinusitis can lead to secondary infections, notably ear infections, and, very occasionally, meningitis. If in doubt seek professional advice immediately.

Methods of use

♡ Nasal decongestants relieve stuffiness and fight infection. Use 2 to 3 drops each of pine or rosemary, peppermint, and eucalyptus oil in a bowl of steaming water, cover the head with a towel, and inhale deeply for 5–10 minutes with the eyes closed. Repeat several times a day.

♡ To ease congestion, massage the back of the neck, chest, and soles of the feet with 3 to 4 drops each of eucalyptus, pine or rosemary, and peppermint oil in 5 tsp (25ml) of a light base oil or cream.

♡ To combat infection, use tea tree, eucalyptus, and/or thyme in a vaporizer or humidifier during the day, and more soothing oils (marjoram, lavender, and/or myrtle) in the bedroom at night. A few drops of essential oil may also be put on a handkerchief for inhalation throughout the day.

♡ Hot baths with 8 to 10 drops of any of the recommended oils (or a combination), aid the body's natural response to infection. This also has a similar effect to steam inhalation.

♡ For inflamed mucous membranes in the nose, mix 2 to 3 drops (in total) of chamomile, lavender, and/or rose oil with 1 tsp (5ml) petroleum jelly (such as Vaseline). Apply a small amount to the nostrils 2–3 times a day.

Aromatherapy oils

Benzoin, cinnamon, ginger, nutmeg, clove, aniseed, marjoram, myrtle, peppermint, hyssop, pine, rosemary, lavender, eucalyptus blue gum, tea tree, bergamot, thyme, camphor, cajeput, Spanish sage, rose, lavender, chamomile.

Earache/otitis

EAR INFECTIONS may affect the outer ear, middle ear, or inner ear. Middle ear infection, causing earache, is a common complaint, especially among children, often in association with a cold. Fever and partial loss of hearing are common symptoms. In some cases, earache can lead to a more serious infection of the inner ear. Earache may be a sign of dental decay, an abscess or boil, or it may herald the onset of mumps. Exposure to cold, damp, high winds, or loud noise can also bring on earache.

DIETARY FACTORS

If there is a cold, influenza, or sinusitis, avoid mucus-inducing foods such as dairy produce and white-flour products. Drink warm lemon and honey, chamomile, or peppermint tea. Eat lots of garlic to combat infection. Echinacea is the most valuable herb for persistent ear infections: drink echinacea tea three times a day.

OTHER MEASURES

Keep the affected ear warm, and protect from wind by wrapping in a warm scarf. Check for dental decay—if necessary see a dentist. See also Abscesses/boils (p. 144), Colds (p. 185), Influenza (p. 226), Sinusitis (p. 191).

CLINICAL NOTES

The anti-inflammatory/analgesic effects of chamomile (especially German chamomile) have been extensively researched.
SEE *DATA BASE*, VOL. 1, PP. 8–10.

Methods of use

♡ A hot compress applied gently to the ear, using a cloth treated with a few drops of lavender or chamomile (a hot water bottle can be used in this way) can help ease the pain.

♡ Massage gently around the painful area using 2 to 3 drops each of lavender, chamomile, and/or tea tree oil diluted in 1 tbsp (15ml) carrier oil.

♡ Soak an absorbent cotton ball in 1 tsp (5ml) warm olive or almond oil to which have been added 3 drops (in total) of lavender and/or chamomile oil, and insert gently into the outer ear.

NOTE: This should be done only after a medical examination to ensure the eardrum is not perforated.

WARNING
Infection (as in a cold) can travel very rapidly from the nose via the Eustachian tube to cause middle ear infection. If untreated, this can damage the eardrum, or spread to the mastoid bone, which projects from the skull. If there is a high temperature, blood, or pus, or if pain is severe or persistent, seek professional advice immediately.

BELOW The middle ear is composed of the eardrum and three interconnecting bones: the hammer, anvil, and stirrup

---

Aromatherapy oils

Chamomile (Roman and German), lavender, tea tree.

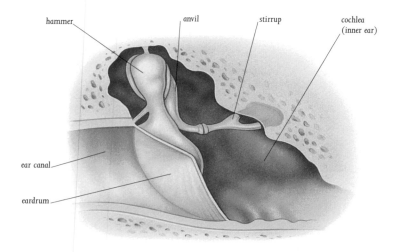

hammer · anvil · stirrup · cochlea (inner ear)

ear canal

eardrum

Throat infections

A SORE THROAT—inflammation of the membranes lining the mouth and throat—can be very painful. Laryngitis—inflammation of the larynx (voice box)—causes hoarseness, or a temporary loss of voice. A sore throat usually accompanies other respiratory infections, such as flu, bronchitis, or the common cold. It is often the first sign of illness, and immediate treatment can prevent further infection from developing—or at least shorten the duration of the disease. Laryngitis is brought on by an infection such as bronchitis or flu, or by overstraining the vocal chords, affecting singers, for example. Cold, damp, or very dry air, smoking, stress, and poor nutrition can all be contributory factors.

DIETARY FACTORS

Eat plenty of fresh fruits and vegetables, especially those high in Vitamin C (including lemons, oranges, and strawberries) and lots of onions and garlic. As a quick, short-term form of treatment, take a course of garlic capsules and Vitamin C tablets. Sage or thyme tea, or lemon and honey are recommended.

OTHER MEASURES

Stop smoking; keep warm, especially the neck and chest area; rest the voice as much as possible, especially for laryngitis. See also Bronchitis (p. 188), Colds (p. 185), Influenza (p. 226).

CLINICAL NOTES

Tea tree is a very effective remedy for sore throats: "... came down with sore throats; we gargled with a few drops in water and within a few days the sore throat was gone." SEE T. LORETTE, AS CITED IN C.W. OLSON, *AUSTRALIAN TEA TREE OIL*, P. 18.

Aromatherapy oils

Bactericidal—tea tree, eucalyptus, thyme, Spanish sage, clary sage, bergamot, peppermint, cajeput, marjoram, myrtle, geranium, hyssop, lavender, pine. **Balsamic**—sandalwood, benzoin, myrrh, cedarwood, frankincense.

Methods of use

♡ Steam inhalation is the most effective treatment for laryngitis, and excellent for sore throats. If the throat is dry, regular steam inhalations will help to soothe irritation. Add 2 to 3 drops each of sandalwood, cedarwood or benzoin, and frankincense to a bowl of steaming hot water and inhale for 5–10 minutes. If there is infection, use 2 to 3 drops each of tea tree, lavender, thyme (or eucalyptus) oil. Repeat at least twice a day.

♡ Add 2 drops each of tea tree, Spanish sage or clary sage, and thyme oil to a glass of warm water, mix well and gargle. Repeat three or more times a day.

♡ For loss of voice, or a dry throat, make up a concentrated massage oil by mixing 3 to 4 drops each of thyme, Spanish sage or clary sage, benzoin, and sandalwood in 5 tsp (25ml) of carrier oil. Apply to the chest and throat. Repeat at least twice a day.

♡ To combat infection, and to soothe the throat, use bactericidal or balsamic oils in a vaporizer or humidifier or on a handkerchief during the day, and more soothing oils (marjoram or myrtle) in the bedroom at night.

THYME

LEFT Sage may be mixed with other oils to make a soothing gargle or massage oil for the chest and throat.

Toothache/tooth abscess

TOOTHACHE is characterized by a persistent pain within the tooth itself. In the case of a tooth abscess, the surrounding gums become swollen, infected, and very painful. Poor dental hygiene, resulting in tooth decay, is the main causative factor in toothache and tooth abscesses. Stress and being run down contribute to the formation of abscesses, as these conditions weaken the immune system.

DIETARY FACTORS

Refined sugar products, candies, and sweet fizzy drinks contribute to tooth decay. Choose low-sugar products whenever possible and educate children to eat candies in moderation only. A sweet tooth, once acquired, can easily become a matter of habit. If an abscess has already developed, the herbs garlic and echinacea are indicated to combat the infection, and a course of Vitamin C will help to encourage healing.

OTHER MEASURES

Improve dental hygiene, and visit a dentist regularly—prevention is better than cure. See also Abscesses/boils (p. 144), Mouth and gum infections (p. 195), Mouth ulcers (p. 196), Stress (p. 236).

References

ABSCESS see TOOTHACHE/ TOOTH ABSCESS page 194
BAD BREATH see HALITOSIS page 197
GUMS see MOUTH AND GUM INFECTIONS page 196
ORAL THRUSH see MOUTH AND GUM INFECTIONS page 196

Aromatherapy oils

Clove, tea tree, thyme, lavender, chamomile (Roman and German), peppermint, myrrh, cinnamon leaf.

Methods of use

♡ As an emergency measure, to ease pain, apply 1 to 2 drops of clove oil directly to the tooth, using the fingertip or a cotton bud.

♡ To ease swelling and aching pain, massage the outer cheek with the following blend: 1 to 2 drops each of chamomile (Roman or German), lavender, and peppermint oil in 1 tbsp (15ml) carrier oil or cream. Teething pain in babies and infants can be relieved by mixing 1 drop of lavender or chamomile (Roman or German) oil in 1 tsp (5ml) of carrier oil, and massaging into the cheek.

♡ As a general measure, and to combat infection, add 5 to 6 drops of tea tree oil to a glass of warm water, mix well, rinse the mouth, and/or gargle once or twice daily, morning and evening, after brushing the teeth.

WARNING

Dental abscesses can be dangerous, as the infection can enter the bloodstream and may spread throughout the body. Seek medical advice, especially if there are signs of fever.

LEFT Increased vitamin C intake, such as through citrus fruits or a course of vitamins, will encourage healing.

ABOVE Clove oil relieves pain when applied directly on to the gums.

Mouth and gum infections

THE MOST COMMON types of mouth and gum infection are thrush and gingivitis. Thrush of the mouth is common among young children, but also sometimes occurs in adults, especially after a course of antibiotics. This appears as small white flecks on the inside of the cheeks or roof of the mouth—the breath is also often offensive. Gingivitis (gum disease) is characterized by a red, spongy swelling of the gums, which bleed easily, especially when cleaning the teeth. Thrush is caused by the fungal organism *Candida albicans*, the same organism that causes vaginal thrush. Gingivitis is caused by buildup of dental plaque. This can harden to form calcium deposits (calculus or tartar), and is aggravated by poor dental hygiene.

DIETARY FACTORS

Reduce refined sugar and processed foods in the diet. Lack of Vitamin C is associated with puffy or bleeding gums, and lack of Vitamin B3 with bad breath. Eat plenty of live yogurt (or take lacto-bacillus tablets) to restore intestinal flora destroyed by antibiotics. To combat infection, the herbal teas of sage, fennel, thyme, and echinacea are especially useful—they may also be used as a mouthwash.

OTHER MEASURES

Improve dental hygiene—correct and regular brushing of the teeth, and flossing are vital; give up smoking; if necessary visit a dentist. See also Candida/thrush (p. 210), Halitosis (p. 197), Mouth ulcers (p. 196), Toothache/tooth abscess (p. 194).

WARNING

If left untreated, gingivitis can develop into periodontitis, which causes loss of teeth.

Aromatherapy oils

Rose, thyme, clove, cinnamon leaf, tea tree, fennel, Spanish sage, clary sage, geranium, lemon eucalyptus, myrrh.

CLARY SAGE

Methods of use

♡ For gingivitis, thrush, or other mouth and gum infections add 4 to 5 drops of tea tree oil (or a blend of the oils listed) to a glass of warm water, mix well, rinse the mouth and/or gargle once or twice daily. Repeat morning and evening, after brushing the teeth.

♡ Alternatively, for thrush, make up a solution containing 6 to 7 drops each of tea tree, geranium, and myrrh or lemon eucalyptus oil, dissolved in 1 tbsp (15ml) witch hazel and added to 2fl oz (50ml) distilled water or lavender water. Put in a small spray bottle and shake well each time before using to spray the mouth.

♡ For gingivitis, massage or rinse the gums before going to bed, using the following blend (it must be diluted): 2 tbsp (30ml) tincture of myrrh, 5 to 6 drops of tea tree, and 2 to 3 drops of lemon eucalyptus, peppermint and/or thyme oils. Add 6 to 8 drops of this mixture to a glass of lukewarm water and stir well before using—two or three times a day.

Mouth ulcers

MOUTH ULCERS are tiny blisters that burst to form painful sores inside the mouth. They may be caused by a mild viral infection, or food sensitivity. They tend to appear when the body is run down.

DIETARY FACTORS
Successful prevention and cure have been achieved by taking 1 to 2 tablets daily of 100mg zinc orotate tablets. Avoid alcohol and very spicy foods as they aggravate the condition. Drink plenty of water, and eat fresh fruit and vegetables. Increase Vitamin C intake to speed healing, and eat plenty of live yogurt (or take lacto-bacillus tablets) to restore intestinal flora destroyed by antibiotics. Drink sage, thyme, or echinacea herbal tea regularly.

OTHER MEASURES
Check dental hygiene—regular brushing and flossing are vital. See also Halitosis (p. 197), Mouth and gum infections (p. 195), Stress (p. 236).

CLINICAL NOTES Research
has shown that tea tree is very effective in the treatment of mouth ulcers or pockets of pus in the gums.
SEE J. LAWLESS, *TEA TREE OIL*, PP. 9–11.

Methods of use

♡ For mouth ulcers, use tea tree oil direct, or dilute to 50% in water (dilute more for children). Mix well, and apply to spots or ulcers with a cotton bud. Repeat the treatment twice daily for three days.

♡ As a general measure, add 5 to 6 drops of tea tree oil to a glass of warm water, mix well, rinse the mouth and/or gargle once or twice daily, morning and evening, after brushing the teeth.

Aromatherapy oils

Cypress, myrrh, tea tree.

CYPRESS

MYRRH

ABOVE To cure mouth ulcers, drink sage, thyme, or echinacea tea regularly.

Halitosis

HALITOSIS, OR offensive breath, is often the first sign of illness. Common causes include smoking, poor dental hygiene, infection, gastric disorders, or faulty diet.

DIETARY FACTORS

Lack of Vitamin B3 is especially associated with bad breath and a coated tongue, while Vitamin C deficiency results in weak gums. Chewing caraway seeds, coriander seeds, cardamoms (which neutralize the smell of garlic), clove buds, or candied ginger root are traditional remedies for sweetening the breath. Parsley, peppermint, spearmint, and basil help to freshen the breath after eating strong-smelling foods.

OTHER MEASURES

Dental hygiene with regular brushing and flossing is vital. See also Mouth and gum infections (p. 195).

Aromatherapy oils

Cardamom, coriander, thyme, clove, cinnamon leaf, tea tree, Spanish sage, clary sage, ginger, fennel.

Methods of use

♥ Add 4 to 5 drops of tea tree (or a blend of antiseptic or germicidal oils) to a glass of lukewarm water. Stir well. Wash the mouth out and gargle with the mixture twice daily.

♥ For general hygiene, dissolve 5 drops each of thyme, tea tree, clove or cinnamon leaf, fennel, and sage oil in 1 tbsp (15ml) vodka, and add to 8fl oz (250ml) distilled water in a dark, well-stoppered container. Shake well. Leave for one month, then filter, using a coffee filter-paper. Use for rinsing the mouth twice daily.

CARDAMOM

ABOVE AND RIGHT Chewing cardamoms or fresh parsley is a traditional remedy for offensive breath. It neutralizes the odors caused by strong-smelling foods, and refreshes the mouth.

PARSLEY

RIGHT Brushing and flossing are essential for healthy teeth and gums, as are regular dental check-ups.

THE DIGESTIVE SYSTEM

Constipation

CONSTIPATION is a condition in which the normal rhythmic functioning of the digestive system breaks down. The stools are hard and compacted, so defecation becomes difficult and infrequent. This causes discomfort, tiredness, and feelings of bloatedness, sometimes with stomach pain. If the body is congested with waste matter for prolonged periods, this can lead to secondary problems, such as hemorrhoids, blemished skin, headaches, or colic. Constipation is not a disease but the symptom of an underlying condition. The principal immediate causes of constipation, however, are lack of dietary fiber and insufficient fluid intake. Lack of exercise, stress, liver congestion, pregnancy, PMS, certain medications, and the long-term use of laxatives, are also common contributory factors.

DIETARY FACTORS
Increase the amount of roughage in the diet—eat plenty of fresh fruit, vegetables, and whole grains, especially bran and oats, and prunes. Avoid refined foods, and drink plenty of liquids, including fennel or ginger tea. Two or three glasses of spring water each morning will benefit the whole digestive system enormously. Lack of inositol or choline (found in wheat germ and yeast) and Vitamin B (especially niacin and thiamin) is also associated with constipation and a sluggish digestive system. Eat meals at regular intervals. The herbal remedies senna and rhubarb root, taken as a tea, are also indicated.

OTHER MEASURES
Exercise regularly and review eating patterns. See also Dyspepsia (p. 200), Liver congestion (p. 202), PMS/PMT (p. 209), Pregnancy (p. 216).

References
COLIC see DYSPEPSIA page 200 and IRRITABLE BOWEL SYNDROME page 203
GASTRIC FLU see DIARRHEA page 199
INDIGESTION see DYSPEPSIA page 200
SICKNESS see NAUSEA/VOMITING page 204

Methods of use

♥ Mix 3 to 4 drops each of rosemary, peppermint, ginger or black pepper with 5 tsp (25ml) almond oil (or other base oil) and massage the abdomen in a gentle, circular movement, in a clockwise direction. Repeat twice daily, or as required.

♥ To reduce stress, boost the circulation and get rid of accumulated toxins in the system, have a full-body massage weekly, using a blend of depurative and digestive oils, such as 7 to 8 drops each of rosemary, neroli or petitgrain, and fennel or geranium oil in 2fl oz (50ml) almond or grapeseed oil.

♥ A warm compress placed over the abdomen, using a flannel soaked in hot water containing a few drops of the above oils, can help relieve pain. A hot water bottle (with the oils sprinkled on it) can be used instead, or the bottle can be placed on top of the compress to keep it warm.

♥ In addition, add 8 to 10 drops of any of the recommended oils to the bathwater on a regular basis.

Aromatherapy oils

Depuratives—carrot seed, celery seed, juniper, bergamot, fennel, dill, aniseed, coriander, angelica, orange, neroli, grapefruit, tangerine, lime, palmarosa, petitgrain, lemon, geranium. **Digestive stimulants**—ginger, rosemary, cinnamon leaf, peppermint, citronella, cardamom, black pepper.

Diarrhea

DIARRHEA is characterized by frequent, loose bowel movements, with or without cramp. Other symptoms that may accompany diarrhea (e.g. with gastric flu) are nausea, vomiting, and fever. Like constipation, diarrhea is not in itself a disorder, but the symptom of an underlying condition, such as bacterial or viral infection, stress, gastric flu, food poisoning, or sudden change in diet. It can also be a side effect of certain medications.

DIETARY FACTORS
Assess the diet for possible causes (such as food poisoning or sudden dietary change). If a bacterial infection is suspected, eat plenty of garlic or take a course of garlic capsules. Avoid dairy products, and keep the diet simple (eat soups, rice, stewed fruits). Castor oil (1–2 tbsp/15–30ml daily), fresh lemon juice, peppermint, meadowsweet, ginger, and cinnamon tea (with honey) are also indicated. Whatever the cause, drink plenty of water or other liquids to prevent dehydration—if severe, take extra salt.

OTHER MEASURES
If there is pain, vomiting, or fever, rest in bed. As a preventive measure, before going on vacation, find out about local customs. For example, it may be advisable to drink only bottled or boiled water, peel all fruit, and avoid uncooked food and ice in drinks. See also Fever (p. 227), Nausea/vomiting (p. 204), Stress (p. 236).

CLINICAL NOTES
Cinnamon and nutmeg oil have been used successfully in treating diarrhea: "...where the active constituent was identified as eugenol, which is also the main constituent of cloves."

SEE M. LIS-BALCHIN, *AROMASCIENCE*, PP. 41, 81.

> **WARNING**
> If symptoms are severe, or if they continue for more than three days, seek medical help.

Methods of use

♡ For stress-related diarrhea, take a warm bath with 3 drops each of geranium, lavender, and ginger oil added. If there is also fever or nausea, take a cool bath with 3 drops each of peppermint, tea tree or thyme, and ginger or nutmeg oil added to the water.

♡ Make a massage oil by mixing 3 to 4 drops each of lavender, ginger or nutmeg, and geranium oil in 5 tsp (25ml) of a light base oil. Rub gently into the abdomen in circular, clockwise movements. If viral or bacterial infection is suspected, add a few drops of tea tree or thyme oil to the blend.

♡ A warm compress placed over the abdomen, using a flannel soaked in hot water containing a few drops of the above oils, can help relieve pain. A hot water bottle can be used instead, or to keep the compress warm.

Aromatherapy oils

Geranium, peppermint, lavender, thyme, ginger, nutmeg, tea tree, cinnamon leaf, clove, chamomile.

RIGHT Cinnamon leaf. Eugenol, one of the principal constituents of cinnamon oil, helps to relieve the symptoms of diarrhea.

Dyspepsia

DYSPEPSIA (INDIGESTION) is a common
complaint. Symptoms include heartburn,
flatulence, colic, abdominal pain, and nausea.
It is often associated with anxiety, stress, or
underlying emotional tension. Eating too
quickly or too much, bad food combinations, and
food allergies are also common causes. Infantile
colic is often caused by an allergy to cow's milk.

DIETARY FACTORS

Assess the diet for possible causes, and, if necessary, check for food allergies. Many herbs traditionally used in cooking aid digestion, notably garlic, rosemary, marjoram, sage, and spices (e.g. black pepper, ginger, coriander, cardamom). Herbs that have a soothing effect on the digestive system, and which may be drunk as a tea for indigestion and wind, include fennel, dill, aniseed, peppermint, and chamomile.

OTHER MEASURES

Wearing tight belts or restrictive clothing can induce stomach pains, as can remaining in a cramped position. Do not eat while feeling anxious or stressed, and relax immediately after eating a heavy meal to allow digestion to take place. See also Anxiety (p. 228), Depression (p. 231), Stress (p. 236).

CLINICAL NOTES

Lavender is especially valuable for all types of digestive disorders, where there is a strong nervous or emotional element involved. In *The British Herbal Pharmacopoeia*, lavender is indicated specifically for "depressive states associated with digestive dysfunction." In clinical cases: "Lavender oil has carminative properties and has been used to treat flatulence and colic, given on a sugar lump or as a compound tincture."
SEE M. LIS-BALCHIN, *AROMASCIENCE*, P. 65.

WARNING

Abdominal pain can be associated with more serious digestive complaints, such as gastritis, gastric ulcers, enteritis, colitis, diverticulitis, or hiatus hernia. Although aromatherapy can offer preventive measures or complementary support for complaints of this type, such conditions require the attention of a medical herbalist, nutritionist or physician.

Internal use of essential oils is not recommended for use at home except on the advice of a qualified physician.

FENNEL

Methods of use

♡ Mix 3 to 4 drops each of lavender, Roman chamomile, and peppermint oil in 5 tsp (25ml) of carrier oil and gently massage the abdomen in a clockwise direction. If there is flatulence, add a few drops of fennel or dill to the blend. Stomach ache or colic in babies, infants, and older children can be eased by mixing 1 to 3 drops (in total) of lavender, Roman chamomile, and dill in 1 tbsp (15ml) carrier oil, and gently massaging the lower back and stomach in a clockwise direction.

♡ For stress-related indigestion, take a warm bath with 8 to 10 drops (in total) of Roman chamomile, lavender, and/or clary sage oil added.

♡ If there is nausea, inhale peppermint oil from a tissue, or put a few drops in a vaporizer.

♡ A warm compress placed over the abdomen, using a facecloth soaked in hot water containing a few drops of lavender, or chamomile, can help relieve pain. A hot water bottle can be used instead, or to keep the compress warm.

Aromatherapy oils

Lavender, Roman chamomile, peppermint, angelica, black pepper, fennel, dill, carrot seed, cardamom, nutmeg, marjoram, melissa, rose, neroli, clary sage, lemongrass, petitgrain, valerian, palmarosa.

Liver congestion

THE LIVER is involved, directly or indirectly, in all the physiological processes of the body. It plays a vital part in digestion—notably in the metabolism of carbohydrates, proteins, fats, and vitamins, as well as in the detoxification of drugs or potential poisons. It also excretes bile, a digestive juice essential for the digestive processes. Any congestion or dysfunction of the liver will thus manifest in all sorts of minor complaints, such as skin problems, digestive disturbances, or a general lack of vitality. Liver congestion can have a variety of causes—alcohol or drug abuse is the most common factor. Rich, fatty, or heavy foods, and chemical additives, also put an undue strain on the liver. In conditions such as jaundice or hepatitis, physical damage and infection can also be causative factors.

DIETARY FACTORS

Avoid all fried and roasted food; reduce all fats and fatty foods to a minimum; cut out or reduce alcohol, and foods containing chemical additives. Use rosemary and garlic in cooking, and drink plenty of liquids. There are many folk remedies (e.g. silver birch sap and fresh lemon juice) that are used as spring tonics for general liverishness, to strengthen the liver and cleanse the body after a winter of heavy food. A good herbal spring tonic is to drink the following tea after each meal: 2 parts each of dandelion and meadowsweet; 1 part each of fringetree and golden seal.

OTHER MEASURES

Stop smoking—tar irritates the digestive system, and it has been shown that nicotine slows the healing of gastric ulcers. Take gentle exercise in the fresh air.

WARNING

Serious liver complaints such as all forms of jaundice and hepatitis, as well as problems related to the gall bladder, such as gall stones, require specialist attention. Liver and pancreatic disorders call for a professional diagnosis before any course of aromatherapy treatment is embarked upon.

Methods of use

♥ If there is pain in the liver area, a low dilution of rosemary oil (0.25%, or 2 drops per 2fl oz/50ml) can be applied to the nape of the neck, solar plexus, and soles of the feet.

♥ Have a regular full-body massage using the following blend: 7 to 8 drops each of rosemary, carrot seed (or celery seed), and grapefruit oil in 2fl oz (50ml) almond oil.

♥ Use 8 to 10 drops of the above blend in baths on a regular basis.

Aromatherapy oils

Rosemary, carrot seed, celery seed, parsley seed, lemon, rose, clary sage, thyme, Spanish sage, chamomile (Roman and German), lavender, geranium, yarrow, tea tree, lemon eucalyptus, grapefruit.

CARROT SEED

ROSEMARY

Irritable bowel syndrome

SYMPTOMS INCLUDE alternating bouts of constipation and diarrhea, stomach pain, colic, and flatulence. General feelings of tiredness and debility are also common. Stress, allergies, and too little fiber, are indicated.

DIETARY FACTORS

Eat fruits, vegetables, whole wheat bread, grains, and cereals—but not wheatbran, as it can irritate a sensitive digestive tract. Avoid or reduce alcohol, tea, and coffee. Take herbal teas, such as lemon balm, peppermint, valerian, chamomile, and hops. Peppermint oil capsules, available from health food stores, can also be helpful.

OTHER MEASURES

Relaxation exercises, massage, yoga, and meditation are beneficial. See also Stress (p. 236).

WARNING

For any sudden change or irregularity in bowel habits in those over 40, seek medical advice.

Aromatherapy oils

Chamomile, lavender, marjoram, peppermint, melissa, rose, neroli, petitgrain.

Methods of use

♡ Mix 3 to 4 drops each of chamomile, peppermint, and lavender oil with 5 tsp (25ml) almond oil (or other base oil) and massage the abdomen in a gentle, circular movement, in a clockwise direction.

♡ To reduce stress, have a full-body massage weekly, using a blend of relaxing and carminative oils—mix 7 to 8 drops each of lavender, neroli, or petitgrain, and peppermint oil in 2fl oz (50ml) almond or grapeseed oil.

♡ A warm compress placed over the abdomen, using a facecloth soaked in hot water containing a few drops of chamomile or lavender, can help relieve pain. A hot water bottle may be used instead, or to keep the compress warm.

♡ Add 8 to 10 drops of any of the recommended oils to the bathwater on a regular basis.

RIGHT AND BELOW Fruit is a good source of fiber and should be a regular part of your diet.

WHOLE WHEAT BREAD

Nausea/vomiting

NAUSEA IS A common complaint that can start as slight queeziness and progress to sickness or vomiting. With motion or travel sickness, the sense of balance, originating in the inner ear, is disturbed by the movement. Nausea can arise from many causes, including motion (as in travel sickness), viral infection, digestive problems, overeating, food poisoning, and emotional anxiety or tension.

DIETARY FACTORS

Do not eat while feeling nauseous. Peppermint, spearmint, lemon balm, and ginger teas relieve nausea. Herbal travel-sickness tablets are also available.

CLINICAL NOTES

Lavender is indicated specifically for sickness due to nerves or emotional upset, especially in combination with other digestive symptoms. Peppermint is used clinically where nausea is associated with fever, diarrhea, dyspepsia, or travel sickness.

Methods of use

♡ Inhale lavender or peppermint directly from a tissue, or use in a vaporizer in the room.

♡ For nausea with indigestion, gently massage the solar plexus or abdomen in a clockwise direction, using 3 to 4 drops of peppermint, ginger, and lavender oils in 5 tsp (25ml) carrier oil.

Aromatherapy oils

Peppermint, ginger, lavender, Roman chamomile, cardamom, coriander, fennel, nutmeg, melissa, aniseed.

BELOW To reduce nausea, use lavender or peppermint in a vaporizer in the home.

LAVENDER

PEPPERMINT

Dysmenorrhea

MILD TO SEVERE cramping pains in the abdominal region, lasting from a matter of minutes to several days at a time. The pain is caused by uterine spasm during menstruation, although the frequency and severity of period pains is variable. Heredity, lack of exercise, being fitted with an intra-uterine device (IUD), underlying emotional problems, and faulty diet can all contribute to this condition.

DIETARY FACTORS

Constipation and poor nutrition are contributing factors, particularly lack of calcium in the diet—extra calcium is required by women using the contraceptive pill. Calcium supplements are recommended, and extra Vitamin E and Vitamin C are also indicated. A very effective long-term remedy for frequent attacks is the herb cramp bark, taken as a tea, three times a day.

OTHER MEASURES

Assess the lifestyle, aiming to reduce stress levels. If pain is severe, rest and keep warm. See also Cramp (p. 175), PMS/PMT (p. 209).

CLINICAL NOTES

Many oils, notably clary sage, chamomile (Roman and German), marjoram, peppermint, lavender, valerian, ginger, and nutmeg, have been demonstrated clinically to have a strong antispasmodic action—valuable in all types of muscular spasm.
SEE *DATA BASE*, VOL. 3, P. 25.

References

CHANGE IN LIFE see MENOPAUSE page 207
HEAVY PERIODS see MENORRHAGIA page 206
LABOR see CHILDBIRTH page 218
MISSING PERIODS see AMENORRHEA page 208
PAINFUL PERIODS see DYSMENORRHEA page 205
THRUSH see CANDIDA/THRUSH page 210
URETHRITIS see CYSTITIS AND URETHRITIS page 212
VAGINAL ITCHING see LEUCORRHEA AND PRURITUS page 213
"WHITES" see LEUCORRHEA AND PRURITUS page 213

WARNING
Very severe or persistent pain may indicate a gynecological disorder such as endometriosis.

Methods of use

♡ Gentle massage to the abdomen and lower back with 4 to 5 drops each of clary sage, marjoram, and lavender in 5 tsp (25ml) of base oil, with 1 tbsp (15ml) evening primrose oil can be very effective.

♡ Hot compresses, using a few drops of any of the oils listed below on a facecloth (or on a hot water bottle) can be placed on the abdomen as an aid to relieving pain.

♡ Relaxing in a hot aromatic bath (using 8 to 10 drops of a relaxant oil) eases pain, and also soothes away stress and tension.

Aromatherapy oils

Chamomile (Roman and German), clary sage, lavender, rose, marjoram, melissa, nutmeg, geranium, neroli, peppermint, ginger, valerian, rosemary, cardamom, cinnamon leaf.

RIGHT Cramp bark is a natural herbal remedy that is often helpful.

Menorrhagia

EXCESSIVE MENSTRUAL flow, often in association with cramping pains. There are many possible causes of these symptoms, including endometriosis, fibroids, stress, poor diet, excessive exercise, and muscular strain.

DIETARY FACTORS
A diet containing too many saturated oils and refined carbohydrates, together with a lack of fresh fruit and vegetables, can contribute to menstrual problems and make the flow congested. To balance the loss of additional blood, a diet rich in iron (or iron supplements) is recommended. Improve the diet, cut down on alcohol, and drink plenty of water and herbal teas—especially raspberry leaf, American cranesbill, lady's mantle, and yarrow.

OTHER MEASURES
Make time for relaxation; take gentle exercise; assess lifestyle and emotional factors. See also Dysmenorrhea (p. 205), Stress (p. 236).

CLINICAL NOTES
Cypress and yarrow are both recognized medicinally for their astringent action: "Tincture of cypress, like that of hamamelis (witch hazel) is given for hemorrhoids, varicose veins, menorrhagia, menopausal problems etc ... "
SEE J. VALNET, *THE PRACTICE OF AROMATHERAPY*, P. 121.

Rose is also helpful for menorrhagia. Case histories show that: "Rose has a regulating effect on the cycle, and is a uterine tonic."
SEE P. DAVIS, *AROMATHERAPY: AN A–Z*, P. 224.

Methods of use

♡ Gently massage the abdomen and lower back with the following blend each day, especially on the days immediately prior to menstruation: 3 to 4 drops of geranium, cypress or yarrow, and rose in 5 tsp (25ml) base oil.

♡ Use 8 to 10 drops of any of the recommended oils in the bathtub regularly, especially on the days just before and during menstruation.

♡ Have a regular massage, using a blend of stress-relieving oils—for example use from 7 to 10 drops of chamomile or rose, geranium, and lavender in 2fl oz (50ml) base oil.

Aromatherapy oils
Cypress, geranium, rose, yarrow, chamomile, lavender.

WARNING
Prolonged or heavy bleeding may indicate a more serious gynecological problem—seek medical advice.

RIGHT Taking a warm, relaxing bath containing a few drops of the recommended oils, prior to and during menstruation, relieves pain associated with menorrhagia.

Menopause

THE MENOPAUSE can sometimes be accompanied by unpleasant emotional and physical symptoms, such as headaches, hot flushes, depression, rapid mood swings, irritability, edema, and the tendency to put on weight. Nevertheless, a recent survey indicates that only 25 percent of women suffer menopausal problems, hot flushes being the most common symptom. Hormonal changes, notably a decrease in estrogen and progesterone levels, are the main physiological causative factors of these symptoms. Underlying psychological attitudes to the change in life also need to be taken into account, since anxiety about the future or fear of growing older can contribute to the discomfort and duration of menopausal symptoms.

DIETARY FACTORS

Nutrition can have a profound influence on the menopausal experience—it is very important to have a healthy, wholesome diet. Supplements of evening primrose oil, minerals, and trace elements (especially calcium, to prevent bones becoming brittle), as well as multivitamin tablets (incorporating especially Vitamins D, E, and the B complex vitamins) can be very helpful. Specifically formulated menopausal herbal supplements (e.g. Phytesterol) are available from some pharmacies/health food stores—ginseng root, sage, and fennel tea are also found to help in many cases.

OTHER MEASURES

Gentle exercise, such as yoga, swimming, or walking, and some form of spiritual nourishment (prayer or meditation) are beneficial. Relaxation techniques, the Bach flower remedies, counseling, psychotherapy, or homeopathy can all be valuable supports at this time. See also Anxiety (p. 228), Depression (p. 231), Edema (p. 184), Faintness/shock (p. 234), Headaches (p. 229), Palpitations (p. 180), Stress (p. 236).

CLINICAL NOTES

Fennel tea helps to regulate hormonal change, and boosts estrogen levels during the menopause. Clinical studies have demonstrated that fennel oil is also estrogenic.
SEE M. LIS-BALCHIN, *AROMASCIENCE*, P. 84.

Trials have also demonstrated the benefits of ginseng root.
SEE B. SALMON, *NATURE'S SECRETS*, P. 72.

Methods of use

♡ Massage is very comforting and relaxing in itself. The following blend has in addition a regulating effect: 4 to 5 drops each of geranium or rose, fennel, and clary sage oils in 5 tsp (25ml) of a light base oil, plus 1 tbsp (15ml) of evening primrose oil or borage oil for their high gamma-linoleic acid (GLA) content.

♡ Choose oils to scent the environment, according to specific moods or symptoms (e.g. lavender for headaches, or to soothe anxiety).

♡ For hot flushes, use cold compresses of chamomile, lavender, or rose water on the face and body.

♡ Add 8 to 10 drops of any of the recommended oils to a warm bath on a daily basis. To help prevent night sweats, take a warm (not hot) bath before retiring, using a blend of grapefruit, clary sage, and geranium (8 to 10 drops in total).

Aromatherapy oils

Geranium, rose, chamomile, bergamot, clary sage, jasmine, lavender, neroli, sandalwood, ylang ylang, fennel, grapefruit.

RIGHT Ginseng root, taken as a tea or in tablet form, has been found by many women to help them overcome the symptoms of the menopause.

Amenorrhea

AMENORRHEA CAN TAKE several forms, ranging from the total absence of menstruation over an extended period, to a scanty or missed period. Amenorrhea is common at the onset of puberty, and during the menopause, when the menstrual cycle is irregular. (Pregnancy also causes menstrual periods to cease.) A woman's menstrual cycle can become irregular as a result of emotional stress, shock, excessive exercise, nutritional deficiency, hormonal imbalance, or a serious illness.

DIETARY FACTORS

Girls and women suffering from anorexia nervosa often stop menstruating, due to lack of the nutrients needed to synthesize the body's hormones. Protein deficiency, and lack of Vitamin B12 and folic acid result in anemia (insufficient red blood corpuscles) and scanty or irregular menstruation. It is therefore important to improve the diet: liver, leafy greens, and yeast products (e.g. spreads such as Marmite) are especially indicated. Avoid tea, coffee, and alcohol, and drink the herb teas yarrow, rose-hip, chasteberry, mugwort, or marigold (all uterine tonics).

OTHER MEASURES

Assess lifestyle, and, if necessary, seek psychotherapeutic help: stress and emotional disharmony are commonly implicated in amenorrhea. See also Menopause (p. 207), Shock (p. 234), Stress (p. 236).

CLINICAL NOTES

Case histories have shown that the use of rose oil can help to promote and reassert a natural rhythm: "Rose is of great help to women who have been trying to conceive, as it makes it possible to predict the time of ovulation more accurately."
SEE P. DAVIS, *AROMATHERAPY: AN A–Z*, P. 224.

WARNING
Amenorrhea can lead to fertility problems—if the condition persists, seek medical advice.

Methods of use

♡ Gently massage the abdomen and lower back with 3 to 4 drops each of carrot seed, clary sage, and myrrh or rose oil in 5 tsp (25ml) carrier oil daily, especially before menstruation is due.

♡ Use a few drops of any of the recommended oils in the bath regularly (best used in combination)—always check contraindications first: see Safety data for each oil on pp. 271–277.

♡ If possible, put aside some time each week to have a professional massage, using a blend of relaxing or stress-relieving oils—e.g. 6 to 7 drops each of marjoram, lavender, rose, and clary sage oil in 2fl oz (50ml) carrier oil.

Aromatherapy oils

Angelica, carrot seed, celery seed, cinnamon leaf, clary sage, dill, sweet fennel, hyssop, juniper, marjoram, myrrh, parsley seed, rose, Spanish sage.

ANGELICA ROOT

PMS/PMT

THE SYMPTOMS of pre-menstrual syndrome or tension are various: on a physical level they may include fluid retention, tender breasts, headaches, weight gain, spots, nausea, or a swollen abdomen; while on an emotional level, symptoms may include depression, sudden mood swings, weepiness, or unpredictable behavior. Onset of symptoms varies from two days to two weeks prior to menstruation. PMS is fundamentally caused by a temporary hormonal imbalance—notably inadequate amounts of progesterone in the body—in the days prior to menstruation. The condition is also aggravated by other factors, including stress, poor diet, viral infection, smoking, and overwork.

DIETARY FACTORS

A nutritional approach to PMS has been found to have a 70 percent success rate. Cut out refined sugar altogether, and reduce dairy products, tea, coffee, chocolate, alcohol, salt, and red meat. Foods containing Vitamin E, magnesium, and the B vitamins (especially B6) are particularly indicated (and these can be taken as supplements). However, the most successful single remedy is evening primrose oil, because it contains essential fatty acids, including GLA (gamma-linoleic acid), which stimulate the body's production of prostaglandins, natural hormone-like substances. Take 2 to 4 capsules daily, or on each day during the ten days prior to menstruation. The herb chaste tree (*Vitex agnus-castus*) can also help to regulate hormonal imbalance (also available in tablet form).

OTHER MEASURES

These depend on the particular symptoms. See also Acne (p. 145), Anxiety (p. 228), Depression (p. 231), Edema (p. 184), Headaches (p. 229), Stress (p. 236).

CLINICAL NOTES

Case studies show that aromatherapy can be a great aid in combating pre-menstrual tension: "I blended the following oils for her: chamomile, lavender, geranium and melissa (to be used in the bath and in a massage oil for two weeks before her period) ... she has now had four periods and says that both mentally and physically it has been a huge success."

SEE J. GINGELL, "P.M.T.," IN *AROMATHERAPY QUARTERLY*, NO. 8, 1985, P. 12.

Methods of use

♡ Use 8 to 10 drops of a chosen oil (see below) in baths during the ten days prior to menstruation, and throughout the duration of the period.

♡ A regular full-body massage treatment can be a great aid in combating PMS. The oils need to be selected according to the specific symptoms (e.g. 7 to 10 drops of lavender, geranium, and chamomile in 2fl oz (50ml) base oil, plus 1 tbsp (15ml) of evening primrose oil, can be very helpful for moodiness/irritability).

♡ For self-treatment to help regulate hormonal imbalance, mix 4 to 5 drops each of rose/lavender, fennel, and geranium in 5 tsp (25ml) light carrier oil, plus 1tbsp (15ml) evening primrose oil. Apply by gentle massage to the abdomen and lower back.

♡ Use any of the recommended oils (according to mood) in burners during the ten days prior to menstruation, and throughout the duration of the menstrual period.

Aromatherapy oils

Fennel, rose, geranium, clary sage, bergamot, nutmeg, grapefruit, jasmine, chamomile, palmarosa, melissa, parsley seed, lavender, neroli, vitiver, ylang ylang.

ROSE

Candida/thrush

THRUSH, ALSO KNOWN as candidiasis or moniliasis, can manifest in several forms. It is caused by the yeastlike fungus *Candida albicans*, which thrives in moist, warm parts of the body. In its most common form, however, thrush affects the vagina, causing severe itching, redness, and a milky white discharge. The organism *Candida albicans* (formerly called *Monila albicans*) causes problems of infection only when it proliferates above a certain level. Some people are more prone to this infection than others, and this can be connected to food allergies, low immunity levels, and stress. Quite commonly, it is a result of antibiotic treatment. This is because antibiotics kill some of the intestinal flora that keep the candida organisms under control. Balanitis (affecting the penis) is usually passed to the male by sexual contact with a woman suffering from vaginal thrush.

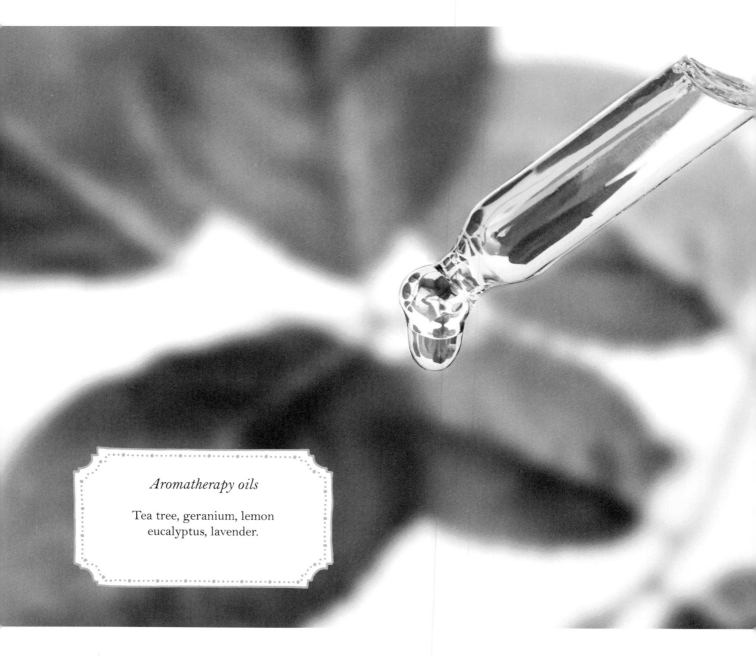

Aromatherapy oils

Tea tree, geranium, lemon
eucalyptus, lavender.

DIETARY FACTORS

To encourage beneficial intestinal flora, eat plenty of live yogurt (or take acidophilus capsules), avoid alcohol, and keep sugary and starchy foods to a minimum. Garlic is also indicated to help build up resistance to infection.

OTHER MEASURES

Do not wear underwear made from synthetic fibers (e.g. nylon or lycra), which do not let the skin breathe, and avoid harsh chemical soaps and toiletries. Both male and female partners must be treated simultaneously before renewing sexual relations to avoid reinfection occurring. See also Eczema (p. 140), Mouth and gum infections (p. 195).

CLINICAL NOTES

Tea tree is very effective for treating thrush, due to its powerful fungicidal action, combined with its mildness on the skin, even when applied to the delicate mucous membranes.

SEE J. LAWLESS, *TEA TREE OIL*, PP. 13, 14.

In clinical tests, Algerian geranium and lemon eucalyptus oil showed very effective fungicidal activity against *Candida albicans*.

SEE M. LIS-BALCHIN, *AROMASCIENCE*, PP. 51, 58.

Methods of use

♡ A simple way of treating vaginal thrush is to soak a tampon in a 1% tea tree/water solution (20 drops of tea tree oil to 3½fl oz (100ml) purified or distilled water) and insert into the vagina. Replace every 8 hours. (This is the routine method employed at the Annandale Women's Centre in Sydney, Australia.)

♡ Alternatively, a pessary can be made with a 1% dilution of tea tree oil in a cocoa butter base, 10 drops of oil to 2fl oz (50ml) melted cocoa butter cooled slightly and formed into pellets, then left to harden. One of these can be inserted into the vagina once or twice a day.

♡ For a vaginal douche, add 20 to 25 drops of tea tree oil to 8fl oz (200ml) of purified or distilled water. This helps reduce infection, irritation, and discomfort, and may be used between the treatments described above.

♡ As a wash, add 8 to 10 drops of tea tree or geranium or lemon eucalyptus oil to a bowl or shallow bath of warm water and soak in this for 5–10 minutes daily.

♡ Balanitis may be treated by washing the area carefully with a 1 percent solution (20 drops to 3½fl oz/100ml water) of tea tree oil in distilled water. Shake well, and apply four times a day.

♡ As an adjunct to treatment, or as a general precautionary measure, add 8 to 10 drops of any recommended oil to the bathwater.

WARNING

Although it is normal to experience a temporary, warm sensation when tea tree is used in the vaginal area, discontinue the treatment if a burning irritation develops.

GERANIUM

Cystitis and urethritis

CYSTITIS IS A bacterial infection causing inflammation of the bladder, more common among women than men. It is characterized by a frequent need to urinate (even when the bladder is empty), a painful, burning sensation while passing water (which is often cloudy), a pain in the groin, and sometimes fever. Many attacks of cystitis start as urethritis—an infection of the urethra. Bacterial infection, inhalation of industrial chemical fumes, a physical injury, catching a chill, or prolonged stressful circumstances can all trigger an attack. Some individuals are more prone than others, especially those who have undergone surgery to the urethra or (in men) who suffer from an enlarged prostate gland. So-called honeymoon cystitis can occur as a result of prolonged sexual activity.

DIETARY FACTORS

Occasionally, food allergies are implicated in chronic cystitis. If in doubt, check with an allergy specialist for possible dietary causes. Whatever the case, drink plenty of water and herbal teas (especially echinacea, fennel, yarrow, golden seal, or thyme) to flush out the kidneys and dilute the urine. In addition, eat lots of garlic (or take as capsules) to build up the immune system.

OTHER MEASURES

Avoid tightly fitting clothes and nylon underwear. Assess the lifestyle, and make appropriate changes if stress could be a causative factor. Rest as much as possible, especially if there is fever. See also Fever (p. 227), Stress (p. 236).

CLINICAL NOTES

Tea tree oil has been successful taken internally as part of treatment for cystitis but this requires clinical prescription and supervision.

WARNING

If symptoms do not improve within a few days, or if there is blood or pus in the urine, seek professional help immediately.

Do not take tea tree oil internally without medical supervision.

Methods of use

♡ Make up a solution of 10 to 12 drops of tea tree oil in 3½fl oz (100ml)of cooled, boiled water. Using soaked absorbent cotton (cotton wool) swab the opening of the urethra frequently and each time after passing water. Shake the solution well before each application.

♡ Bathe frequently, using bactericidal oils, as a general disinfectant and preventive measure. Add 8 to 10 drops of a recommended oil (or a combination) to the bathwater.

♡ Make up a massage oil using 3 to 4 drops each of tea tree, sandalwood, bergamot (or lavender) in 5 tsp (25ml) of a light carrier oil (such as sweet almond or grapeseed) and rub gently into the lower abdomen and back. Repeat at least twice daily.

Aromatherapy oils

Bergamot, lavender, chamomile, tea tree, sandalwood, juniper, frankincense, parsley seed, celery seed, thyme, yarrow.

FENNEL

Leucorrhea and pruritus

THE MAIN SYMPTOM of leucorrhea is a thick white or yellow discharge, and severe itching of the vaginal area. Pruritus, or itching, generally accompanies any type of mild vaginal infection. Leucorrhea is an inflammation of the vagina caused by a proliferation of a variety of bacteria or fungi (e.g. candida or other nonspecified organisms). Infections of this kind often occur during times of stress.

DIETARY FACTORS
Boost intake of Vitamin C and B complex vitamins. Take garlic capsules, and keep consumption of tea, coffee, alcohol, and spices to a minimum.

OTHER MEASURES
Avoid tight clothing, nylon underwear, and harsh bubble baths. See also Cystitis (p. 212), Genital herpes (p. 214), Stress (p.236), Thrush (p. 210).

CLINICAL NOTES
Tea tree has been found to be very effective for the treatment of these conditions.

GERANIUM LEAVES

Methods of use

♡ Add 8 to 10 drops of tea tree or lavender oil to a bowl or shallow bath of warm water and soak for 5–10 minutes daily to treat the condition.

♡ Add 8 to 10 drops of any of the recommended oils to the bathwater on a daily basis as a general preventive and antiseptic measure.

Aromatherapy oils

Tea tree, lavender, geranium, lemon eucalyptus, myrrh.

GARLIC CAPSULES

RIGHT A dietary supplement of garlic capsules and a few drops of lavender oil in the bath are a good preventative measure.

LAVENDER

Genital herpes

GENITAL HERPES is an infection transmitted by sexual contact. The first attack is generally the worst: the skin of the genital region becomes red and itchy and then erupts into small, very painful blisters that can last for several weeks. This tends to be followed by recurrent attacks that take a milder form, often precipitated by stress, sexual activity, or an infection, and lasting only a few days. This is caused by the virus Herpes simplex II, which, like Herpes simplex I (the cause of cold sores), often lies dormant in the body, flaring up during times of stress.

DIETARY FACTORS
Take garlic and Vitamin C and B complex vitamins in the diet or as supplements.

OTHER MEASURES
Avoid sexual activity during attacks. Reduce stress levels. See also Chicken pox (p. 223), Cold sores (p. 157), Stress (p. 236).

WARNING
Although it is normal to experience a temporary, warm sensation in using tea tree oil, discontinue this method if irritation occurs.

Aromatherapy oils
Lavender, bergamot (bergapten-free), tea tree, chamomile, yarrow, peppermint, geranium, melissa, myrrh, eucalyptus blue gum, bergamot.

Methods of use

♡ At the very first signs of infection, make a concentrated solution by mixing 10 to 12 drops of tea tree oil with 3½fl oz (100ml) of warm water. Using this solution to douche or wash the genital area frequently will soothe irritation and prevent the infection from developing. Shake or stir well before use.

♡ Use neat tea tree oil to dab any blisters as soon as they begin to develop—check for sensitivity first. Repeat frequently over a period of several days, or until the condition has cleared.

♡ Add 8 to 10 drops of tea tree oil to the bathwater as a general disinfectant measure.

BELOW Use a solution of water and tea tree oil to wash the affected area frequently.

MELISSA

Sexual problems

DEBILITY, FRIGIDITY, impotence, inability to conceive, and lack of confidence are all commonly encountered. Many physical problems, such as frigidity or impotence, have a psychological basis, and may be accompanied by depression, anxiety, or other stress-related conditions.

DIETARY FACTORS

A wholesome, nutritious diet is required for optimum health and the maintenance of sexual vitality. Although alcohol can act as an aphrodisiac in small doses, in excess it is soporific, depressant, and damaging to the whole system. Zinc and beta carotene are specifically indicated to increase sexual vigor. Ginseng is also recommended as a general sexual stimulant, due to its ability to increase the production of hormones, and can be taken as capsules.

OTHER MEASURES

Make time for relaxation; adequate exercise is also a basic requirement for a healthy body. Psychotherapy, hypnotherapy, Bach flower remedies, and nutritional advice may also be valuable aids. See also Stress (p. 236).

WARNING

Essential oils should not be allowed to come into contact with condoms, as they can have a detrimental effect on the rubber.

Deep-seated sexual problems may require professional help.

Methods of use

♥ Wear essential oils such as rose, ylang ylang, or sandalwood (or a personalized blend) as a perfume to create a sensual mood.

♥ Make up a massage oil using 5 to 7 drops each of rose, sandalwood, and ylang ylang in 2fl oz (50ml) of a light base oil. Massage between partners can be a very intimate experience and a means of enhancing sexual communication.

♥ Aromatic bathing can be a mood-setting sensual experience in itself—select a favorite scent (or a blend) from the recommended oils.

♥ Set the scene for seduction by using aphrodisiac oils in a vaporizer, or light a scented candle, and simply enjoy the erotic aroma.

Aromatherapy oils

Aphrodisiacs—rose, neroli, clary sage, patchouli, ylang ylang, jasmine, black pepper, cardamom, sandalwood.

Regulators—lavender, geranium.

GINSENG ROOT

LEFT Neroli oil can help to relieve psychological tension and is said to be aphrodisiac.

Pregnancy

PROBLEMS DURING pregnancy can arise for all kinds of reasons, both physical and psychological. Common complaints include edema, lower back pain, constipation, fatigue, hemorrhoids, morning sickness, leg cramps, and feelings of anxiety or depression.

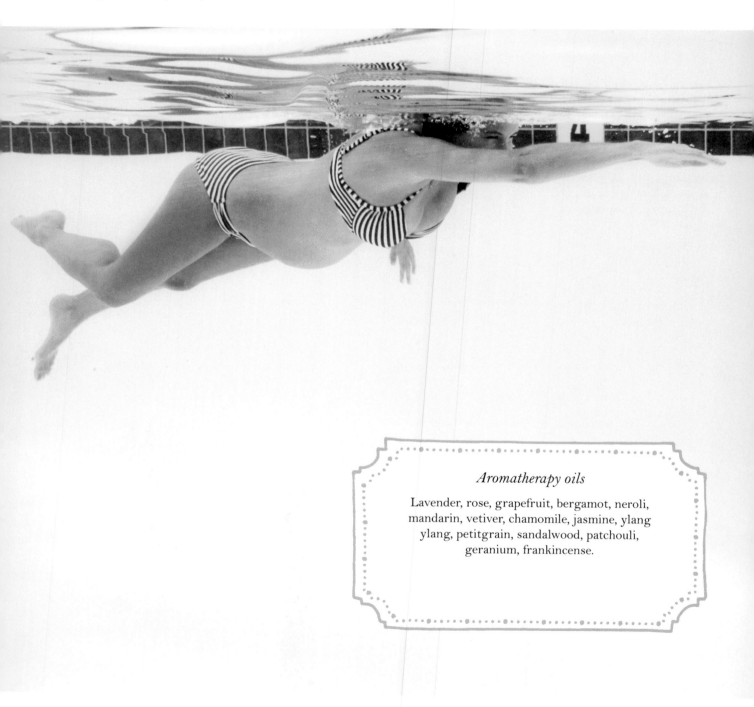

Aromatherapy oils

Lavender, rose, grapefruit, bergamot, neroli, mandarin, vetiver, chamomile, jasmine, ylang ylang, petitgrain, sandalwood, patchouli, geranium, frankincense.

DIETARY FACTORS

Eat nourishing food—everything that goes into the body directly affects the growing child, whether it is carbohydrates, fats, minerals, vitamins, or toxic chemicals, alcohol, or tobacco. It is now recognized that the nutritional foundations of good health are laid down during prenatal life. Although it is common to have specific food fads during the early stages of pregnancy, it is important to establish good eating habits—eat plenty of fresh fruit and vegetables, whole grains, adequate protein, and cold-pressed vegetable oils on a daily basis. Avoid refined products, and cut down on tea, coffee, and alcohol.

OTHER MEASURES

Do not overwork—adequate rest is essential for the health of the growing child, and relaxation ensures that the mother and child enjoy their prenatal togetherness. Nonstrenuous daily exercise is also important, such as stretching, walking, yoga, or swimming. Stop smoking. See also Anxiety (p. 228), Constipation (p. 198), Childbirth (p. 218), Debility (p. 232), Depression (p. 231), Edema (p. 184), Hemorrhoids (p. 182), Muscular pain (p. 173), Nausea/vomiting (p. 204), Stress (p. 236).

Methods of use

♡ To prevent stretch marks (or to get rid of existing stretch marks), prepare the following blend: 1 tbsp (15ml) each of wheat germ, borage, and/or rose-hip seed oil in 5 tsp (25ml) jojoba or grapeseed or sweet almond oil. A few drops (not more than 10 drops in total) of rose, neroli, frankincense, and lavender (singly, or in combination) may also be added. Use this twice daily for light massage to the belly and breasts, especially after the fourth month. The blend can also be rubbed into the perineum for 5–10 minutes daily in the last six weeks before the birth.

♡ Aromatic bathing is a great pleasure and relief, especially toward the end of pregnancy. Add 4 to 5 drops of any of the recommended oils to a warm bath, according to mood, and relax in the aromatic vapors. For weary muscles, use equal amounts of chamomile and lavender oil.

♡ Gentle massage, using mild essential oils such as rose, neroli, petitgrain, lavender, or chamomile can help with a wide variety of problems, such as back pain, anxiety, depression, or fatigue. Keep the concentration of the blend low (10 to 12 drops of essential oil to 2fl oz (50ml) base oil).

♡ Cooling compresses of lavender, chamomile, or rose water can be very refreshing during the latter stages of pregnancy. Alternatively, add the flower water to a fine mist spray for regular application throughout the day.

♡ Postnatal depression can be helped by the use of rose, bergamot, neroli, lavender, mandarin, vetivert, or ylang ylang in burners or worn as a perfume.

WARNING

All essential oils should be used in half the usual quantities, or less, during pregnancy.

Some essential oils should be avoided altogether during pregnancy. These include basil, clove, cinnamon leaf, hyssop, juniper, marjoram, myrrh, Spanish sage, and thyme. The following oils are best avoided during the first four months of pregnancy: fennel, rose, peppermint, Atlas cedarwood, and rosemary.

Childbirth

CHILDBIRTH (LABOR) is one of the most moving yet demanding experiences that a woman can undergo. More and more women are choosing a natural or active birth, whether it is in a hospital or at home. Whatever the case, good preparation is the key to coping with the experience, and playing an active role in the birth. There are many problems that can arise during childbirth, but the key point is to be prepared. Breech birth, methods for coping with severe pain or a long labor, the possible need for Caesarean section or an episiotomy (cutting the perineum), are all options that need to be discussed in advance.

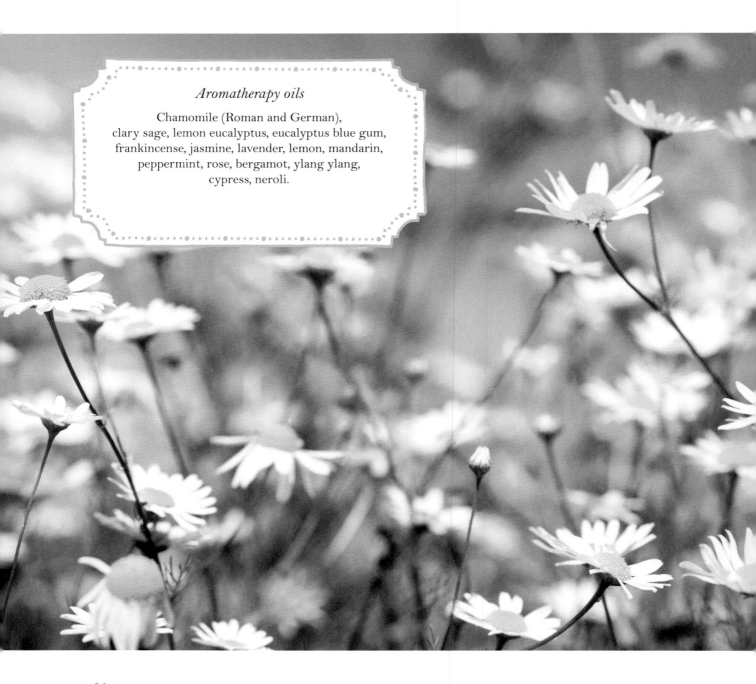

Aromatherapy oils

Chamomile (Roman and German),
clary sage, lemon eucalyptus, eucalyptus blue gum,
frankincense, jasmine, lavender, lemon, mandarin,
peppermint, rose, bergamot, ylang ylang,
cypress, neroli.

DIETARY FACTORS

It is vital to have a nourishing diet throughout pregnancy. In addition, in preparation for childbirth, take raspberry leaf tea 2–3 times daily during the final three months of pregnancy. It is a marvelous aid to easy childbirth, toning the whole reproductive system and the uterine muscles. Use 1oz (30g) of dried herb to 18fl oz (500ml) boiled water, infused for 15 minutes (tablets are also available). This also makes an excellent postnatal tonic to restore normal function and tone. An adequate milk supply can be ensured by drinking plenty of fennel, dill, or aniseed tea immediately prior to the birth and afterward.

CLINICAL NOTES

Many mothers, midwives, and nurses are now using essential oils during pregnancy and for childbirth. Aromatherapy is well regarded as a noninvasive aid to natural birth and of great benefit in promoting rapid recovery. In hospital trials, over a six-month period, the use of essential oils during labor was studied and recorded. The trials involved over five hundred women. The essential oils used were chamomile, clary sage, eucalyptus, frankincense, jasmine, lavender, lemon, mandarin, peppermint, and rose, used in different combinations and at different stages. The results showed "a high degree of overall satisfaction by mothers and midwives on the use of aromatherapy during labor/delivery." SEE BURNS AND BLAMEY, "USING AROMATHERAPY IN CHILDBIRTH," CITED IN *DATA BASE*, VOL. 3, P. 24.

Methods of use

♡ Two weeks prior to the delivery, use the following blend daily to help prepare for the birth and strengthen the uterine muscles: 2 to 3 drops each of rose, jasmine, and black pepper or nutmeg in 5 tsp (25ml) light carrier oil, rubbed into the lower abdomen.

♡ During labor, a firm massage to the lower abdomen, and to the whole lower back region, between contractions can be very comforting and can provide good pain relief. Make the following blend in preparation: 2 to 3 drops each of clary sage, rose or lavender, and ylang ylang or nutmeg oils in 5 tsp (25ml) carrier oil.

♡ A hot compress applied to the lower abdomen, using warm water and a few drops of clary sage oil—frequently replaced—can act as a natural anesthetic during labor.

♡ Relaxing in an aromatic bath during the early stages of labor and/or soon after the birth can be a great aid and comfort.

♡ During the birth, and in preparing to bring the baby home, the use of vaporized oils (such as bergamot, chamomile, or lavender) to scent the environment can be very conducive to creating an uplifting or relaxing mood. These oils also help to prevent the spread of airborne bacteria.

♡ To help heal the perineum after the birth, add a few drops of rose, cypress, or lavender to a sitz bath, or a shallow bath and soak for at least 10 minutes. Up to a handful of sea salt added to the water will aid healing and prevent infection.

♡ After the birth, the breasts can become engorged by the sudden flow of milk. Massage the hard, swollen lumps with a mixture of 3 to 4 drops (in total) of geranium, rose, or peppermint oil in 1 tbsp (15ml) carrier oil or a nonallergenic cream.

Immune system

THE IMMUNE SYSTEM is supported by and closely related to other body systems, especially the lymphatic and nervous systems. Recent research suggests that emotional and psychological factors play a vital role in the efficiency of immune response. This may help to account for the fact that viral infections and conditions involving suppressed immune systems are becoming an increasing problem today. The immune response is orchestrated by three distinct groups of cells—the phagocytes, the T cells, and the B cells. These all originate from white blood cells in the bone marrow, and serve to protect the body from infection. If this defensive barrier breaks down for some reason, the body becomes vulnerable to invasion from all sorts of pathogenic organisms. There are many factors that lead to a damaged immune system—notably the overuse of antibiotics.

DIETARY FACTORS

Insecticides and other additives found in many food products can contribute to the breakdown of the immune system. In extreme cases, this can lead to all types of allergies and sensitization reactions, with symptoms such as headaches, stomach pains, or general fatigue. To maintain optimum health, it is important to follow an organic and additive-free diet as much as possible. To boost the immune system, a course of garlic capsules, Vitamin E, and Vitamin C are also indicated.

OTHER MEASURES

Since stress contributes to a depressed immune system, it is vital to assess general lifestyle, including work and emotional environment. Psychotherapy, counseling, yoga, meditation, and even allergy testing can all be valuable aids in this field.

CLINICAL NOTES

Many essential oils, particularly tea tree oil, stimulate the immune system and assist the body in resisting and fighting infection.

References
EPIDEMIC PAROTITIS see MUMPS page 221
FLU see INFLUENZA page 226
GERMAN MEASLES (RUBELLA) see MEASLES page 226
PERTUSSIS see WHOOPING COUGH page 222
ZONA (SHINGLES) see CHICKEN POX page 223

ABOVE A vitamin-rich diet, including a course of vitamins, can boost immunity.

Methods of use

♡ To help build up resistance levels, use 8 to 10 drops of tea tree oil in the bathwater at least twice a week.

♡ To strengthen the immune system, have a massage once a week using 7 to 8 drops each of tea tree and rosemary, and 2 to 3 drops of cinnamon leaf oil in 2fl oz (50ml) base oil. If this is not possible, make up a 5% tea tree concentrated massage oil blend (50 drops per 2fl oz/50ml base oil), and rub this firmly into the palms of the hands and soles of the feet once a day.

♡ Use tea tree and any of the other essential oils listed above as room fragrancers on an everyday basis.

Aromatherapy oils

Tea tree, cinnamon leaf, clove, eucalyptus, thyme, rosemary, lavender, pine.

Mumps

NORMALLY A childhood illness, mumps (*epidemic parotitis*) is often preceded by a slight fever and a sore throat. This is followed by an egglike swelling of one or both of the salivary glands in front of the ears. High fever, earache, and headache can accompany the main swelling, and these symptoms usually subside after a few days. Mumps is caused by an airborne virus that can be passed via saliva or the breath. It is contagious from one day before symptoms appear to one week after all swelling has gone, and the disease has an incubation period of two to three weeks.

DIETARY FACTORS
Give soft, easily eaten foods since the pain is made worse by chewing and swallowing. Do not give acids such as vinegar, oranges, or lemons. Rinse the mouth with water to prevent dryness.

CLINICAL NOTES
Due to its low toxicity, lavender is especially suited to the treatment of childhood complaints such as mumps.
SEE J. LAWLESS, *LAVENDER OIL*, PP. 31–38.

Methods of use

♡ Use lavender and tea tree, or eucalyptus and myrtle in vaporizers, or on a handkerchief or pillow.

♡ Give a daily hot bath, with a few drops of lavender (for older children), or chamomile (for young children) in the water. This soothes aching limbs and acts as a steam inhalation. A high temperature can be reduced by immersing the whole body in a lukewarm bath to which a few drops of lavender or tea tree oil have been added.

♡ Apply a warm lavender or chamomile compress to the swollen cheeks.

♡ Gargle with 2 drops of tea tree or lemon oil, and 2 drops Roman chamomile in a glass of distilled water (children over six only).

Aromatherapy oils

Tea tree, lavender, coriander, lemon, cajeput, chamomile, eucalyptus, myrtle.

WARNING

Mumps can cause complications in adults, as the infection can spread to other glands such as the testes, ovaries, or pancreas. Seek medical help immediately.

BELOW Use a small amount of lavender and tea tree, or myrtle and eucalyptus, on a pillow.

Whooping cough

WHOOPING COUGH is characterized by a sudden intake of breath or "whoop" after a bout of coughing. Coughing is sudden, frequent, and violent; there may also be vomiting. It is highly infectious and can last up to 12 weeks. It usually affects children under eight. Despite immunization, it is possible to contract a mild form of this viral disease, especially after an infection such as a cold or influenza. It is contagious for at least two weeks after the onset of symptoms.

DIETARY FACTORS

Cut out dairy products and red meats, which encourage formation of mucus. Give a diet that is light, nutritious, and easy to digest, with vegetable soups, chicken broth, fruit juices, mineral water, and herb teas—especially mouse ear, sundew, coltsfoot, thyme, and white horehound. Give additional Vitamin C and cod liver oil.

WARNING

Whooping cough can be extremely dangerous, especially for babies and children under five years of age. Always seek medical advice.

Methods of use

♥ Use a few drops of lavender, thyme, or hyssop in vaporizers in the bedroom during the course of the illness, and in steaming hot inhalations to soothe bouts of coughing. A humid atmosphere is essential.

♥ Apply a hot compress to the chest, using a few drops of lavender oil on a cotton pad (this can be kept warm with a hot water bottle), to facilitate breathing.

♥ Make up a blend of lavender, thyme (white), and tea tree oil (dilution according to age, see Safety Data, p. 375) and rub onto the child's throat and chest.

♥ Add a few drops of lavender and/or tea tree oil to the bathwater (according to age).

Aromatherapy oils

Thyme, hyssop, cinnamon leaf, cypress, cajeput, tea tree, lavender.

RIGHT Hyssop is beneficial for respiratory problems.

THYME

CINNAMON LEAF

Chicken pox

CHICKEN POX is a highly contagious viral infection, most commonly affecting children. A fever develops, and itchy spots appear in crops, progressing to blisters and then to crusts. Eruption usually starts on the trunk, and spreads to face and limbs, beginning one day after the onset of symptoms and lasting for one to two weeks. In the related shingles (zona), the virus affects the sensory nerves and clusters of blisters appear along the line of a nerve, often in the form of a band around the torso. The condition can be accompanied by severe pain, usually beginning before the rash appears, and there may be fever.

Chicken pox is caused by the same virus as shingles, *Herpes zoster*. It usually occurs in epidemics and spreads through contact at school or playgroups. Its incubation period (the time from first contact to appearance of symptoms) is two to three weeks, and it is contagious from one day before symptoms appear, until all lesions have crusted over. The virus can also lie dormant and return as shingles later in life.

DIETARY FACTORS
It is vital to drink plenty of liquids—water, fruit juices, peppermint, yarrow, chamomile, or elderflower tea (with honey)—to avoid dehydration. Fever is usually accompanied by loss of appetite. As the fever subsides, light, nutritious foods such as soup, rice, or fruit are recommended. Garlic and Vitamin C increase resistance to infection and aid in recovery. See also Fever (p. 227).

CLINICAL NOTES
Tea tree is a very effective remedy for chicken pox due to its combined properties. It soothes itching and promotes rapid healing of spots, thus helping to prevent possible infection or scarring due to scratching. German chamomile oil can be added for its soothing qualities.

WARNING
In adults, chicken pox or shingles can be dangerous, with high temperatures and pain. Seek medical advice immediately.

Methods of use

♡ Soak frequently for 10–15 minutes in tepid water, every few hours if possible. For babies, add 2 drops of tea tree and 1 drop of chamomile or lavender oil dissolved in 1 tsp (5ml) of alcohol or witch hazel; for children add 3 drops of tea tree and 2 drops of chamomile or lavender oil in 1 tsp (5ml) alcohol or witch hazel); for adults add 5 drops of tea tree and 5 drops of chamomile or lavender oil in 1 tsp (5ml) alcohol or witch hazel. A handful of colloidal oatmeal (available from most pharmacies), may also be added to the bathwater to soothe the skin and encourage healing.

♡ Dissolve 20 (10 for children) drops of tea tree and 10 (5 for children) drops each of lavender and chamomile oils in 2 tsp (10ml) alcohol, and mix with 2fl oz (50ml) rose water and 2fl oz (50ml) witch hazel. Apply the lotion frequently to the spots. Shake well before each use.

NOTE: This treatment is not suitable for young babies.

Aromatherapy oils
Tea tree, lavender, chamomile, yarrow, peppermint, eucalyptus blue gum, bergamot.

BELOW Elderflower tea helps against dehydration—important during fevers and loss of appetite.

Measles and rubella

MEASLES IS A common childhood illness. Its symptoms include fever; barking cough; sensitivity to light; white spots in the mouth, and a blotchy rash on the face and behind the ears. The rash begins three to five days after the appearance of the first symptoms, and lasts up to a week, spreading downward. The symptoms of German measles include fever, catarrh, headache, swollen, tender lymph nodes behind the ears, and a rash of pink spots, which begin on the face and neck, and then spread. The rash appears on the first or second day and lasts for up to three days. Both conditions are spread by the rubella virus. Measles is contagious five days before and after the first appearance of the rash, and the incubation period is one to two weeks. German measles is contagious from one day before the appearance of the symptoms until one day after the disappearance of the rash; incubation is two to three weeks.

Aromatherapy oils

Chamomile (Roman and German), lemon eucalyptus, eucalyptus blue gum, lavender, cajeput, tea tree, myrtle.

CHAMOMILE TEA

DIETARY FACTORS

It is vital to drink plenty of liquids to avoid dehydration. Give water, fruit juices, or lukewarm peppermint, yarrow, chamomile, or elderflower tea (with honey). There is usually loss of appetite, but as the fever subsides, light, nutritious foods such as soup, rice, or fruit are recommended. Garlic and Vitamin C increase resistance to infection and aid recovery.

OTHER MEASURES

During the fever stage, bed rest is advisable. Keep lighting dim in cases of measles. See also Fever (p. 227), Sore throat (p. 193).

CLINICAL NOTES

Lavender is a useful children's remedy during any infectious illness, due to its ability to ease both physical and psychological discomfort, and its balancing nature or two-way effect, which is both calming and stimulating.

This effect is put to use simultaneously at signs of the onset of an infection, such as fever, sore throat, headache, aches and pains, and unrest. Lavender's calming actions as an anti-inflammatory, analgesic, antipyretic, and nervous system sedative will relieve these symptoms early. However, its stimulating actions as a diaphoretic, antiinfective and antiseptic will work directly on the source of the infection itself.

WARNING

German measles can be dangerous to unborn babies. Pregnant women who have not had rubella should seek immediate medical advice if they have been exposed to the disease. Measles in adults can also lead to serious complications. Medical advice should always be sought.

Methods of use

♡ Use lavender and tea tree, or eucalyptus and myrtle, in vaporizers throughout the duration of the illness, or add a few drops to a handkerchief for inhalation throughout the day, and to the pillow at night.

♡ Give a daily hot bath with a few added drops of lavender (for older children) or chamomile (for young children) to the water. This soothes aching limbs and also acts as a steam inhalation. A high temperature can be reduced by immersing the whole body in a lukewarm bath to which a few drops of lavender or tea tree oil have been added.

♡ For a sore throat, add 3 to 4 drops of lavender or tea tree to a glass of warm water, mix well and use the mixture as a gargle. Repeat at least two or three times a day.

♡ If the fever is very high, it can be reduced by applying cold compresses, and sponging the body at regular intervals, using 3½ fl oz (100ml) distilled water, with 2fl oz (50ml) witch hazel, and 5 drops each of tea tree, lavender, and chamomile oil.

♡ For older children, regular steam inhalations will help to soothe coughing. Add 3 to 6 drops (in total) of tea tree or eucalyptus or myrtle oil to a bowl of steaming hot water and get the child to inhale for 5–10 minutes.

Influenza

INFLUENZA IS THE most common single cause of fever, although the term is often used to include various unidentified viral infections. All are characterized by a raised temperature, aching limbs, fatigue, sore throat, and other respiratory symptoms, such as catarrh or a dry cough. Flu is caused by a virus, and often occurs in epidemics during the winter. New strains of the virus seem to emerge each year, despite the availability of flu vaccines.

DIETARY FACTORS

Drink plenty of liquids, especially peppermint or elderflower teas, and sliced ginger or lemon and honey in hot water. Once the fever has subsided, eat foods which are easy to digest such as soups, rice, or steamed vegetables. Garlic and Vitamin C increase resistance to infection and aid recovery.

OTHER MEASURES

Stay in bed and keep warm. Contact with other people should be kept to a minimum as influenza is highly contagious (incubation is from 12 to 24 hours; contagion lasts for the first three days of symptoms). See also Headaches (p. 229), Coughs (p. 186), Fever (p. 227), Throat infections (p. 193).

CLINICAL NOTES

Essential oils can do much to prevent an attack of flu, or to reduce the severity of the illness. The most effective is tea tree through its powerful antiviral, bactericidal, and immunostimulant qualities. It is also a diaphoretic in cases of fever, and helps the body to sweat out the fever. (However, when the body is in its normal state, these diaphoretic qualities are absent.)

SEE J. LAWLESS, *TEA TREE OIL*, P. 69.

Methods of use

♥ Use tea tree, eucalyptus, and/or rosemary oils, or another recommended oil, in vaporizers, especially at the onset of influenza. Sprinkle a few drops of marjoram or bergamot oil onto the pillow at night.

♥ At the very first sign of infection, take a hot bath with 8 to 10 drops of tea tree added to the water, and go straight to bed. Repeated each evening, this is often enough to avert a fullblown attack. Lavender, marjoram, or chamomile oil can also be used in the bathtub to soothe aching limbs and encourage restful sleep.

♥ To combat respiratory infection, add 2 to 3 drops each of tree tree, Spanish sage or clary sage, and thyme oil to a glass of warm water, mix well and gargle. Repeat the treatment at least two or three times a day.

♥ Massage the back of the neck, chest and soles of the feet with 4 to 5 drops each of tea tree, lemon eucalyptus, and cinnamon or clove oil in 5 tsp (25ml) base oil. Repeat twice daily.

Aromatherapy oils

Lemon eucalyptus, peppermint, lavender, bergamot, tea tree, rosemary, thyme, basil, citronella, ginger, marjoram, lemongrass, lemon, cinnamon, yarrow, cajeput, Spanish sage, camphor, clove, nutmeg.

WARNING

Influenza can be dangerous in that bacterial pneumonia may develop.

Fever

A FEVER IS ANY condition in which the body temperature is higher than normal (i.e. above 37°C/98.4°F). A raised temperature is a vital and healthy response to infection because it speeds up the body's metabolic rate and strengthens its defense systems. In many instances, a fever should be allowed to take its course. This process often includes shivering or feelings of cold, and culminates in a period of profuse sweating that eventually subsides at the same time as a lowering of the fever. Fever can result from numerous viral or bacterial infections, ranging from influenza—the most common cause—to tropical diseases such as malaria or typhoid.

DIETARY FACTORS

Eating is not beneficial while the fever is high because vital energy can be diverted into the digestive process—as opposed to fighting the infection. Feverish people rarely feel like eating anything anyway. However, it is vital to drink plenty of liquids—water, fruit juices, peppermint or elderflower tea—to avoid dehydration. As the fever subsides, light, nutritious foods such as soup, rice, or fruit are recommended. Garlic and Vitamin C increase resistance to infection and aid recovery.

OTHER MEASURES

A feverish person must be kept in bed—rest is essential for the body to recuperate. Eat plenty of live yogurt afterward, if antibiotic treatment has been necessary.

WARNING

If the fever remains high, or rises to a dangerous level, seek professional medical advice immediately. Use no more than 3 drops of the spice oils, eucalyptus, camphor, or peppermint in the bath.

Methods of use

♡ Use tea tree, eucalyptus (lemon or blue gum) and/or rosemary (or another recommended oil) in vaporizers throughout the duration of the illness.

♡ To help control a high temperature, immerse the whole body in a tepid bath containing 3 to 10 drops in total of the following cooling oils: peppermint, basil, tea tree, or eucalyptus (lemon or blue gum). If the person is too weak to get into a bathtub, sponge the body using a facecloth soaked in tepid water to which a few drops of the above oils have been added.

♡ Massage the back of the neck, chest, and soles of the feet with 4 to 5 drops each of tea tree, lemon eucalyptus, cinnamon or clove oil in 5 tsp (25ml) base oil. Repeat twice daily.

Aromatherapy oils

Eucalyptus blue gum, peppermint, lavender, bergamot, tea tree, rosemary, thyme, basil, lemon eucalyptus, citronella, lemongrass, lemon, cinnamon, yarrow, cajeput, Spanish sage, camphor, clove.

EUCALYPTUS BLUE GUM

CITRONELLA

THE NERVOUS SYSTEM

Anxiety

ANXIETY IS ONE of the most common stress-related conditions encountered today. It is accompanied at the physical level by such symptoms as high blood pressure and palpitations, and at the mental level by insomnia, and irritability. Some people are more prone to worrying than others, although a certain degree of anxiety can also be a natural response to a stressful situation. Anxiety becomes a problem when it is not expressed or released, and when the psychological factors underlying the anxiety are not addressed. Food allergies or the side effects of certain drugs can promote anxiety.

DIETARY FACTORS
Cut down on stimulants such as tea, coffee, alcohol, and on sweet carbonated drinks and refined sugar products. Drink herb teas such as chamomile, lemon balm, lime flowers (linden), hops, or verbena. Oatmeal or porridge oats as a regular part of the diet is one of the best tonics for the nerves.

OTHER MEASURES
Gentle exercise, yoga, meditation, and, if necessary, psychotherapy can all be helpful. Bach flower remedies can be beneficial for chronic worriers or those prone to unpredictable panic attacks. See also Depression (p. 231), High blood pressure (p. 178), Insomnia (p. 230), Stress (p. 236).

References
LISTLESSNESS see DEPRESSION page 231

MIGRAINE see HEADACHES page 229

NERVE PAIN see NEURALGIA page 237

NERVOUS FATIGUE see DEBILITY page 232

SHOCK see FAINTNESS/SHOCK page 234

WARNING
If the state of anxiety is allowed to persist over a prolonged period, it can lead to secondary, more serious complaints, such as stomach ulcers or heart failure. Chronic anxiety requires professional help.

Methods of use

♡ Add 8 to 10 drops of lavender (or any combination of the recommended oils) to a warm evening bath to relieve insomnia, restlessness, anxiety, and tension.

♡ Regular massage can dramatically reduce anxiety levels. A suitable blend of oils would be 7 to 8 drops each of clary sage, ylang ylang, and lavender in 2fl oz (50ml) base oil.

♡ For self-treatment, blend 2 to 3 drops of lavender or chamomile oil with 1 tsp (5ml) sweet almond oil, and massage the oil into the hands and the soles of the feet.

♡ For a soothing room fragrance, use lavender, frankincense, or bergamot oil in a vaporizer. Put a few drops of any of these oils on a handkerchief for inhalation throughout the day. Use rose, ylang ylang, or neroli oil (or a blend) neat as a perfume.

Aromatherapy oils

Bergamot, chamomile, neroli, ylang ylang, lavender, valerian, vetiver, rose, clary sage, frankincense, cedarwood, melissa.

Headaches

HEADACHES ARE a common complaint among both adults and children. They can vary in intensity from a mild ache to severe and lasting pain. Headaches can be caused, or aggravated, by sinus congestion, nervous stress, muscular spasm, physical injury, structural misalignment, inhaling toxic fumes, eye strain, too much sun, or too much alcohol.

DIETARY FACTORS

Recurrent headaches may be related to food allergies. Migraine is most commonly a food-related complaint, and is often triggered by foods containing tyramine. These include chocolate, citrus fruits, cheese, caffeine, alcohol, peanut butter, vinegar, yogurt, yeast, and cured meats. Relaxing herbal remedies such as chamomile, hops, linden, lemon balm, or verbena can help soothe tension headaches when taken as tea. Peppermint tea can help ease congested headaches. Feverfew is recommended for migraine headaches.

OTHER MEASURES

Try to identify the cause of the headache and treat accordingly. This may involve assessing lifestyle, aiming to reduce stress; avoiding the sun; visiting an osteopath or chiropractor to check for structural misalignment; consulting an allergy specialist; avoiding fumes and odors which trigger an attack. See also Anxiety (p. 228), High blood pressure (p. 178), Sinusitis (p. 191), Stress (p. 236).

CLINICAL NOTES

Clinical evidence and CNV data (contingent negative variation curve—a device for measuring electrical brainwave patterns created by anticipation) have demonstrated that several essential oils have a combined sedative and antispasmodic effect that can help in reducing nervous tension. These include lavender, Roman chamomile, marjoram, and melissa.

SEE M. LIS-BALCHIN, *AROMASCIENCE*, PP. 38, 65, 74.

WARNING
Persistent headaches and migraines require professional diagnosis and treatment.

Methods of use

♡ For tension headaches, inhale a few drops of lavender or rose and/or melissa oil from a tissue, or apply a drop direct to the temples. Nasal decongestants can relieve stuffiness and congested headaches.

♡ Use 2 to 3 drops each of peppermint and/or eucalyptus oil in a bowl of steaming water, cover the head with a towel, and inhale deeply for 5–10 minutes, keeping the eyes closed.

♡ Headaches brought on by tension or stress can be eased by a firm neck and shoulder massage, using 4 to 5 drops each of lavender, peppermint and marjoram oil in 5 tsp (25ml) carrier oil.

♡ For eye strain, apply a cold compress of rose water, chamomile, water, or lavender water (not the essential oil) to the eyelids. A cold compress may also be applied to the forehead or the back of the neck to soothe tension headaches and sunstroke. Relax in a warm aromatic bath to ease away tension, using 8 to 10 drops (in total) of lavender, chamomile, and/or rose oil; to promote decongestion, use a few drops of peppermint, eucalyptus, and/or marjoram oil.

Aromatherapy oils

Rose, lavender, melissa, chamomile, peppermint, eucalyptus, marjoram.

Insomnia

INABILITY TO SLEEP (insomnia) is another common stress-related complaint that everyone suffers from at some time. When insomnia continues over a period of time, however, it can lead to secondary problems such as reduced concentration, irritability, depression, and chronic fatigue.

DIETARY FACTORS
Reduce intake of stimulants such as tea or coffee, especially in the evening, and do not eat a heavy meal just before retiring. Lack of Vitamin B is associated with poor sleep patterns. Three of the B group are known as antistress vitamins, because they are especially required during periods of stress. A Vitamin B complex supplement, and chamomile, hops, skullcap, or valerian taken as a tea (or in tablet form) last thing at night can help induce relaxation.

OTHER MEASURES
Make sure the bedroom is neither too cold nor too stuffy; assess lifestyle and work patterns, aiming to reduce stress levels—yoga, meditation, relaxation exercises or tapes can be useful. See also Anxiety (p. 228), Debility (p. 232), High blood pressure (p. 178), Stress (p. 236).

CLINICAL NOTES
Several studies in hospitals have shown that vaporized lavender oil helps to induce sleep—in some cases with better effect than night medication.
SEE J. LAWLESS, *LAVENDER OIL*, PP. 22–25.

WARNING
Do not use valerian oil for more than two weeks at a stretch, since it is a depressant to the central nervous system.

Aromatherapy oils
Lavender, chamomile, vetiver, valerian, marjoram, neroli, clary sage.

LEFT A few drops of neat lavender or chamomile oil, massaged into the soles of the feet, are quickly absorbed into the bloodstream, where they act as a sedative.

Methods of use

♥ Massage a few drops of neat lavender or chamomile oil into the soles of the feet before retiring. This will quickly be absorbed into the bloodstream to act as a natural sedative. For more stubborn cases of insomnia, valerian oil can be used instead.

♥ To encourage relaxation or a restful night (also excellent during pregnancy, and for children), put a few drops of lavender oil on the pillow or on pajamas. Scenting the sheets with lavender oil also helps to induce sleep. Alternatively, use the vaporized oil of lavender, marjoram, valerian, and/or chamomile in the bedroom.

♥ Relax for at least 10 minutes before retiring for the night in a warm bath to which you have added 8 to 10 drops of lavender, or one of the other recommended oils. Restlessness, hyperactivity, and insomnia in babies, infants, and older children can be helped by adding a few drops of lavender or chamomile oil to the bathtub at bedtime.

♥ A regular massage, using soothing oils such as lavender, chamomile, clary sage, and marjoram is also very beneficial in reducing stress and helping to induce sleep.

Depression

DEPRESSION CAN TAKE many forms: it is often associated with lack of energy and listlessness, but can also be accompanied by restlessness or agitation, and sometimes alternates between the two. It can be triggered by a traumatic event such as a bereavement, a divorce, or even moving house. It may also be caused by ongoing problems such as emotional or financial difficulties.

DIETARY FACTORS
To speed recovery, it is vital to eat balanced, nutritious food when suffering from depression. It is easy to slip into bad food habits, or simply not to eat enough, during such times. A course of good multimineral and multivitamin supplements (especially the B complex vitamins) can be helpful. Ginseng or damiana (taken as a tea or as tablets) are valuable restorative herbal remedies.

DIETARY FACTORS
Bach flower remedies, yoga, meditation, and psychotherapy, counseling or attending support groups can all help. See also Anxiety (p. 228), Debility (p. 232), Faintness/shock (p. 234), Stress (p. 236).

WARNING

Chronic depression, or deep depression that has no apparent cause, requires professional treatment.

CLINICAL NOTES
Mild depression responds well to aromatherapy treatment, as does depression arising from having to cope with difficult life situations involving grief, loss, or fear. In one case history, a doctor describes her own reasons for using aromatherapy after the death of her mother as follows:

"I didn't want tranquilizers and didn't feel antidepressants were needed as mine was a perfectly normal reaction to the stress I was living through. I didn't want to take alcohol and yet craved relief from what I was experiencing. I knew these pharmacological treatments did not work for real-life situations of stress … [whereas] a combination of massage and essential oils is more powerful than either one alone, and [makes for] a valuable form of relaxation therapy."

SEE DR. ANN COXON, "PRESCRIBING AROMATHERAPY," *AROMATHERAPY QUARTERLY*, 1991, NO. 31, P. 9.

Aromatherapy oils

Basil, bergamot, neroli, jasmine, melissa, rose, sandalwood, lavender.

Methods of use

♥ Add 8 to 10 drops of lavender oil and any of the other recommended oils in the bath.

♥ Receiving a regular professional massage, using a blend of antidepressant oils, can help encourage feelings of self-worth and well-being. A suitable blend would be 7 to 8 drops (in total) of lavender, neroli or petitgrain, and bergamot in 2fl oz (50ml) base oil.

♥ For an uplifting or soothing room fragrance use oils such as bergamot or lavender in a vaporizer. Wear rose, jasmine, or neroli oil as a perfume.

SANDALWOOD

GINSENG TEA

Debility

DEBILITY (NERVOUS FATIGUE) is often characterized by both physical and mental languor. Symptoms include low spirits, feeling constantly tired, dizziness or faintness, and a general sense of malaise. The causes of debility are various: common contributing factors include emotional or physical exhaustion due to long working hours, VDU strain (low-level radiation from computer screens), a severe or longterm illness, or emotional pressure.

DIETARY FACTORS

Nervous fatigue and weakness are associated with insufficient folic and pantothenic acid (both found in liver and yeast) and Vitamin B1 (thiamine), which regulates the release of energy in the body. Eat plenty of unrefined carbohydrates and complete proteins that produce energy gradually, since excessively high or low blood sugar levels ultimately lead to exhaustion and depression—as in diabetes. Drink fresh ginger root tea with honey for an excellent restorative herbal remedy.

OTHER MEASURES

Assess lifestyle and work patterns; take gentle exercise; perform deep breathing in the fresh air; consider psychotherapy; if necessary, take a complete break to rest and recuperate. See also Anxiety (p. 228), Depression (p. 231), Faintness/shock (p. 234), Stress (p. 236).

CLINICAL NOTES

Rosemary is still specific in *The British Herbal Pharmacopoeia* for "depressive states with general debility." Dr. Valnet recommended rosemary in "fortifying morning baths," especially for children, and for adults with general fatigue. Lemon, grapefruit, and lime oils have been used as an air spray in Japanese offices to increase concentration levels: "… typing mistakes were reduced by 54% when lemon oil was disbursed in the room."
SEE J. LAWLESS, *AROMATHERAPY AND THE MIND*, P. 172.

Methods of use

♡ Add 8 to 10 drops of rosemary or pine oil to the daily bath, or to a footbath, as a reviving "pick-me-up."

♡ Inhaling eucalyptus, lemon, or rosemary from a tissue can help counteract feelings of weakness or nervous fatigue. Alternatively, use any of the recommended oils in a vaporizer, at home or in the workplace.

♡ Use fortifying oils for massage to strengthen the whole nervous system. For example, 7 to 8 drops each of rosemary, pine, and black pepper or basil in 2fl oz (50ml) base oil.

GRAPEFRUIT

BLACK PEPPER

Aromatherapy oils

Peppermint, pine, geranium, rosemary, basil, ginger, eucalyptus, angelica, lavender, lemon, grapefruit, bergamot, orange, and most spice oils.

Epilepsy

EPILEPSY IS THE most common serious neurological disorder. Epileptic fits can vary from momentary attacks (inattention), without loss of consciousness (minor epilepsy) to muscular spasm and convulsions (major epilepsy). Caused by a disturbance in the central nervous system, epilepsy is associated with brief disruptions in the normal electrical activity of the brain. It may start in childhood, or may come on unexpectedly, but the precipitating factor is often a traumatic or stressful life event with high anxiety levels.

DIETARY FACTORS

Certain substances, when ingested in significant doses, are known to promote epilepsy because they are neurotoxic: these are notably ketones found in herbs such as tansy, mugwort, rue, thuja, pennyroyal, and wormwood (and, to a lesser degree, in common sage, fennel, hyssop, and rosemary). Relaxing herbs such as hops, chamomile, and lemon balm (melissa) are beneficial taken as a tea.

OTHER MEASURES

Do not try to restrain, move, or wake an individual during an epileptic fit. On regaining consciousness after an attack, the person needs to rest quietly for a period, in order to establish equilibrium.

CLINICAL NOTES

One patient using chamomile oil in a series of clinical trials "showed a 90 percent reduction in seizures" and it was found that: "Intervention with the use of essential oils in individuals who have epilepsy can significantly reduce seizure rates, although maintenance of treatments might be necessary."
SEE *INTERNATIONAL JOURNAL OF AROMATHERAPY*, P. 23, CITED IN T. CLOUSTON, OILS FOR EPILEPSY.

Methods of use

♡ If you suffer from epilepsy, if possible, have a full-body massage once a week using a chosen oil (from the list below) diluted to 2.5% in sweet almond oil (25 drops per 2fl oz/50ml base oil). Alternatively, practice self-massage on the hands and feet with a similar blend.

♡ Inhale neat lavender oil (or other chosen oil) from a tissue, or use in a vaporizer. Wearing neroli or rose oil as a perfume can help allay anxiety and provide comfort.

♡ Add 8 to 10 drops of lavender, chamomile, or ylang ylang oil to a warm bath to help restore equilibrium and cope with the emotional after effects of an attack.

Aromatherapy oils

Chamomile, lavender, melissa, ylang ylang, rose, neroli.

RIGHT *During an epileptic seizure, the normal electrical activity of the brain is interrupted. This brain scan shows one such episode.*

Faintness/shock

THIS CAN VARY from a mild feeling of faintness to complete collapse. Symptoms may include nausea, vomiting, restlessness, a pale and clammy skin, and a racing pulse. Slight faintness or dizziness can result from a number of causes, such as sunstroke, hangover, nervous exhaustion, or very low blood pressure. It is common during the menopause and with PMS. Shock can cause faintness due to a reduced volume of blood or body fluid through either physical injury or fear.

DIETARY FACTORS
Faintness may also be due to anemia (low red blood corpuscle count), anorexia, bulimia, hunger, or poor nutrition. It is important to eat regular, balanced meals.

OTHER MEASURES
Rest, keep warm and loosen any tight clothing. Breathe deeply, remain calm.

WARNING
Traumatic (injury) shock is a serious condition that requires immediate medical attention.

Aromatherapy oils

Lavender, neroli, rose, geranium, palmarosa, ylang ylang, clary sage, jasmine.

Methods of use

♡ Inhale neat lavender oil from a tissue, or use in a vaporizer. Neroli, jasmine, or rose oil can be inhaled to help allay anxiety and provide comfort.

♡ Add 8 to 10 drops of lavender, clary sage, or geranium oil to a warm bath to help restore equilibrium and cope with the emotional after effects of a shock.

♡ Rose, lavender, or orange flower water applied to the temples and face is reviving to the spirits and helpful in cases of emotional shock, as well as good for hangovers, nervous exhaustion, and sunstroke.

RIGHT Neroli can be used to help with problems of an emotional origin.

RIGHT Jasmine can help to allay anxiety.

Jetlag

THE SYMPTOMS OF JETLAG after a long flight are well recognized: sleep disturbance, swollen ankles, disorientation, nervous fatigue, and dehydration. The problems are caused by disruption of the body's biological clock due to crossing time zones; change in altitude; being in a pressurized atmosphere, and, often, anxiety or nausea brought on by traveling.

DIETARY FACTORS
Drink plenty of bottled water or other liquids (not alcohol) to avoid dehydration during the flight. If stress is involved, take extra Vitamins C and B complex to aid recovery.

OTHER MEASURES
Keep the feet raised as much as possible to avoid swollen ankles. See also Anxiety (p. 228), Edema (p. 184), Nausea/vomiting (p. 204), Stress (p. 236).

Methods of use

♡ To prevent jetlag, freshen up frequently during the flight using a little lavender water, or inhale lavender or geranium oil from a tissue.

♡ Use a lavender or rose moisturizing cream on the face and hands to prevent skin dryness.

♡ On arrival, if possible, take a long bath containing 8 to 10 drops of lavender or geranium or chamomile oil for relaxing, or rosemary or bergamot or grapefruit oil for an enlivening effect. This helps readjust physiological and psychological rhythms.

Aromatherapy oils

Lavender, chamomile, geranium, rosemary, bergamot, grapefruit, peppermint, lemon, clary sage.

BELOW After travel, jetlag can manifest itself in disturbed sleep, disorientation, lethargy, and swollen ankles.

BELOW To prevent jetlag, inhale lavender or geranium oil from a tissue during the flight.

Stress

STRESS IS A multidimensional syndrome that can cause a wide range of physical ailments and psychological problems, from high blood pressure, headaches, or digestive complaints, to feelings of constant tiredness, depression, or nervous anxiety. Stress weakens the immune system, and, in the long term, makes an individual more susceptible to all kinds of disease.

It occurs when excessive demands are placed on an individual's physical, mental, or emotional resources. The body reacts by boosting levels of adrenaline—the hormone that prepares us for fight or flight in situations of danger. Many potentially stressful events are dealt with on a day-to-day basis and can provide interest and challenge in life. When unresolved demanding situations build up over a period of time, this causes what we call stress.

DIETARY FACTORS

There may be a deficiency in trace elements such as copper, cobalt, manganese or iron, in minerals such as phosphorus and potassium, or in vitamins, and especially Vitamin B6 (pyridoxine) and Vitamin B3 (niacin). It is important to have a wholesome mixed diet, containing adequate protein, fats, carbohydrates, vitamins, and minerals, and to avoid processed foods and foods containing chemical additives. Nervine and relaxant herbs such as chamomile (suitable for children), valerian, hops, or skullcap are recommended, taken as teas or in tablets.

OTHER MEASURES

Take regular exercise, if possible in the fresh air, as this helps work out physical and emotional tension, and aids relaxation. Find time to practice yoga, meditation, deep breathing, and pleasurable hobbies. Make clear boundaries between work and free time. Assess work and lifestyle—psychotherapeutic help or counseling may be beneficial. See also Anxiety (p. 228), Debility (p. 232), Depression (p. 231), High blood pressure (p. 178), Insomnia (p. 230), Palpitations (p. 180).

CLINICAL NOTES

Clinical research has shown that the synergistic combination of smell and touch can have a profoundly nourishing and comforting effect on the psyche.

Several oils have been shown in clinical tests to have destressing effects, including valerian, nutmeg, neroli, rose, and lavender.

SEE R. TISSERAND, *INTERNATIONAL JOURNAL OF AROMATHERAPY*, VOL. 4, NO. 2, P. 16.

Methods of use

♥ Add 8 to 10 drops of lavender (or any combination of the recommended oils) to a warm evening bath to relieve insomnia, restlessness, anxiety, and nervous tension.

♥ Receiving a regular professional massage can dramatically reduce stress levels. A blend of oils such as clary sage, ylang ylang, and lavender is often found to be helpful.

♥ For self-treatment, mix 2 to 3 drops of lavender or Roman chamomile oil with 1 tsp (5ml) sweet almond oil, and massage the blend into the hands and the soles of the feet.

♥ For a soothing room fragrance, use lavender, frankincense, or bergamot oil in a vaporizer or put a few drops on a handkerchief for inhalation throughout the day. In addition, rose, ylang ylang, or neroli oil may be used as a perfume.

Aromatherapy oils

Lavender, chamomile, valerian, bergamot, clary sage, marjoram, frankincense, melissa, nutmeg, neroli, rose, jasmine.

RIGHT Neroli can be used to help with problems of an emotional origin.

Neuralgia

NERVE PAIN or neuralgia can take many forms. It may run the whole length of a nerve, or may affect a localized point on the skin's surface. Sciatica is a form of neuralgia that is characterized by an intense shooting pain or tenderness felt along the length of the sciatic nerve, which runs from the back of the thigh to the lower calf. The term is also often used to describe nerve pain that radiates from the lower back to the thigh. This distressing condition can result from a variety of causes, including an infection, an accident, or an osteopathic problem, but more commonly it occurs through general debility, poor diet, lack of exercise, and stress. Facial neuralgia can be triggered by cold wind. Although sciatica is often associated with a misalignment of the hips or lower spine, causing pressure on the sciatic nerve, the root cause of the problem frequently lies in abdominal congestion and constipation.

DIETARY FACTORS

It is vital to tackle the root of the problem, and this often means a change of diet. Include plenty of roughage, green vegetables, fruit, oats, and a course of Vitamin B complex. Relaxant herbs, and nervines such as hops, skullcap, valerian, and peppermint, taken as a tea (or as tablets) are also recommended.

OTHER MEASURES

Assess lifestyle to reduce stress levels; if necessary, consult an osteopath or chiropractor; take gentle exercise. See also Constipation (p. 198), Debility (p. 232), Stress (p. 236).

CLINICAL NOTES

Rosemary can be of great relief to those suffering from sciatica or neuralgia. It also acts as a stimulant for the whole system, including the abdominal region, thus helping to relieve any congestion in this area. Case studies have also shown that: "Where there is neuralgia or nerve pain, relaxing nervines and tonics will help … massage of the lower back and legs may help a lot."
SEE D. HOFFMAN, *THE HOLISTIC HERBAL*, P. 85.

Methods of use

♥ Simply soaking in a hot bath is an easy and effective way of bringing pain relief. Use 8 to 10 drops of any of the above oils added to the bathwater to increase the benefits.

♥ Gentle massage is itself very helpful for sciatica and neuralgia. Add about 25 drops (in total) of rosemary, lavender, marjoram, and/or peppermint to 2fl oz (50ml) of St. John's wort oil and rub gently into the affected area.

Aromatherapy oils

Lavender, peppermint, rosemary, marjoram, chamomile, ginger.

MARJORAM

BELOW Valerian tea is recommended for relaxation.

PART FOUR

♡

*Index of
Essential Oils*

Index of essential oils

IN THE FOLLOWING PAGES a profile is given for each of the oils in the four groups listed on pages 32–33 and mentioned in the uses, remedies, and treatments suggested throughout this book. Each profile describes the plant from which the oil is derived, the quality of the oil in appearance and scent, its general actions, and the ways in which it is used.

The profile of each oil explains the scent properties of the oil and the general effect it has in use, both physiologically and psychologically. These are a useful guide to understanding the nature of the oil, but the qualities and effects of essential oils are extremely subtle, and vary both according to the particular source and also with the physical and emotional state of the person using them. Intuition and experience can be used in selecting oils for use. Symbols at the top right corner of the pages indicate the part of the plant used for extraction of the oil. An additional symbol highlights

oils that can be used for children. There is a key to these symbols on page 242.

The oil profiles are arranged in botanical name order to emphasize related groups, but an alphabetical index of oils can be found on page 396 for reference.

All essential oils are very strong and some can be toxic in various ways if incorrectly used. Before using any oil, check its profile, look out especially for Safety data and Warning boxes, which describe ways in which the oil must be used, and give contraindications for its use.

Key to symbols

Icons in the top right corner of every page in this section indicate the parts of plants that each oil is extracted from. There is also a symbol to indicate oils that are recommended for children.

TREE

FLOWERS

PARTS OF PLANTS

RESIN

LEAVES

FRUIT

SEEDS

ROOTS

WHOLE PLANT

GOOD FOR CHILDREN

Fir needle, silver

ABIES ALBA FAMILY PINACEAE

Description A relatively small coniferous tree, with a regular pyramidal shape and a silvery white bark, grown chiefly for timber and as Christmas trees.

Actions Analgesic, antiseptic (pulmonary), antitussive, deodorant, expectorant, rubefacient, stimulant, tonic.

Extraction Essential oil by steam distillation from the needles and young twigs, or from the fir cones and broken up pieces (templin oil).

Characteristics A colorless or pale yellow liquid of pleasing, rich, sweet-balsamic odor. It blends well with galbanum, labdanum, lavender, rosemary, lemon, pine, and marjoram.

SAFETY DATA
Nontoxic, nonirritant (except in high concentration), nonsensitizing.

Perfume

Scent: Rich, sweet-balsamic, orange-like.
Key qualities: Antibiotic, antiseptic, balsamic, sedative, tonic. **Odor intensity:** Medium.

Aromatherapy use

Circulation muscles and joints: Arthritis, muscular aches and pains, rheumatism.
Respiratory system: Bronchitis, coughs, sinusitis, etc.
Immune system: Colds, fever, flu.
Other: Employed as an ingredient in some cough and cold remedies and rheumatic treatments. Used as a fragrance component in deodorants, room sprays, disinfectants, bath preparations, soaps, and perfumes.

MAINLY USED FOR RESPIRATORY COMPLAINTS, FEVER, MUSCULAR, AND RHEUMATIC PAIN.

Mimosa

ACACIA DEALBATA FAMILY *MIMOSACEAE*

Description An attractive small tree up to 40ft (12m) high, having a grayish-brown bark with irregular longitudinal ridges, delicate foliage, and clusters of ball-shaped, fragrant yellow flowers.

Actions Antiseptic, astringent.

Extraction A concrete and absolute by solvent extraction from the flowers and twig ends.

Characteristics The concrete is a hard wax-like yellow mass with a sweet-woody, deep floral fragrance. The absolute is an amber-colored viscous liquid with a slightly green, woody-floral scent. It blends well with lavandin, lavender, ylang ylang, violet, styrax, citronella, Peru balsam, cassie, floral, and spice oils.

SAFETY DATA
Nontoxic, nonirritant, nonsensitizing.

Perfume

Scent: Sweet, floral, woody, honey-like, leathery. **Key qualities:** Calming, warming, soothing, relaxing, uplifting, balancing. **Odor intensity:** Medium.

Aromatherapy use

Skin care: Oily, sensitive, general skin care.
Nervous system: Anxiety, nervous tension, over-sensitivity, stress.

THE BARK OF MIMOSA HAS HISTORICALLY BEEN USED TO TREAT DIARRHEA.

Yarrow

FAMILY ASTERCEAE (COMPOSITAE)

Description A perennial herb with simple stems, up to 3ft/1m high, with finely dissected leaves, and bearing numerous, pinky white, dense flower heads.

Actions Anti-inflammatory, antipyretic, antirheumatic, antiseptic, antispasmodic, astringent, carminative, cicatrizant, diaphoretic, digestive, expectorant, hemostatic, hypotensive, stomachic, tonic.

Extraction The oil is extracted by steam distillation from the dried herb.

Characteristics A dark blue or greenish-olive liquid, with a fresh, green, sweet, herbaceous, slightly camphoraceous odor. It blends well with cedarwood, pine, chamomile, valerian, vetivert, and myrrh.

SAFETY DATA
Nontoxic, nonirritant, but there is possible sensitization in some individuals. The oil can cause skin irritation in concentration.

Perfume

Scent: Warm, fresh, green, sweet, herbaceous, slightly camphoraceous. **Key qualities:** Balancing, restorative, tonic (nerve), strengthening, opening, grounding, revitalizing, mildly stimulating. **Odor intensity:** High.

Aromatherapy use

Skin care: Acne, burns, cuts, eczema, hair rinse, inflammation, rashes, scars, wounds. **Circulation, muscles, and joints:** Arteriosclerosis, high blood pressure, rheumatoid arthritis, thrombosis, varicose veins. **Digestive system:** Constipation, cramp, flatulence, hemorrhoids, indigestion. **Reproductive system:** Amenorrhea, dysmenorrhea. **Immune system:** Colds, fever, flu. **Urinary system:** Cystitis, and other infections. **Nervous system:** Hypertension, insomnia, stress-related conditions.

Fragonia

AGONIS FRAGRANS FAMILY *MYRTACEAE*

Description The species generally have fibrous, brown bark, dull green leaves, and inflorescences of small, white flowers. They are best known and most readily identified by the powerful peppermint or eucalyptus-like odor emitted when the leaves are crushed or torn.

Actions Analgesic (mild), antibacterial, anti-inflammatory, antifungal, antimicrobial, anti-infectious, antiseptic, expectorant, immuno-tonic, nervine, regulating.

Extraction An essential oil by steam distillation from the stems, twigs, and leaves.

Characteristics A pale, watery liquid with a pleasant slightly citrus, fresh-clean, and faintly medicinal top note, mixed with a slight spicy, earthy, and balsamic undertone: more pleasing than tea tree. It blends well with niaouli, eucalyptus, myrtle, lemon myrtle, rosemary, and tea tree.

Perfume

Scent: Citrus, spicy, earthy, balsamic.
Key qualities: Antimicrobial, anti-inflammatory, soothing, calming. **Odor intensity:** Medium.

Aromatherapy use

Skin care: Cuts, bites, stings and general skin care. **Circulation muscles and joints:** Aching muscles and joints, arthritis, rheumatism.
Respiratory system: Asthma, bronchitis, coughs, colds, influenza, sinusitis, tonsillitis.
Genitourinary system: Candida (thrush), menstrual pain and breast tenderness, vaginitis. **Immune system:** Powerful immune-system tonic and restorative.
Nervous system: Anxiety, depression, emotional blockages, grief, insomnia, nervous debility and tension, mood swings, stress.

SAFETY DATA
Nontoxic, nonirritant and nonsensitizing: an extremely mild oil when applied to the skin and safe for children.

Verbena, lemon

AMYRIS BALSAMIFERA FAMILY *RUTACEAE*

Description A handsome deciduous perennial shrub up to 16ft (5m) high with a woody stem, very fragrant, delicate, pale green, lanceolate leaves arranged in threes, and small, pale purple flowers. Often grown as an ornamental bush in gardens.

Actions Antiseptic, antispasmodic, carminative, detoxifying, digestive, febrifuge, hepatobiliary stimulant, sedative (nervous), stomachic.

Extraction Essential oil by steam distillation from the freshly harvested herb.

Characteristics A pale olive or yellow mobile liquid with a sweet, fresh, lemony, fruity-floral fragrance. It blends well with neroli, palmarosa, olibanum, Tolu balsam, elemi, lemon, and other citrus oils.

SAFETY DATA
Possible sensitization; phototoxicity due to high citral levels. However, true verbena oil is virtually nonexistent. Most so-called "verbena oil" is either from the Spanish verbena (an inferior oil), or a mix of lemongrass, lemon, citronella, etc.

Perfume

Scent: Sweet, fresh, lemony, fruity-floral. **Key qualities:** Antiseptic, cleansing, uplifting, refreshing, reviving, energizing. **Odor intensity:** Medium.

Aromatherapy use

Digestive system: Cramps, indigestion, liver congestion. **Nervous system:** Anxiety, insomnia, nervous tension and stress-related conditions.

LEMON VERBENA IS USEFUL FOR SOOTHING UPSET STOMACHS AND HANGOVERS, AS WELL AS FOR A REFRESHING, UPLIFTING "PICK-ME-UP."

Amyris

AMYRIS BALSAMIFERA FAMILY RUTACEAE

Description A small bushy tree with compound leaves and white flowers, which grows wild in thickets all over the island of Haiti.

Actions Antiseptic, balsamic, sedative, decongestant, emollient.

Extraction Essential oil by steam distillation from the broken-up wood and branches. Best if the wood is seasoned first. It provides a very plentiful yield.

Characteristics A pale yellow, slightly viscous liquid with a musty, faintly woody scent, quickly fading away. It blends well with lavandin, citronella, oakmoss, sassafras, cedarwood, and other wood oils.

Perfume

Scent: Soft-woody, oily-sweet, lightly spicy. **Key qualities:** Balsamic, soothing, calming, pleasing. **Odor intensity:** Low.

Aromatherapy use

Ideally used in perfumes or massage oils.

SAFETY DATA
Generally nontoxic, and nonirritant, nonsensitizing.

LOCALS CALL IT "CANDLE WOOD" BECAUSE OF ITS HIGH OIL CONTENT; IT BURNS LIKE A CANDLE. IT IS USED AS A TORCH BY FISHERMEN AND TRADERS. IT ALSO MAKES EXCELLENT FURNITURE WOOD.

Dill seed

ANETHUM GRAVEOLENS FAMILY APIACEAE (UMBELLIFERAE)

Description Annual or biennial herb, up to 3ft (1m) high, with a smooth stem, feathery leaves, and umbels of yellowish flowers followed by flat, small seeds.

Actions Antispasmodic, bactericidal, carminative, digestive, emmenagogue, galactagogue, hypotensive, stimulant, stomachic.

Extraction The oil is extracted by steam distillation (sometimes water) from the seeds.

Characteristics Seed oil is a colorless to pale yellow, mobile liquid, with a light, fresh, warm-spicy scent. Weed oil is a colorless or pale yellow, mobile liquid, with a powerful, sweet-spicy aroma. It blends well with mint, nutmeg, spice, and the citrus oils.

SAFETY DATA
Nontoxic, nonirritant, nonsensitizing.

Perfume

Scent: Herbaceous, fresh, peppery, spicy, warm. **Key qualities (mind):** Reviving, clearing, tonic. **Odor intensity:** Medium.

Aromatherapy use

Digestive system: Colic, dyspepsia, flatulence, indigestion. **Reproductive and endocrine systems:** Amenorrhea, galactagogue.

Angelica root

ANGELICA ARCHANGELICA FAMILY APIACEAE (UMBELLIFERAE)

Description A large, hairy plant with rhizome-like roots, ferny leaves, and umbels of white flowers. The whole plant has a strong, aromatic scent.

Actions Antispasmodic, carminative, depurative, diaphoretic, digestive, diuretic, emmenagogue, expectorant, febrifuge, nervine, stimulant, stomachic, tonic, bactericidal, fungicidal.

Extraction The essential oil is produced by steam distillation from the roots.

Characteristics The root oil is colorless, or pale yellow, turning yellowy-brown with age. It has a rich, herbaceous-earthy body note. The seed oil is a colorless liquid, with a fresher, spicy top note. Blends well with patchouli, clary sage, vetivert, and citrus oils.

> ### SAFETY DATA
> Not to be used during pregnancy or by young children or people with diabetes. The root oil is phototoxic. Use with care, in low dilutions only (1%).

Perfume

Scent: Balsamic, musky, herbaceous, bitter-sweet, powerful, earthy, spicy, long-lasting. Acts as a fixative. **Key qualities:** Restorative, revitalizing, tonic, purifying, comforting, stimulating (in small quantities), sedating (in large quantities), warming, grounding, aphrodisiac. **Odor intensity:** High.

Aromatherapy use

Skin care: Dull and congested skin, irritated conditions, psoriasis. **Circulation, muscles, and joints:** Accumulation of toxins, arthritis, gout, rheumatism, water retention. **Respiratory system:** Bronchitis, colds, coughs. **Digestive system:** Anemia, anorexia, flatulence, indigestion. **Nervous system:** Fatigue, migraine, nervous tension, stress-related disorders.

Rosewood/bois de rose

ANIBA ROSAEODORA, FAMILY *LAURACEAE*

Description
Medium-size, tropical, evergreen tree, with a reddish bark and heartwood, bearing yellow flowers; used extensively for timber.

Actions
Mildly analgesic, anticonvulsant, antidepressant, antimicrobial, antiseptic, aphrodisiac, bactericidal, cellular stimulant, cephalic, deodorant, immune system stimulant, tissue regenerator, tonic.

Extraction
The oil is extracted by steam distillation of the wood chippings.

Characteristics
Colorless to pale yellow liquid, with a very sweet, woody-floral fragrance that has a spicy hint. Blends well with most oils, especially citrus, woods, and florals; it helps give body, and rounds off sharp edges.

SAFETY DATA
Nontoxic, nonirritant, nonsensitizing.

Perfume

Scent: Rosy, woody, dry, floral, slightly green, fresh, mild. **Key qualities (mind):** Warming, comforting, pleasing. **Odor intensity:** Low.

Aromatherapy use

Skin care: Acne, dermatitis, scars, wounds, wrinkles, and good for general skin care of all skin types. **Immune system:** Colds, coughs, fever, infections, immune system stimulant. **Nervous system:** Frigidity, headaches, nausea, nervous tension, stress-related conditions.

Celery seed

APIUM GRAVEOLENS FAMILY *APIACEAE (UMBELLIFERAE)*

Description A familiar biennial plant, 2–3ft (30–60cm) high, with a grooved, fleshy, erect stalk, shiny pinnate leaves, and umbels of white flowers.

Actions Antioxidant, antirheumatic, antiseptic (urinary), antispasmodic, aperitif, depurative, digestive, diuretic, carminative, cholagogue, emmenagogue, galactagogue, hepatic, nervine, sedative (to nervous system), stimulant (uterine), stomachic, tonic (digestive).

Extraction The oil is extracted by steam distillation from the whole or crushed seeds.

Characteristics A pale yellow, or orange, spicy-warm, sweet, long-lasting odor. It blends well with lavender, pine, tea tree, coriander, and other spices.

Perfume

Scent: Spicy-warm, sweet, long-lasting.
Key qualities (mind): Warming, refreshing, reviving. **Odor intensity:** Medium.

Aromatherapy use

Circulation, muscles, and joints: Arthritis, build-up of toxins in the blood, gout, rheumatism. **Digestive system:** Dyspepsia, flatulence, indigestion, liver congestion, jaundice. **Reproductive and endocrine systems:** Amenorrhea, glandular problems, increases milk flow. **Urinary system:** Cystitis. **Nervous system:** Neuralgia, sciatica.

WARNING
Avoid using during pregnancy.

Nontoxic, nonirritant, possible sensitization.

Frankincense/olibanum

BOSWELLIA CARTERI FAMILY *BURSERACEAE*

Description A small tree or shrub, with pinnate leaves, and white or pale pink flowers. It yields a natural oleo-gum resin.

Actions Anti-inflammatory, antiseptic, astringent, carminative, cicatrizant, cytophylactic, digestive, diuretic, emmenagogue, expectorant, sedative, tonic, uterine, vulnerary.

Extraction The oil is extracted by steam distillation from selected oleo-gum resin (around 3–10% oil to 60–70% resin).

Characteristics A pale yellow or greenish, mobile liquid, with a fresh terpeney top note, and a warm, rich, sweet-balsamic undertone. It blends well with sandalwood, pine, vetivert, geranium, lavender, neroli, orange, bergamot, and other citrus oils, camphor, basil, pepper, cinnamon, and other spice oils.

Perfume

Scent: Balsamic, long-lasting, woody, slightly camphoraceous, resinous, rich, sweet, incense-like, dry. This oil is a fixative, and preservative.
Key qualities: Clearing, purifying, restorative, warming, sedative, uplifting, tonic, cephalic, revitalizing. **Odor intensity:** High.

Aromatherapy use

Skin care: Blemishes, dry and mature complexions, scars, wounds, wrinkles. **Respiratory system:** Asthma, bronchitis, catarrh, colds, coughs, flu, laryngitis.
Genitourinary system: Cystitis, dysmenorrhea, leukorrhea, metrorrhagia. **Nervous system:** Anxiety, nervous tension, stress-related conditions. Frankincense has the ability to slow down, and deepen, the breath—very conducive to prayer and meditation.

SAFETY DATA
Nontoxic, nonirritant, nonsensitizing.

Linaloe

BURSERA GLABRIFOLIA FAMILY *BURSERACEAE*

Description A tall, bushy tropical shrub or tree, with a smooth bark and bearing fleshy fruit. The wood is only used for distillation purposes when the tree is 20 or 30 years old. The oil is partially a pathological product since its production is stimulated by lacerating the trunk—which apparently must be wounded on the night of the full moon for the tree to produce any oil!

Actions Anticonvulsant, anti-inflammatory, antiseptic, bactericidal, deodorant, gentle tonic.

Extraction Essential oil by steam distillation from the wood, seeds, and husk. (An essential oil is also occasionally produced from the leaves and twigs.)

Characteristics A pale yellow liquid with a sweet-woody, floral scent, similar to rosewood. It blends well with rose, sandalwood, cedarwood, rosewood, frankincense, floral, and woody fragrances.

SAFETY DATA
Nontoxic, nonirritant, nonsensitizing.

Perfume

Scent: Sweet-woody, floral.
Key qualities: Relaxing, calming, soothing, aphrodisiac, sedative, anti-infectious, anti-inflammatory, purifying, uplifiting. **Odor intensity:** Low.

Aromatherapy use

Skin care: Acne, cuts, dermatitis, wounds, etc. **Nervous system:** Nervous tension and stress-related conditions.

THE SEED OIL IS KNOWN IN INDIA AS "INDIAN LAVENDER OIL."

Ylang ylang

CANANGA ODORATA, FORMA GENUINA FAMILY *ANNONACEAE*

Description A tall tropical tree up to 68ft (20m) high, with large, tender, fragrant flowers, that can be pink, mauve, or yellow.

Actions Aphrodisiac, antidepressant, anti-infectious, antiseborrheic, antiseptic, euphoric, hypotensive, nervine, regulator, sedative (nervous), stimulant (to the circulatory system), tonic.

Extraction The oil is extracted by water or steam distillation from freshly picked flowers. Yellow flowers yield the best oil.

Characteristics A colorless to pale yellow liquid with a light, fresh balsamic, slightly spicy scent. A good oil has a creamy, rich top note. A very intriguing perfume oil in its own right, it also blends well with sandalwood, jasmine, bois de rose, vetiver, bergamot, rose, and floral and oriental bases. It is also an excellent fixative.

SAFETY DATA
Nontoxic, nonirritant, but a few cases of sensitization have been reported. Use in moderation, since the oil's heady scent can cause headaches or nausea.

Perfume

Scent: Exotic, sweet, balsamic, floral, slightly spicy, sensual, heady, oriental, rich, voluptuous.
Key qualities: Powerfully sedative, soothing, calming, regulating, euphoria-inducing, and narcotic when used in large quantities; aphrodisiac. **Odor intensity:** High.

Aromatherapy use

Skin care: Acne, hair growth, hair rinse, insect bites, irritated and oily skin, general skin care.
Circulation: High blood pressure, hyperpnoea (abnormally fast breathing), tachycardia, palpitations. **Nervous system:** Depression, frigidity, impotence, insomnia, nervous tension, and stress-related disorders.

Elemi

CANARIUM LUZONICUM FAMILY *BURSERACEAE*

Description A tropical tree up to 100ft (30m) high, which yields a resinous exudation from its trunk. This has a green, pungent odor, and although it is called a gum, it is made up almost entirely of resin and essential oil.

Actions Antiseptic, balsamic, cicatrizant, expectorant, fortifying, regulator, stimulant, stomachic, tonic.

Extraction The oil is extracted by steam distillation from the resin.

Characteristics A colorless to pale yellow liquid, with a light, fresh, balsamic-spicy, lemon-like odor. It blends well with myrrh, frankincense, rosemary, lavender, sage, cinnamon, and other spices.

Perfume

Scent: Light, fresh, soft, balsamic, slightly camphoraceous, incense-like, spicy, green, diffusive. **Key qualities:** Restorative, stimulating, drying, fortifying, warming, refreshing. **Odor intensity:** High.

Aromatherapy use

Skin care: Aging skin, infected cuts and wounds, inflammation, wrinkles (rejuvenator). **Respiratory system:** Bronchitis, catarrhal conditions, unproductive coughs. **Nervous system:** Nervous exhaustion, stress-related conditions.

SAFETY DATA
Nontoxic, nonirritant, nonsensitizing.

Caraway

CARUM CARVI FAMILY *APIACEAE (UMBELLIFERAE)*

Description A biennial herb up to 2.5ft (75cm) high with a much-branched stem, finely cut leaves and umbels of white flowers, with a thick and tapering root. The small seeds are curved with five distinct pale ridges.

Actions Antihistaminic, antimicrobial, antiseptic, aperitif, astringent, carminative, diuretic, emmenagogue, expectorant, galactagogue, larvicidal, stimulant, spasmolytic, stomachic, tonic, vermifuge.

Extraction Essential oil by steam distillation from the dried ripe seed or fruit (approx. 2–8 percent yield).

Characteristics Crude caraway oil is a pale yellowish-brown liquid with a harsh, spicy odor. The redistilled oil is colorless to pale yellow, with a strong, warm, sweet-spicy odor, like rye bread. It blends well with jasmine, cinnamon, cassia, and other spices; however, it is very overpowering.

SAFETY DATA
Nontoxic, nonsensitizing, may cause dermal irritation in concentration.

Perfume

Scent: Strong, warm, sweet-spicy.
Key qualities: Warming, stress-relieving, stimulating, antiseptic, expectorant.
Odor intensity: High.

Aromatherapy use

Respiratory system: Bronchitis, coughs, laryngitis. **Digestive system:** Dyspepsia, colic, flatulence, gastric spasm, nervous indigestion, poor appetite. See also sweet fennel and dill. **Immune system:** Colds.

Cedarwood, Atlas

CEDRUS ATLANTICA FAMILY PINACEAE

Description Pyramidal evergreen tree, with a majestic stature, up to 130ft (40m) high. The wood is hard, and strongly aromatic, due to its high essential oil content.

Actions Antiseptic, antiputrescent, antiseborrheic, astringent, diuretic, expectorant, fungicidal, mucolytic, sedative (to nervous system), stimulant (to circulatory system), tonic.

Extraction The oil is extracted by steam distillation from the wood, stumps, and sawdust.

Characteristics A yellow, orange, or deep amber, viscous oil with a warm, camphoraceous top note, and a sweet, tenacious, woody balsamic undertone. It blends well with bois de rose, bergamot, cypress, jasmine, juniper, neroli, mimosa, frankincense, clary sage, vetiver, rosemary, ylang ylang, oriental, and floral bases.

WARNING
Avoid using during pregnancy.

Perfume

Scent: Balsamic, sweet, smoky, slightly camphoraceous, dry-woody, tenacious, turpentine-like, long-lasting, and acts as a fixative. **Key qualities:** Aphrodisiac, warming, tonic, uplifting, elevating, grounding, opening, comforting, reviving. **Odor intensity:** Medium–low.

Aromatherapy use

Skin care: Acne, dandruff, dermatitis, eczema, fungal infections, greasy skin, hair loss, skin eruptions, ulcers. **Circulation, muscles, and joints:** Arthritis, rheumatism. **Respiratory system:** Bronchitis, catarrh, congestion, coughs. **Genitourinary system:** Cystitis, leukorrhea, pruritus. **Nervous system:** Nervous tension, stress-related conditions. **Other:** Insect repellent (moths).

Chamomile, Roman

CHAMAEMELUM NOBILIS/ANTHEMIS NOBILIS FAMILY ASTERACEAE (COMPOSITAE)

Description A small, stocky, perennial herb, up to 10in (25cm) high, with a much-branched, hairy stem, half spreading or creeping. It has feathery, pinnate leaves, and daisy-like, white flowers.

Actions Analgesic, antianemic, antineuralgic, antiphlogistic, antiseptic, antispasmodic, bactericide, carminative, cholagogue, cicatrizant, digestive, emmenogogue, febrifuge, hepatic, hypnotic, nerve sedative, stomachic, sudorific, tonic, vermifuge, vulnerary.

Extraction The oil is produced by steam distillation from the flower heads.

Characteristics A pale blue liquid (turning yellow on keeping), with a warm, sweet, fruity, herbaceous scent. It blends well with bergamot, clary sage, jasmine, neroli, rose, geranium, and lavender.

Perfume

Scent: Slightly fruity, sweet, fresh, warm, herbaceous, rich, grassy, fragrant, apple-like.
Key qualities: Restorative, calming, sedative, relaxing, soothing, warming, balancing, comforting, mild, slightly soporific or hypnotic in large doses. **Odor intensity:** High.

Aromatherapy use

Skin care: Acne, boils, burns, cuts, chilblains, dermatitis, earache, eczema, inflammation, insect bites, rashes, sensitive skin, wounds.
Circulation, muscles, and joints: Arthritis, inflamed joints, muscular pain, neuralgia, rheumatism, sprains. **Digestive system:** Dyspepsia, colic, indigestion, nausea.
Reproductive system: Dysmenorrhea, menopausal problems, menorrhagia. **Nervous system:** Headache, insomnia, nervous tension, migraine, and stress-related complaints.

Chamomile, German/blue

CHAMOMILLA MATRICARIA/MATRICARIA RECUTITA FAMILY ASTERACEAE

Description A strongly aromatic annual herb, up to 2ft (60cm) tall, with a hairless, erect, branching stem. It has delicate feathery leaves and daisy-like, white flowers.

Actions Analgesic, anti-allergenic, anti-inflammatory, antiphlogistic, antispasmodic, bactericide, calminative, cicatrizant, cholagogue, digestive, febrifuge, fungicidal, hepatic, nerve sedative, stimulant of leukocyte production, stomachic, sudorific, vermifuge, vulnerary.

Extraction The oil is extracted by steam distillation from the flower heads.

Characteristics An inky-blue, viscous liquid, with a strong, sweetish, warm-herbaceous odor. It blends well with geranium, lavender, patchouli, rose, benzoin, neroli, bergamot, marjoram, lemon, ylang ylang, jasmine, and clary sage.

SAFETY DATA
Generally nontoxic, nonirritant, but causes dermatitis in some individuals.

Perfume

Scent: Warm, herbaceous, sweet, slightly bitter, green. **Key qualities:** Relaxing, soothing, balancing, calming, tonic (nerve). **Odor intensity:** Very high.

Aromatherapy use

Skin care: Acne, allergies, boils, burns, cuts, chilblains, dermatitis, earache, eczema, hair care, inflammation, insect bites, rashes, sensitive skin, teething pain, toothache, wounds. **Circulation, muscles, and joints:** Arthritis, inflamed joints, muscular pain, neuralgia, rheumatism, sprains. **Digestive system:** Dyspepsia, colic, indigestion, nausea. **Reproductive system:** Dysmenorrhea, menopausal problems, menorrhagia. **Nervous system:** Headache, insomnia, nervous tension, migraine, stress-related complaints.

Camphor, white

CINNAMOMUM CAMPHORA FAMILY LAURACEAE

Description A tall, handsome, evergreen tree, up to 100ft (30m) high. It has many branches, bearing clusters of small white flowers followed by red berries.

Actions Anti-inflammatory, antiseptic, antiviral, bactericidal, counterirritant, diuretic, expectorant, stimulant, vermifuge.

Extraction Crude camphor is collected from the trees in crystalline form. The essential oil is produced by steam distillation from the wood, rootstumps, and branches.

Characteristics White camphor is the lightest (lowest boiling) fraction, and is a colorless to pale yellow liquid, with a sharp, pungent, camphoraceous odor. Brown camphor is the middle fraction, and yellow camphor, a blue-green or yellowish liquid, is the heaviest. Camphor blends with herb and spice oils.

Perfume

Scent: Clear, sharp, penetrating, camphoraceous, pungent. **Key qualities:** Anaphrodisiac, restorative, balancing, refreshing. **Odor intensity:** High.

Aromatherapy use

Skin care: Acne, inflammation, oily conditions, spots. **Circulation, muscles, and joints:** Arthritis, muscular aches and pains, rheumatism, sprains. **Respiratory system:** Bronchitis, chills, coughs. **Immune system:** Colds, fever, flu, infectious disease. **Other:** Insect prevention (flies, moths).

SAFETY DATA
White camphor, which does not contain safrole, is relatively nontoxic, nonsensitizing, and nonirritant. Avoid using it for children, however.

WARNING
Brown and yellow camphor (containing safrole) are toxic and carcinogenic. They should not be used in therapy, either internally or externally.

Ho wood

CINNAMOMUM CAMPHORA CT LINALOL FAMILY LAURACEAE

Description A tall, tropical evergreen tree, quite dense with small white flowers and black berries, which grows up to 100ft (30m) in height. This is the same tree that produces camphor, which comes from the wood of the tree.

Actions Analgesic, antifungal, anti-infectious, anti-inflammatory, antioxidant, antiseptic, antispasmodic, bactericidal, immune support, sedative, tonic. It is also believed to be a mild aphrodisiac.

Extraction Steam distilled from the leaves (ho leaf oil) and wood (ho wood oil).

Characteristics Ho wood oil is a pale yellow liquid with a soft, warm, floral, spicy-woody scent with a slightly camphor-like undertone. The leaf oil has a sweet-fresh, green-floral, and woody scent. It blends well with basil, bergamot, cedarwood, chamomile, lavender, lime, geranium, juniper, neroli, petitgrain, myrtle, sandalwood, ylang ylang, and spice oils.

SAFETY DATA
Nontoxic and nonirritant, but with possible sensitization in some individuals.

Perfume

Scent: Soft, warm, floral, spicy, woody. **Key qualities:** Calming, relaxing. **Odor intensity:** Medium.

Aromatherapy use

Skin care: Acne, cuts, dermatitis, stretch marks, scars, wounds and general skin care: dry, oily, mature and sensitive skin. **Circulation, muscles and joints:** Aches and pains caused by inflammation. **Respiratory system:** Chills, coughs and colds, flu. **Immune system:** Low libido: boosts vitality. **Nervous system:** Anxiety, depression, insomnia, nervous tension, stress. **Other:** An effective insect repellent.

Cinnamon leaf

CINNAMOMUM ZEYLANICUM FAMILY LAURACEAE

Description A tropical evergreen tree, up to 50ft (15m) high, with stiff sharp spines, smooth ovate leaves, and small white flowers and bluish-white berries.

Actions Anthelmintic, antidiarrheal, antidote, antimicrobial, antiseptic, antispasmodic, antiputrescent, astringent, digestive, emmenagogue, hemostatic, parasiticide, refrigerant, spasmolytic, stimulant, stomachic, vermifuge.

Extraction Essential oil is extracted by water or steam distillation from the leaves and twigs.

Characteristics Leaves and twigs yield a yellow to brownish oil, with a warm-spicy, somewhat harsh odor. It blends well with frankincense, ylang ylang, orange, mandarin, and benzoin.

SAFETY DATA
The leaf oil is relatively nontoxic, though possibly a skin irritant. Its major component, eugenol, causes irritation to the mucous membrane. Use in moderation. The bark oil should not be used on the skin.

Perfume

Scent: Sweet-spicy, peppery, hot, dry, tenacious, slightly woody, herbaceous, diffusive, powerful, oriental, warm. **Key qualities (mind):** Warming, reviving, tonic, strengthening, aphrodisiac, restorative, uplifting. **Odor intensity:** High.

Aromatherapy use

Skin care: Lice, scabies, tooth and gum care, warts, wasp stings. **Circulation, muscles, and joints:** Poor circulation, rheumatism. **Digestive system:** Anorexia, colitis, diarrhea, dyspepsia, intestinal infection, sluggish digestion, spasm. **Reproductive system:** Childbirth (stimulates contractions), frigidity, leukorrhea, metrorrhagia (scanty periods). **Immune system:** Chills, colds, flu, infectious diseases. **Nervous system:** Debility, nervous exhaustion, stress-related conditions.

Labdanum

CISTUS LADANIFERUS FAMILY *CISTACEAE*

Description A small sticky shrub up to 10ft (3m) high with lance-shaped leaves which are white and furry on the underside, and fragrant white flowers. Labdanum gum, a dark brown solid mass, is a natural oleoresin which is obtained by boiling the plant material in water.

Actions Antimicrobial, antiseptic, antitussive, astringent, balsamic, emmenagogue, expectorant, tonic.

Extraction The oil is extracted by steam distillation from the crude gum, the absolute, or from the leaves and twigs of the plant directly.

Characteristics A dark yellow or amber viscous liquid with a warm, sweet, dry-herbaceous, musky scent. It blends well with oakmoss, clary sage, pine, juniper, calamus, opopanax, lavender, lavandin, bergamot, cypress, vetiver, sandalwood, patchouli, olibanum, chamomile maroc, and oriental bases.

SAFETY DATA
Generally nontoxic, nonirritant, nonsensitizing. Avoid during pregnancy.

Perfume

Scent: Amber, warm, sweet, herbaceous, musky.
Key qualities: Calming, soothing, uplifting, rejuvenating. **Odor intensity:** High.

Aromatherapy use

Skin care: Mature skin, wrinkles.
Respiratory system: Coughs, bronchitis, rhinitis, etc. **Immune system:** Colds.

Lime

CITRUS AURANTIFOLIA FAMILY RUTACEA

Description A small evergreen tree, up to 15ft (4.5m) high, with stiff, sharp spines, smooth, ovate leaves, and small white flowers. The bitter fruit is a pale green color, about half the size of a lemon.

Actions Antirheumatic, antiscorbutic, antiseptic, antiviral, aperitif, bactericidal, febrifuge, restorative, tonic.

Extraction The oil is extracted by cold expression from the peel of the unripe fruit, or by steam distillation of the whole, ripe, crushed fruit.

Characteristics The peel oil is a pale yellow or olive-green liquid, with a fresh, sweet citrus-peel odor. The fruit oil is a water-white or pale yellow liquid, with a fresh, sharp, fruity-citrus scent. It blends well with neroli, citronella, lavender, rosemary, clary sage, and other citrus oils.

SAFETY DATA
Generally nontoxic, nonirritant, nonsensitizing. The expressed peel oil (not the steam-distilled whole fruit oil) is phototoxic.

Perfume

Scent: Fresh, bitter, citrus, penetrating, green, fruity, clean. **Key qualities (mind):** Refreshing, uplifting, active. **Odor intensity:** High.

Aromatherapy use

Skin care: Acne, anemia, brittle nails, boils, chilblains, corns, cuts, greasy skin, herpes, insect bites, mouth ulcers, spots, warts **Circulation, muscles, and joints:** Arthritis, cellulitis, high blood pressure, nosebleeds, obesity (congestion), poor circulation, rheumatism. **Respiratory system:** Asthma, bronchitis, catarrh. **Digestive system:** Dyspepsia. **Immune system:** Colds, flu, fever, throat infections, infections.

Petitgrain, orange

CITRUS AURANTIUM, VAR. AMARA FAMILY RUTACEAE

Description The oil of orange petitgrain is produced from the leaves and twigs of the same tree that produces both bitter orange oil and neroli oil (see below).

Actions Antiseptic, antispasmodic, deodorant, digestive, nervine, stimulant (to both digestive, and nervous systems), stomachic, tonic.

Extraction The oil is extracted by steam distillation from the leaves and twigs.

Characteristics A pale yellow to amber liquid, with a fresh-floral citrus scent, and a woody, herbaceous undertone. It blends well with rosemary, lavender, geranium, bergamot, orange, neroli, clary sage, jasmine, benzoin, palmarosa, and clove, and is a classic ingredient in eau-de-Cologne and toilet waters.

Perfume

Scent: Citrus and floral. **Key qualities:** Calming and refreshing. **Odor intensity:** Medium.

Aromatherapy use

Skin care: Acne, excessive perspiration, greasy skin and hair, toning. **Digestive system:** Dyspepsia, flatulence. **Nervous system:** Convalescence, insomnia, nervous exhaustion, stress-related conditions.

SAFETY DATA
Nontoxic, nonirritant, nonsensitizing, nonphototoxic.

Neroli

CITRUS AURANTIUM VAR. AMARA FAMILY *RUTACEAE*

Description An evergreen tree, up to 33ft (10m) high, with dark green, glossy, oval leaves, paler beneath, and with long, but not very sharp, spines. It has a smooth, grayish trunk and branches, and very fragrant white flowers. The fruits are smaller and darker than those of the sweet orange.

Actions Antiseptic, antispasmodic, bactericidal, carminative, cicatrizant, cordial, deodorant, digestive, mildly fungicidal, stimulant (nervous), tonic.

Extraction Essential oil is extracted by steam distillation from the freshly picked flowers.

Characteristics The oil is a pale yellow, mobile liquid, with a light, sweet-floral fragrance and terpeney top note. Blends well with virtually all oils, especially jasmine, lavender, rose, lemon, and other citrus oils.

SAFETY DATA
Nontoxic, nonirritant, nonsensitizing, nonphototoxic.

Perfume

Scent: Floral, soft, delicate, pervasive, sweet, warm, rich. **Key qualities:** Aphrodisiac, hypnotic, sedative, soothing, tonic, restorative, uplifting, antidepressant. **Odor intensity:** Medium–high.

Aromatherapy use

Skin care: Scars, stretch marks, thread veins, mature and sensitive skin, wrinkles, tones the complexion. **Circulatory system:** Palpitations, poor circulation. **Digestive system:** Diarrhea(chronic), colic, flatulence, spasm, nervous dyspepsia. **Nervous system:** Anxiety, depression, nervous tension, PMS, shock, stress-related conditions, and especially problems of emotional origin.

Bergamot

CITRUS BERGAMIA FAMILY RUTACEAE

Description A small tree, about 15ft (4.5m) high, with smooth, oval leaves, bearing small, round fruit that ripens from green to yellow.

Actions Analgesic, anthelmintic, antiseptic, antispasmodic, antitoxic, carminative, digestive, diuretic, deodorant, febrifuge, laxative, parasiticide, rubefacient, stimulant, stomachic, tonic, vermifuge, vulnerary, insecticide.

Extraction Bergamot oil is extracted from the peel of the nearly ripe fruit by cold expression. Bergapten-free oil is produced by a process known as fractionation.

Characteristics A light greenish-yellow liquid, with a fresh, sweet-fruity scent, and slightly spicy-balsamic undertone. It blends well with lavender, neroli, jasmine, cypress, geranium, clary sage, chamomile, juniper, coriander, and other citrus oils.

WARNING
Phototoxic: extreme care must be taken when using the oil in dermal applications, or a rectified, bergapten-free oil should be substituted.

Perfume

Scent: Fresh, citrus, sweet, light, warm, slightly spicy-floral, green. **Key qualities:** Reviving, refreshing, calming, soothing, uplifting, sedative, regulating, balancing, antidepressant. **Odor intensity:** Low.

Aromatherapy use

Skin care: Acne, boils, cold sores, eczema, insect bites, oily complexion, psoriasis, scabies, spots, varicose ulcers, wounds.

Lemon

CITRUS LIMON FAMILY RUTACEAE

Description A small evergreen tree, up to 20ft (6m) high, with serrated oval leaves, stiff thorns, and fragrant flowers. The fruit ripens from green to yellow.

Actions Antianemic, antimicrobial, antirheumatic, antisclerotic, antiseptic, antispasmodic, antitoxic, astringent, bactericide, carminative, cicatrizant, depurative, diaphoretic, diuretic, febrifuge, hemostatic, hypotensive, insecticide, rubefacient, tonic, vermifuge.

Extraction The oil is extracted by cold expression from the outer part of the fresh peel.

Characteristics A pale greeny-yellow liquid, with a light, fresh, citrus scent. It blends well with lavender, neroli, ylang ylang, rose, sandalwood, olibanum, chamomile, benzoin, fennel, geranium, eucalyptus, juniper, elemi, and other citrus oils.

WARNING
This oil is phototoxic—do not use on skin before exposing to direct sunlight or sun beds. May cause irritation or sensitization. Use in moderation.

Perfume

Scent: Fresh, clean, lemony, light, penetrating, fruity, diffusive. **Key qualities:** Refreshing, mental stimulant, cephalic, purifying, reviving, strengthening, soothing. **Odor intensity:** Medium.

Aromatherapy use

Skin care: Acne, anemia, brittle nails, boils, chilblains, corns, cuts, greasy skin, herpes, insect bites, mouth ulcers, spots, throat infections, warts. **Circulation, muscles, and joints:** Arthritis, cellulitis, high blood pressure, nosebleeds, obesity (congestion), poor circulation, varicose veins, rheumatism. **Respiratory system:** Asthma, bronchitis, catarrh. **Digestive system:** Dyspepsia. **Immune system:** Colds, flu, fever, infections.

Grapefruit

CITRUS X PARADISI FAMILY RUTACEAE

Description A cultivated tree, often over 33ft (10m) high, with glossy leaves, and familiar large yellow fruits.

Actions Antiseptic, antitoxic, astringent, bactericidal, diuretic, depurative, stimulant (to lymphatic and digestive systems), tonic.

Extraction The oil is extracted by cold expression from the fresh peel.

Characteristics A yellow or greenish, mobile liquid, with a fresh, sweet, citrus aroma. It blends well with lemon, palmarosa, bergamot, neroli, rosemary, cypress, lavender, geranium, cardamom, and other spice oils.

SAFETY DATA
Nontoxic, nonirritant, nonsensitizing, but slightly phototoxic. This oil has a short shelf life—it oxidizes quickly.

Perfume

Scent: Citrus, fruity, bitter, powerful, lemony, fresh. **Key qualities (mind):** Cleansing, stimulating, refreshing, uplifting. **Odor intensity:** Medium.

Aromatherapy use

Skin care: Acne, congested and oily skin, promotes hair growth, tones the skin and tissues. **Circulation, muscles, and joints:** Cellulitis, exercise preparation, muscle fatigue, obesity, stiffness, water retention. **Immune system:** Chills, colds, flu. **Nervous system:** Depression, headaches, nervous exhaustion, performance stress.

Mandarin

CITRUS RETICULATA FAMILY RUTACEAE

Description
A small evergreen tree, up to 20ft (6m) high, with glossy leaves, fragrant flowers, and bearing fleshy fruit. The tangerine is larger than the mandarin, and is rounder, with a more yellowy skin.

Actions
Antiseptic, antispasmodic, carminative, digestive, diuretic (mild), laxative (mild), sedative, stimulant (to digestive and lymphatic systems), tonic.

Extraction
The oil is extracted by cold expression from the outer peel.

Characteristics
Mandarin oil is a yellowy-orange, mobile liquid with a blue-violet hint. It has a sweet, almost floral, citrus scent. It blends well with other citrus oils, especially neroli, and spice oils such as nutmeg, cinnamon, and clove.

SAFETY DATA
Nontoxic, nonirritant, nonsensitizing, but slightly phototoxic.

Perfume

Scent: Fresh, warm, sweet, fruity, soft, mild. **Key qualities (mind):** Warming, comforting, soothing, uplifting. **Odor intensity:** Low.

Aromatherapy use

Skin care: Acne, congested and oily skin, scars, spots, stretch marks, toner.
Circulatory system: Fluid retention, obesity.
Digestive system: Digestive problems, dyspepsia, hiccoughs, intestinal problems.
Nervous system: Insomnia, nervous tension, restlessness.

Orange, sweet

CITRUS SINENSIS/CITRUS AURANTIUM, VAR . DULCIS FAMILY *RUTACEAE*

Description An evergreen tree, smaller than the bitter variety, less hardy, and with fewer, or no, spines. The fruit has a sweet pulp, and nonbitter membranes.

Actions Antidepressant, anti-inflammatory, antiseptic, bactericidal, carminative, choleretic, digestive, fungicidal, hypotensor, sedative (to the nervous system), stimulant, stomachic, tonic.

Extraction The oil is extracted by cold expression (by hand or machine), or by steam distillation, of the fresh, ripe, or almost ripe outer peel.

Characteristics The oil is a yellowy-orange or dark orange, mobile liquid, with a sweet, fresh-fruity scent. It blends well with lavender, neroli, lemon, clary sage, myrrh, and spice oils such as nutmeg, cinnamon, and cloves.

WARNING
Distilled orange oil should not be used on the skin before exposure to sunlight or use of a sun bed.

Perfume

Scent: Sweet, warm, sensual, radiant, fresh, citrus, fruity, tangy. **Key qualities:** Tonic (to the nervous system), refreshing, warming, uplifting, soothing, sedative, comforting. **Odor intensity:** Medium–low.

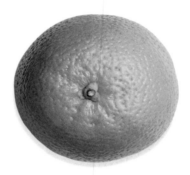

Aromatherapy use

Skin care: Dull and oily complexions (nonirritant, generally nonsensitizing, but can cause dermatitis in some individuals). **Circulatory system:** Obesity, palpitations, water retention. **Respiratory system:** Bronchitis, chills, colds, flu. **Digestive system:** Constipation, dyspepsia, spasm. **Nervous system:** Nervous tension, stress-related conditions. **Other:** Used to treat mouth ulcers.

Myrrh

COMMIPHORA MYRRH FAMILY *BURSERACEAE*

Description Shrubs or small trees up to 33ft (10m) high, with knotted branches, aromatic leaves, and small white flowers The trunk yields oleo-resin (myrrh).

Actions Anti-inflammatory, antimicrobial, antiphlogistic, antiseptic, astringent, balsamic, carminative, cicatrizant, expectorant, fungicidal, sedative, stimulant, stomachic, tonic, uterine, vulnerary.

Extraction Resinoid (and resin absolute) are obtained by solvent extraction from the crude myrrh. The oil is extracted by steam distillation.

Characteristics The essential oil is a pale yellow to amber, oily liquid with a warm, slightly spicy, medicinal odor. It blends well with frankincense, sandalwood, benzoin, cypress, juniper, mandarin, geranium, patchouli, thyme, mints, lavender, and pine.

WARNING
This oil is not to be used during pregnancy. Do not use in high concentrations.

Perfume

Scent: Bitter-spicy, rich, balsamic, resinous, long-lasting. **Key qualities:** Purifying, uplifting, revitalizing, sedative (to nervous system), restorative, soothing. **Odor intensity:** High.

Aromatherapy use

Skin care: Athlete's foot, chapped and cracked skin, eczema, ringworm, wounds, wrinkles, mature complexions (nonirritant, nonsensitizing). **Circulation, muscles, and joints:** Arthritis. **Respiratory system:** Asthma, bronchitis, catarrh, colds, coughs, sore throat, voice loss. **Digestive system:** Diarrhea, dyspepsia, flatulence, hemorrhoids, loss of appetite. **Genitourinary system:** Amenorrhea, leukorrhea, pruritus, thrush. **Other:** Treats gum infections, mouth ulcers.

Coriander/cilantro

CORIANDRUM SATIVUM FAMILY APIACEAE (UMBELLIFERAE)

Description A strongly aromatic annual herb, about 3ft (1m) high, with bright green, delicate leaves, and umbels of lace-like, white flowers, followed by a mass of green (turning brown) round seeds.

Actions Analgesic, aperitif, antioxidant, antirheumatic, antispasmodic, bactericidal, depurative, digestive, carminative, cytotoxic, fungicidal, larvicidal, lipolytic activity, stimulant, stomachic.

Extraction The oil is extracted by steam distillation from the crushed ripe seeds.

Characteristics
A colorless to pale yellow liquid, with a sweet, woody-spicy, slightly musky fragrance. It blends well with clary sage, bergamot, jasmine, frankincense, neroli, petitgrain, citronella, sandalwood, cypress, pine, ginger, cinnamon, and other spice oils.

Perfume

Scent: Fresh, herbal, sweet-spicy, bitter, woody, slightly musky, diffusive. **Key qualities:** Aphrodisiac, stimulating, soporific (in excess), refreshing, warming, comforting, revitalizing, strengthening, purifying, soothing, active. **Odor intensity:** Medium.

Aromatherapy use

Circulation, muscles, and joints: Accumulation of fluids or toxins, arthritis, gout, muscular aches and pains, poor circulation, rheumatism, stiffness. **Digestive system:** Anorexia, colic, diarrhea, dyspepsia, flatulence, nausea, piles, spasm. **Immune system:** Colds, flu, infections (general), measles. **Nervous system:** Debility, migraine, neuralgia, nervous exhaustion.

SAFETY DATA
Generally nontoxic, nonirritant, nonsensitizing, but stupefying in large doses. Use in moderation.

Cumin

CUMINUM CYMINUM FAMILY APIACEAE (UMBELLIFERAE)

Description A small, delicate, annual herb about 20in (50cm) high with a slender stem, dark green feathery leaves and small pink or white flowers followed by small oblong seeds.

Actions Antioxidant, antiseptic, antispasmodic, antitoxic, aphrodisiac, bactericidal, carminative, depurative, digestive, diuretic, emmenagogue, larvicidal, nervine, stimulant, tonic.

Extraction Essential oil by steam distillation from the ripe seeds.

Characteristics A pale yellow or greenish liquid with a warm, soft, spicy-musky scent. It blends well with lavender, lavandin, rosemary, galbanum, rosewood, cardamom, and oriental-type fragrances.

SAFETY DATA
Nontoxic, nonirritant, and nonsensitizing; however the oil is phototoxic, so do not expose treated skin to direct sunlight. Avoid during pregnancy.

Perfume

Scent: Warm, soft, spicy-musky.
Key qualities: Antiseptic, tonic, relaxing, soothing, cleansing.
Odor intensity: Medium.

Aromatherapy use

Circulation, muscles, and joints: Accumulation of fluids or toxins, poor circulation.
Digestive system: Colic, dyspepsia, flatulence, indigestion, spasm.
Nervous system: Debility, headaches, migraine, nervous exhaustion.
Other: Used in veterinary medicine in digestive preparations. As a fragrance component in cosmetics and perfumes, and a flavor ingredient in many foods and drinks, especially meat products and condiments.

Cypress

CUPRESSUS SEMPERVIRENS FAMILY *CUPRESSACEAE*

Description A tall evergreen tree, with slender branches and a statuesque, conical shape. It bears small flowers, and round, brownish-gray cones or nuts.

Actions Antirheumatic, antiseptic, antispasmodic, antisudorific, astringent, deodorant, diuretic, hepatic, styptic, tonic, vasoconstrictive.

Extraction The oil is extracted by steam distillation from the needles and twigs. An oil from the cones is available occasionally.

Characteristics A pale yellow to greenish-olive, mobile liquid, with a smoky, sweet-balsamic, tenacious odor. It blends well with cedarwood, pine, lavender, mandarin, clary sage, lemon, cardamom, juniper, benzoin, bergamot, orange, marjoram, and sandalwood.

Perfume

Scent: Smoky, sweet, balsamic, tenacious, woody, dry, slightly nutty, austere, spicy. **Key qualities:** Refreshing, purifying, relaxing, warming, reviving, restorative, comforting, protective, soothing. **Odor intensity:** Medium–low.

Aromatherapy use

Skin care: Oily, and over-hydrated skin, perspiration, wounds, bruises. **Circulation, muscles, and joints:** Hemorrhoids, varicose veins, cellulitis, muscular cramp, edema, poor circulation, rheumatism. **Respiratory system:** Asthma, bronchitis, spasmodic coughing. **Reproductive system:** Dysmenorrhea, menopausal problems, menorrhagia. **Nervous system:** Nervous tension, stress-related conditions. **Other:** Treats pyorrhea (inflamed/bleeding gums); insect repellent.

SAFETY DATA
Nontoxic, nonirritant, nonsensitizing.

Turmeric

CURCUMA LONGA FAMILY *ZINGIBERACEAE*

Description
A perennial tropical herb up to 3ft (1m) high, with a thick rhizome root, deep orange inside, lanceolate root leaves tapering at each end, and dull yellow flowers.

Actions
Analgesic, anti-arthritic, anti- inflammatory, antioxidant, bactericidal, cholagogue, digestive, diuretic, hypotensive, insecticidal, laxative, rubefacient, stimulant.

Extraction
Essential oil by steam distillation from the "cured" rhizome—boiled, cleaned, and sun-dried. (An oleoresin, absolute, and concrete are also produced by solvent extraction.)

Characteristics
A yellowy-orange liquid with a faint blue fluorescence and a fresh spicy-woody odor. It blends well with cananga, labdanum, elecampane, ginger, orris, cassie, clary sage, and mimosa.

SAFETY DATA
The ketone "tumerone" is moderately toxic and irritant in high concentration. Possible sensitization problems. Use with moderation and care.

Perfume
Scent: Fresh, spicy, woody, warm. **Key qualities:** Anti-inflammatory, soothing, protective, detoxifying, antioxidant, immune-boosting, soothing. **Odor intensity:** Medium.

Aromatherapy use
Circulation, muscles, and joints: Arthritis, muscular aches and pains, rheumatism.
Digestive system: Anorexia, sluggish digestion, liver congestion.

Lemongrass, West Indian

CYMBOPOGON CITRATUS FAMILY *POACEAE (GRAMINACEAE)*

Description A fast-growing, tall, aromatic, perennial grass, up to 5ft (1.5m) high, producing a network of roots and rootlets that rapidly exhaust the soil.

Actions Analgesic, antidepressant, antimicrobial, antioxidant, antipyretic, antiseptic, astringent, bactericidal, carminative, deodorant, febrifuge, fungicidal, galactagogue, insecticide, nervine, sedative (nervous system), tonic.

Extraction The oil is extracted by steam distillation from the fresh, and partially dried, leaves (grass), finely chopped.

Characteristics A yellow, amber, or reddish-brown liquid, with a fresh, grassy-citrus scent, and an earthy undertone. Blends well with geranium, bergamot, and the other citrus oils.

SAFETY DATA
Nontoxic, but possible dermal irritation and/or sensitization in some individuals—use with care.

Perfume

Scent: Citrus, clean, green, hay-like, slightly bitter, lemony, pungent. **Key qualities (mind):** Refreshing, active, stimulating, soothing. **Odor intensity:** High.

Aromatherapy use

Skin care: Acne, athlete's foot, excessive perspiration, open pores, pediculosis, scabies, tissue toner. **Circulation, muscles, and joints:** Muscular pain, poor circulation and muscle tone, slack tissue. **Digestive system:** Colitis, indigestion, gastroenteritis. **Immune system:** Fevers, infectious diseases. **Nervous system:** Headaches, nervous exhaustion, stress-related conditions. **Other:** Insect repellent (fleas, lice, ticks).

Palmarosa

CYMBOPOGON MARTINII VAR . MARTINII FAMILY GRAMINACEAE

Description A wild herbaceous plant, with long, slender stems and terminal flowering tops; the grassy leaves are very fragrant.

Actions Antiseptic, bactericidal, cicatrizant, digestive, febrifuge, hydrating, stimulant (to the digestive and circulatory systems), tonic.

Extraction The oil is extracted by steam or water distillation of the fresh or dried grass.

Characteristics A pale yellow or olive liquid, with a sweet, floral, rosy, geranium-like scent. It blends well with ylang ylang, rose geranium, bois de rose, sandalwood, cypress, cedarwood, and floral oils.

Perfume

Scent: Rosy, sweet, fresh, warm, slightly-green, floral. **Key qualities (mind):** Refreshing, balancing, comforting. **Odor intensity:** Medium–high.

Aromatherapy use

Skin care: Acne, dermatitis and minor skin infections, scars, sores, wrinkles: valuable for all types of treatment for the face, hands, feet, neck, and lips (moisturizes the skin, stimulates cellular regeneration, regulates sebum production). **Digestive system:** Anorexia, digestive atonia, intestinal infections. **Nervous system:** Nervous exhaustion, stress-related conditions.

SAFETY DATA
Nontoxic, nonirritant, nonsensitizing.

Citronella

CYMBOPOGON NARDUS FAMILY *POACEAE (GRAMINACEAE)*

Description A tall, cultivated, aromatic, perennial grass, derived from the wild managrass found in Sri Lanka.

Actions Antiseptic, antispasmodic, bactericidal, deodorant, diuretic, emmenagogue, febrifuge, fungicidal, insecticide, stomachic, tonic, vermifuge.

Extraction The oil is extracted by steam distillation of the fresh, part-dried, or dried grass. Java citronella yields twice as much oil as the Sri Lanka type.

Characteristics
A yellowy-brown, mobile liquid, with a fresh, powerful, lemony scent. The Java oil is colorless to pale yellow, with a fresh, woody-sweet fragrance; it is considered of superior quality in perfumery work. It blends well with geranium, lemon, bergamot, orange, cedarwood, and pine.

WARNING
Avoid using this oil during pregnancy.

Nontoxic, generally nonirritant, but may cause dermatitis in some individuals.

Perfume

Scent: Fresh, lemony, slightly herbaceous, green, powerful. **Key qualities (mind):** Refreshing, active, penetrating. **Odor intensity:** High.

Aromatherapy use

Skin care: Excessive perspiration, oily skin. **Immune system:** Colds, flu, minor infections. **Nervous system:** Fatigue, headaches, migraine, neuralgia. **Other:** Insect repellent. Mixed with Virginia cedarwood oil, it is a popular remedy against mosquitoes.

Carrot seed

DAUCUS CAROTA FAMILY APIACEAE (UMBELLIFERAE)

Description Annual or biennial herb, with a small, inedible, tough whitish root. It has a much-branched stem, up to 5ft (1.5m) high, with hairy leaves, and umbels of white, lacy flowers.

Actions Anthelmintic, antiseptic, carminative, depurative, diuretic, emmenagogue, hepatic, stimulant, tonic, vasodilatory, smooth muscle relaxant.

Extraction The oil is extracted by steam distillation from the dried seeds.

Characteristics A yellow or amber liquid, with a warm, dry, woody-earthy odor. It blends well with cedarwood, geranium, citrus, and with the spice oils.

SAFETY DATA
Nontoxic, nonirritant, nonsensitizing.

Perfume

Scent: Woody-earthy, herbaceous, slightly spicy, strong, warm. **Key qualities (mind):** Clearing, comforting, reviving. **Odor intensity:** Medium–high.

Aromatherapy use

Skin care: Dermatitis, eczema, oily skin, psoriasis, rashes, wrinkles, mature complexions—revitalizing and toning.
Circulation, muscles, and joints: Anemia, accumulation of toxins, arthritis, gout, edema, rheumatism. **Digestive system:** Anorexia, colic, indigestion, liver congestion.
Reproductive and endocrine system: Amenorrhea, dysmenorrhea, glandular problems, PMS.

Cardamom

ELETTARIA CARDAMOMUM FAMILY *ZINGIBERACEAE*

Description
A reed-like perennial herb, up to 13ft (4m) high, with long, silky, blade-shaped leaves. Its long, sheathing stems bear small, yellowish flowers with purple tips, which are followed by oblong red-brown seeds.

Actions
Antiseptic, antispasmodic, carminative, digestive, diuretic, orexigenic, sialagogue, stimulant, stomachic, tonic.

Extraction
The oil is extracted by steam distillation from the dried ripe seeds.

Characteristics
A colorless to pale yellow liquid, with a sweet-spicy, warming fragrance, and a woody-balsamic undertone. It blends well with rose, frankincense, orange, bergamot, cinnamon, cloves, ylang ylang, cedarwood, neroli, and with oriental bases in general.

SAFETY DATA
Nontoxic, nonirritant, nonsensitizing.

Perfume

Scent: Pleasing, camphoraceous, warm, sweet, spicy, powerful, soft, rich, oriental. Has a high odor intensity—easily overshadows other smells. **Key qualities (mind):** Cephalic, aphrodisiac, warming, comforting, refreshing, uplifting, penetrating, soothing. **Odor intensity:** Very high.

Aromatherapy use

Digestive system: Anorexia, colic, cramp, dyspepsia, flatulence, griping pains, halitosis (bad breath), heartburn, indigestion, vomiting. **Nervous system:** Mental fatigue, nervous strain.

Lemon eucalyptus

EUCALYPTUS CITRIODORA FAMILY *MYRTACEAE*

Description An attractive, tall evergreen tree, with a smooth, dimpled bark, blotched in gray, cream, and pink, cultivated as an ornamental plant. The trunk grows fast, straight, and to considerable height, and is used for timber. The young leaves are oval, while the mature leaves are narrow and tapering.

Actions Antiseptic, antiviral, bactericidal, deodorant, expectorant, fungicidal, insecticide.

Extraction The oil is extracted by steam distillation from the leaves and twigs.

Characteristics A colorless or pale yellow, mobile liquid, with a strong, fresh, citronella-like odor, and sweet, balsamic undertone. It blends well with both citrus and floral oils.

SAFETY DATA
Nontoxic, nonirritant, but there is possible sensitization in some individuals.

Perfume

Scent: Lemony, fresh, clean, penetrating. **Key qualities (mind):** Invigorating, active, stimulating. **Odor intensity:** High.

Aromatherapy use

Skin care: Athlete's foot and other fungal infections (such as candida), cuts, dandruff, herpes, infectious skin conditions (such as chicken pox), scabs, sores, wounds. **Respiratory system:** Asthma, laryngitis, sore throat. **Immune system:** Colds, fevers, infectious diseases. **Other:** Insect repellent.

Eucalyptus blue gum

EUCALYPTUS GLOBULUS VAR. GLOBULUS FAMILY MYRTACEAE

Description An evergreen tree, up to 50ft (15m) high. Mature trees have long, narrow, yellowish leaves, creamy-white flowers, and a smooth, pale gray bark often covered in a white powder.

Actions Analgesic, antineuralgic, antiseptic, antiviral, cicatrizant, decongestant, deodorant, depurative, diuretic, expectorant, febrifuge, hypoglycemic, parasiticide, prophylactic, rubefacient, stimulant, vermifuge, vulnerary, insecticide.

Extraction The oil is extracted by steam distillation from the leaves and young twigs.

Characteristics A colorless, mobile liquid that yellows on aging, with a somewhat harsh, camphoraceous odor, and woody-sweet undertone. It blends well with thyme, rosemary, lavender, marjoram, pine, cedarwood, and lemon.

Perfume

Scent: Woody-camphoraceous, penetrating, fresh, slightly sweet. **Key qualities:** Stimulating, refreshing, clearing, purifying, balsamic, regulating. **Odor intensity:** High.

Aromatherapy use

Skin care: Burns, blisters, cuts, herpes, insect bites, lice, skin infections, wounds. **Circulation, muscles, and joints:** Muscular aches and pains, poor circulation, rheumatoid arthritis, sprains. **Respiratory system:** Asthma, bronchitis, catarrh, coughs, sinusitis, throat infections. **Immune system:** Chicken pox, colds, epidemics, flu, measles. **Genitourinary system:** Cystitis, leukorrhea. **Nervous system:** Debility, headaches, neuralgia. **Other:** Insect repellent.

WARNING
Apply in dilution only: in concentration, eucalyptus oil can irritate the skin. The oil should not be used on young children. When taken internally eucalyptus oil is toxic.

Oakmoss

EVERNIA PRUNASTRI FAMILY *USNEACEAE*

Description A light green lichen found growing primarily on oak trees, but sometimes other species.

Actions Antiseptic, demulcent, expectorant, fixative.

Extraction A range of products is produced: a concrete and an absolute by solvent extraction from the lichen that has often been soaked in lukewarm water prior to extraction; an absolute oil by vacuum distillation of the concrete; resins and resinoids by alcohol extraction of the raw material. Most important of these products is the absolute.

Characteristics The absolute is a dark green or brown, very viscous liquid with an extremely tenacious, earthy-mossy odor and a leather-like undertone. The absolute oil is a pale yellow or olive viscous liquid with a dry-earthy, bark-like odor, quite true to nature. The concrete, resin, and resinoids are a very dark-colored semi-solid or solid mass with a heavy, rich-earthy, extremely tenacious odor. They have a high fixative value and blend with virtually all other oils: they are extensively used in perfumery to lend body and rich natural undertones to all perfume types.

Perfume

Scent: Green, woody, slightly fruity, earthy.
Key qualities: Soothing, restorative, antiseptic, anti-aging, refreshing, reinvigorating. **Odor intensity:** High.

Aromatherapy use

As a fixative.

ALSO CALLED OAK LUNGS, LUNG MOSS, LUNGWORT OR "LUNGS OF OAK" BY SOME NORTH AMERICAN INDIGENOUS PEOPLES WHO USE IT FOR RESPIRATORY COMPLAINTS.

SAFETY DATA
Extensively compounded or "bouqueted" by cutting or adulteration with other lichen or synthetic perfume materials.

Galbanum

FERULA GUMBOSA FAMILY APIACEAE (UMBELLIFERAE)

Description A large perennial herb, with a smooth stem, shiny leaflets, and small flowers. It contains resin ducts that exude a milky juice, an oleoresin.

Actions Analgesic, anti-inflammatory, antimicrobial, antiseptic, antispasmodic, aphrodisiac, balsamic, carminative, cicatrizant, digestive, diuretic, emmenagogue, expectorant, hypotensive, restorative, tonic.

Extraction The oil is extracted by water or steam distillation from the oleoresin (gum). Only the Levant or soft type is used for oil production.

Characteristics A colorless, pale yellow, or olive liquid with a fresh, green top note, and woody-dry balsamic undertone. It blends well with lavender, geranium, pine, frankincense, and oriental bases.

Perfume

Scent: Sharp, green-woody, penetrating, turpentine-like, balsamic, musky, earthy, herbaceous, spicy, bitter, clean, powerful.
Key qualities: Uplifting, clearing, purifying, soothing. **Odor intensity:** Very high.

Aromatherapy use

Skin care: Abscesses, acne, boils, cuts, scar tissue, inflammation, mature skin, wrinkles, wounds—tones, softens, and preserves the skin. **Circulation, muscles, and joints:** Poor circulation, muscular aches and pains, rheumatism. **Respiratory system:** Asthma, bronchitis, catarrh, chronic coughs. **Digestive system:** Cramp, flatulence, indigestion. **Nervous system:** Nervous tension, stress-related complaints. **Other:** Insect repellent.

SAFETY DATA
Nontoxic, nonirritant, nonsensitizing.

Fennel, sweet

FOENICULUM VULGARE FAMILY APIACEAE (UMBELLIFERAE)

Description Biennial or perennial herb, up to 6ft 6in (2m) high, with feathery leaves, and golden yellow flowers. There are two varieties of fennel: bitter and sweet. Bitter fennel is not recommended for aromatherapy use.

Actions Aperitif, anti-inflammatory, antimicrobial, antiseptic, antispasmodic, carminative, depurative, diuretic, emmenagogue, expectorant, galactagogue, laxative, stimulant (to circulation), splenetic, stomachic, tonic, vermifuge.

Extraction The oil is extracted by steam distillation from the crushed seeds.

Characteristics Sweet fennel is a colorless to pale yellow liquid, with a very sweet, anise-like, slightly earthy-peppery scent. It blends well with rose geranium, lavender, rose, and sandalwood.

WARNING
Use in moderation—this oil should not be used by people who suffer from epilepsy, children under six, or pregnant women.

Perfume

Scent: Sweet, anise-like, earthy, peppery. The name derives from the Latin *foenum*, meaning hay, descriptive of the plant's musty fragrance. **Key qualities:** Stimulating, balancing, restorative, revitalizing, purifying, cleansing.
Odor intensity: High.

Aromatherapy use

Skin care: Bruises; dull, oily, mature complexions. **Circulation, muscles, and joints:** Cellulitis, obesity, edema, rheumatism. **Respiratory system:** Asthma, bronchitis. **Digestive system:** Anorexia, colic, constipation, dyspepsia, flatulence, hiccoughs, nausea. **Reproductive system:** Amenorrhea, insufficient milk in nursing mothers, menopausal problems. **Other:** Treats pyorrhea.

Immortelle

HELICHRYSUM ANGUSTIFOLIUM FAMILY ASTERACEAE (COMPOSITAE)

Description A strongly aromatic herb, up to 2ft (60cm) high with a much-branched stem, woody at the base. The brightly colored, daisy-like flowers become dry as the plant matures, yet retain their color.

Actions Anti-allergenic, anti-inflammatory, antimicrobial, antitussive, antiseptic, astringent, cholagogue, cicatrisant, diuretic, expectorant, fungicidal, hepatic, nervine.

Extraction The oil is extracted by steam distillation from the fresh flowers and flowering tops.

Characteristics A pale yellow to red oily liquid with a powerful, rich honey-like scent with a delicate tea-like undertone. It blends well with chamomile, boronia, labdanum, lavender, mimosa, oakmoss, geranium, clary sage, rose, Peru balsam, clove, and citrus oils.

Perfume

Scent: Rich, honey, tea-like.
Key qualities: Healing, nourishing, beautifying, balancing, relaxing, uplifting.
Odor intensity: High.

Aromatherapy use

Skin care: Abscess, acne, allergic conditions, boils, burns, cuts, dermatitis, eczema, inflammation, spots, wounds etc. **Circulation, muscles, and joints:** Muscular aches and pains, rheumatism, sprains, strained muscles. **Respiratory system:** Asthma, bronchitis, chronic coughs, whooping cough. **Digestive system:** Liver congestion, spleen congestion. **Immune system:** Bacterial infections, colds, flu, fever. **Nervous system:** Depression, debility, lethargy, nervous exhaustion, neuralgia, stress-related conditions.

SAFETY DATA
Nontoxic, nonirritant, nonsensitizing.

Hyssop

HYSSOPUS OFFICINALIS FAMILY LAMIACEAE (LABIATAE)

Description An attractive perennial, almost evergreen, sub-shrub, up to 2ft (60cm) high, with a woody stem, small, lance-shaped leaves, and purplish-blue flowers.

Actions Astringent, antiseptic, antispasmodic, antiviral, bactericide, carminative, cephalic, cicatrizant, digestive, diuretic, emmenagogue, expectorant, febrifuge, hypertensive, nervine, sedative, sudorific, tonic (to heart and circulation), vermifuge, vulnerary.

Extraction The oil is extracted by steam distillation from the leaves and flowering tops.

Characteristics
A colorless to pale yellowy-green liquid, with a sweet, camphoraceous top note, and warm, spicy-herbaceous undertone. It blends well with lavender, rosemary, myrtle, bay, sage, clary sage, geranium, and the citrus oils.

WARNING
This oil should be used only in moderation, and should be avoided in pregnancy, and by people suffering from epilepsy. Do not use on children.

Perfume

Scent: Sweet, warm, herbaceous, slightly camphoraceous. **Key qualities:** Tonic, cephalic, nervine, warming, calming, purifying, cleansing, aphrodisiac, mental stimulant, balancing. **Odor intensity:** High.

Aromatherapy use

Skin care: Bruises, cuts, dermatitis, eczema, inflammation, wounds (nonirritant, nonsensitizing). **Circulatory system:** Low or high blood pressure, rheumatism. **Respiratory system:** Asthma, bronchitis, catarrh, cough, flu, sore throat, tonsillitis, whooping cough. **Digestive system:** Colic, indigestion. **Reproductive system:** Amenorrhea, leukorrhea. **Nervous system:** Anxiety, fatigue, nervous tension, stress-related conditions.

Elecampane

INULA HELENIUM FAMILY ASTERACEAE (COMPOSITAE)

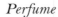

Description A handsome perennial herb up to 5ft (1.5m) high, with a stout stem covered in soft hairs. It has oval pointed leaves, which are velvety underneath, large, yellow, daisy-like flowers, and large, fleshy rhizome roots.

Actions Alterative, anthelmintic, anti-inflammatory, antiseptic, antispasmodic, antitussive, astringent, bactericidal, diaphoretic, diuretic, expectorant, fungicidal, hyperglycaemic, hypotensive, stomachic, tonic.

Extraction Essential oil by steam distillation from the dried roots and rhizomes.

Characteristics A semi-solid or viscous dark yellow or brownish liquid with a dry, soft, woody, honey-like odor, often containing crystals. It blends well with cananga, cinnamon, labdanum, lavender, mimosa, frankincense, orris, tuberose, violet, cedarwood, patchouli, sandalwood, cypress, bergamot, and oriental fragrances.

Perfume

Scent: Soft, woody, honey.
Key qualities: Antiseptic, astringent, stimulating. **Odor intensity:** Medium.

Aromatherapy use

Skin care: Wrinkles, age spots, acne, dull complexions. **Circulation, muscles, and joints:** Accumulation of fluids or toxins, poor circulation. **Digestive system:** Stimulates the metabolism, and has diuretic properties.

SAFETY DATA
Nontoxic, nonirritant; however it is a severe dermal sensitizer. In clinical tests it caused extremely severe allergic reactions in 23 out of 25 volunteers. On the basis of these results it is recommended that the oil should not be used on the skin at all.

ELECAMPANE ROOT IS ONE OF THE RICHEST NATURAL SOURCES OF THE PROBIOTIC INULIN.

Jasmine

JASMINUM OFFICINALE FAMILY OLEACEAE

Description An evergreen shrub or vine up to 33ft (10m) high, with delicate, bright green leaves, and star-shaped, very fragrant white flowers.

Actions Analgesic (mild), anti-inflammatory, antiseptic, antispasmodic, carminative, cicatrizant, expectorant, galactagogue, parturient, sedative, tonic (uterine).

Extraction A concrete is produced from the flowers by solvent extraction. The absolute is obtained from the concrete by separation with alcohol. A second essential oil is produced by steam distillation of the absolute.

Characteristics
The absolute is a dark orange-brown, viscous liquid, with an intensely rich, warm, floral scent, and a tea-like undertone. It blends well with rose, sandalwood, clary sage, and all citrus oils.

Perfume

Scent: Rich, warm, floral, sweet, tealike, exquisite, exotic, long-lasting. **Key qualities:** Intoxicating, uplifting, antidepressant, euphoric, aphrodisiac, tonic, balancing, warming. **Odor intensity:** High.

Aromatherapy use

Skin care: Dry, greasy, irritated, sensitive skin. **Circulation, muscles, and joints:** Muscular spasm, sprains. **Respiratory system:** Catarrh, coughs, hoarseness, laryngitis. **Reproductive system:** Dysmenorrhea, frigidity, labor pains, uterine disorders. **Nervous system:** Depression, nervous exhaustion, stress-related conditions.

SAFETY DATA
Nontoxic, nonirritant, generally nonsensitizing, although an allergic reaction has been known to occur in some individuals.

Juniper

JUNIPERUS COMMUNIS FAMILY *CUPRESSACEAE*

Description An evergreen shrub or tree, up to 20ft (6m) high, with bluish-green, narrow, stiff needles. It has small flowers, and little round, black berries.

Actions Antirheumatic, antiseptic, antispasmodic, antitoxic, aphrodisiac, astringent, carminative, cicatrizant, depurative, diuretic, emmenagogue, nervine, parasiticide, rubefacient, sedative, stomachic, sudorific, tonic, vulnerary.

Extraction The oil is extracted by steam distillation from the berries, the needles or the wood.

Characteristics Juniper berry oil is a water-white or pale yellow, mobile liquid, with a sweet, fresh, woody-balsamic odor. It blends well with vetiver, sandalwood, cedarwood, galbanum, elemi, cypress, clary sage, pine, lavender, rosemary, benzoin, geranium, and citrus oils.

Perfume

Scent: Sweet, fresh, woody, balsamic, turpentine-like, peppery, smoky. **Key qualities:** Aphrodisiac, purifying, clearing, depurative, tonic (nerve), reviving, protective, restorative. **Odor intensity:** Medium.

Aromatherapy use

Skin care: Acne, dermatitis, eczema, hair loss, hemorrhoids, wounds, tonic for oily complexions (nonsensitizing, but may be slightly irritating). **Circulation, muscles, and joints:** Accumulation of toxins, arteriosclerosis, cellulite, gout, obesity, rheumatism. **Immune system:** Colds, flu, infections. **Genitourinary system:** Amenorrhea, cystitis, dysmenorrhea, leukorrhea. **Nervous system:** Anxiety, nervous tension, stress-related conditions.

> **WARNING**
> This oil stimulates the uterine muscle (an abortifacient) and must not be used during pregnancy. It should not be used by those with kidney disease, as it is nephrotoxic. It is not suitable for young children. Use in moderation.

Cedarwood, Virginian

JUNIPERUS VIRGINIANA FAMILY *CUPRESSACEAE*

Description A slow-growing, evergreen coniferous tree, up to 180ft (33m) high, with a narrow, dense, and pyramidal crown, a reddish heartwood, and brown cones.

Actions Abortifacient, antiseborrheic, antiseptic (pulmonary, genitourinary), antispasmodic, astringent, balsamic, diuretic, emmenagogue, expectorant, insecticide, sedative (to the nervous system), stimulant (to the circulation).

Extraction The oil is extracted by steam distillation from lumber waste, sawdust, and shavings.

Characteristics A pale yellow, or orange, oily liquid, with a mild, sweet-balsamic, pencilwood scent. It blends well with sandalwood, rose, juniper, cypress, vetiver, patchouli, and benzoin.

WARNING
Use this oil in dilution only, with care, and in moderation. The oil is a powerful abortifacient—avoid during pregnancy.

Perfume

Scent: Sweet-balsamic, pencilwood, tenacious, tobacco, clean, sporty.
Key qualities (mind): Restorative, uplifting, warming. **Odor intensity:** Medium–low.

Aromatherapy use

Skin care: Acne, dandruff, eczema, greasy hair, oily skin, psoriasis (can cause acute local irritation in some individuals). **Circulation, muscles, and joints:** Arthritis, rheumatism. **Respiratory system:** Bronchitis, catarrh, congestion, coughs, sinusitis. **Genitourinary system:** Cystitis, leukorrhea. **Nervous system:** Nervous tension, stress-related disorders. **Other:** Insect repellent.

Laurel

LAURUS NOBILIS FAMILY *LAURACEAE*

Description An evergreen tree up to 65ft (20m) high with dark green, glossy leaves and black berries; often cultivated as an ornamental shrub.

Actions Antirheumatic, antiseptic, bactericidal, diaphoretic, digestive, diuretic, emmenagogue, fungicidal, hypotensive, sedative, stomachic.

Extraction Essential oil by steam distillation from the dried leaf and branchlets. (An oil from the berries is produced in small quantities.)

Characteristics A greenish-yellow liquid with a powerful, spicy-medicinal odor. It blends well with pine, cypress, juniper, clary sage, rosemary, olibanum, labdanum, lavender, citrus, and spice oils.

SAFETY DATA
Relatively nontoxic and nonirritant; can cause dermatitis in some individuals. Use in moderation due to possible narcotic properties. Should not be used during pregnancy.

Perfume

Scent: Spicy, medicinal, sweet, floral.
Key qualities: Uplifting, confidence-inspiring, energizing, analgesic, antiseptic.
Odor intensity: Medium.

Aromatherapy use

Digestive system: Dyspepsia, flatulence, loss of appetite. **Genitourinary system:** Scanty periods. **Immune system:** Colds, flu, tonsillitis, and viral infections.

Lavender, true

LAVANDULA ANGUSTIFOLIA/L. OFFICINALIS FAMILY *LAMIACEA (LABIATAE)*

Description An evergreen, woody shrub, up to 3ft (1m) tall, with gray-green, narrow, linear leaves, and blue flower spikes.

Actions Analgesic, anticonvulsive, antimicrobial, antirheumatic, antiseptic, antispasmodic, antitoxic, carminative, cholagogue, choleretic, cytophylactic, deodorant, diuretic, emmenagogue, hypotensor, insecticide, nervine, parasiticide, rubefacient, sedative, stimulant, sudorific, tonic, vermifuge, vulnerary.

Extraction The oil is extracted from the fresh flowering tops by steam distillation.

Characteristics The oil is colorless to pale yellow, with a sweet, floral-herbaceous scent, and balsamic-woody undertone. Blends well with most oils, especially citrus, florals, cedarwood, clove, clary sage, pine, geranium, vetivert, and patchouli.

SAFETY DATA
Nontoxic, nonirritant, nonsensitizing.

Perfume

Scent: Light, floral, classic, soft, mellow. **Key qualities:** Soothing, sedative, antidepressant, calming, relaxing, balancing, restorative, cephalic, appeasing, cleansing, purifying. **Odor intensity:** Medium.

Aromatherapy use

Skin care: Abscess, acne, allergies, athlete's foot, boils, bruises, burns, dermititis, eczema, inflammation, insect bites and stings, lice, psoriasis, ringworm, scabies, spots, sunburn, wounds. **Circulation, muscles, and joints:** Lumbago, rheumatism, sprains. **Respiratory system:** Asthma, bronchitis, catarrh, flu, halitosis, throat infections, whooping cough. **Digestive system:** Colic, dyspepsia, flatulence, nausea. **Genitourinary system:** Cystitis, dysmenorrhea, leukorrhea. **Nervous system:** Depression, headache, hypertension, insomnia, migraine, nervous tension, stress.

Lavandin

LAVANDULA X INTERMEDIA FAMILY *LAMIACEAE (LABIATAE)*

Description A hybrid plant developed by crossing true lavender (*L. angustifolia*) with spike lavender or aspic (*L. latifolia*). Due to its hybrid nature, lavandin has a variety of forms: in general, it is a larger plant than true lavender, with woody stems. Its flowers may be blue like true lavender, or grayish like aspic.

Actions Analgesic, anticonvulsive, antimicrobial, antirheumatic, antiseptic, antispasmodic, antitoxic, carminative, cholagogue, choleretic, cytophylactic, deodorant, diuretic, emmenagogue, hypotensor, insecticide, nervine, parasiticide, rubefacient, sedative, stimulant, sudorific, tonic, vermifuge, vulnerary.

Extraction Essential oil by steam distillation from the fresh flowering tops; it has a higher yield of oil than either true lavender or aspic.

Characteristics A colorless or pale yellow liquid with a fresh camphoraceous topnote (which should not be too strong in a good-quality oil), and a woody herbaceous undertone. It blends well with clove, bay leaf, cinnamon, citronella, cypress, pine, clary sage, geranium, thyme, patchouli, rosemary, and citrus oils, especially bergamot and lime.

Perfume

Scent: Camphor, woody, herbaceous.
Key qualities: Rejuvenating, soothing, antidepressant, calming, relaxing, restorative, cephalic, appeasing, cleansing, purifying.
Odor intensity: Medium.

Aromatherapy use

Lavandin has similar uses to true lavender, but it is more penetrating and rubefacient with a sharper scent—good for respiratory, circulatory, or muscular conditions.

SAFETY DATA
Nontoxic, nonirritant, nonsensitizing.

Manuka

LEPTOSPERMUM SCOPARIUM FAMILY MYRTACEAE

Description The Manuka plant is an elegant, bushy evergreen shrub with deep green small spiky leaves that bears small flowers of white to pink in color. The blossom is produced from September to February and most profusely in the later months. Its size ranges from a creeping plant to a small tree—trees can reach heights of up to 26ft (8m), especially when found within dense woodland. The leaves and flowers are strongly aromatic.

Actions Analgesic, antibacterial, antibiotic, antifungal, antihistamine, anti-inflammatory, anti-infectious, antimicrobial, antiseptic, astringent, deodorant, digestive, expectorant, immune stimulant, insecticide, sedative, vulnerary.

Extraction Steam distilled from the leaves, twigs, and branches.

Characteristics A mobile liquid with a distinctive fresh, spicy, herbaceous aroma with a honey-like sweetness. It blends well with bay leaf, bergamot, black pepper, cajuput, cedarwood atlas, cinnamon, clove bud, elemi, ginger, juniper, lavender, nutmeg, peppermint, rose, rosemary, sandalwood, thyme, vetiver, and ylang ylang.

Perfume

Scent: Spicy, herbaceous, fresh, tea tree-like.
Key qualities: Relaxing, soothing, protective, antiseptic, antimicrobial, cleansing, uplifting, balancing. **Odor intensity:** Medium.

Aromatherapy use

Skin care: Acne, abscesses, athlete's foot, bed sores, blisters, boils, burns, carbuncles, cold sores, cracked skin, dandruff, dermatitis, eczema, fungal infections, insect bites and stings, lice, nail infections, oily skin, pimples, ringworm, sores, sunburn, tinea, and ulcers. **Circulation, muscles, and joints:** Aches and pains, muscular tension, sprains and stiffness in joints, rheumatism. **Respiratory system:** Coughs, cold, flu congestion, as well as asthma and hayfever. **Immune system:** Tonic. **Nervous system:** Nervous debility.

SAFETY DATA
Generally it is thought to be nonsensitizing, nontoxic, and nonirritant. Avoid use during pregnancy.

Lovage

LEVISTICUM OFFICINALE FAMILY APIACEAE (UMBELLIFERAE)

Description A large perennial herb up to 7ft (2m) high with a stout hollow stem and dense ornamental foliage. It has a thick fleshy root and greenish-yellow flowers. The whole plant has a strong aromatic scent.

Actions Antimicrobial, antiseptic, antispasmodic, diaphoretic, digestive, diuretic, carminative, depurative, emmenagogue, expectorant, febrifuge, stimulant (digestive), stomachic.

Extraction Essential oil by steam distillation from the fresh roots, and the fresh leaves and stalks of the herb.

Characteristics Oil from the roots is amber or olive-brown liquid with a rich, spicy-warm, root-like odor. Oil from the herb is a very pale yellow mobile liquid with a spicy, warm odor and sweet-floral undertone. It blends well with rose, galbanum, costus, opopanax, oakmoss, bay, lavandin, and spice oils.

SAFETY DATA
Nontoxic, nonirritant, possible sensitization/phototoxic effects. Use with care. Avoid during pregnancy.

Perfume

Scent: Herbaceous, floral, bitter, celery, fresh, warm, sweet, spicy.
Key qualities: Anti-allergenic, anti-inflammatory, soothing, cooling, healing.
Odor intensity: High.

Aromatherapy use

Circulation, muscles, and joints: Accumulation of toxins, congestion, gout, edema, poor circulation, rheumatism, water retention.
Digestive system: Anaemia, flatulence, indigestion, spasm. **Genitourinary system:** Amenorrhoea, dysmenorrhoea, cystitis.

LOVAGE WAS TRADITIONALLY BELIEVED TO BE GOOD FOR THE SIGHT.

Styrax, levant

LIQUIDAMBAR ORIENTALIS FAMILY HAMAMELIDACEAE

Description A deciduous tree up to 50ft (15m) high with a purplish-gray bark, leaves arranged into 5 three-lobed sections, and white flowers. The styrax is a pathological secretion produced by pounding the bark, which induces the sapwood to produce a liquid from beneath the bark. It hardens to form a semi-solid greenish-brown mass with a sweet balsamic odor.

Actions Anthelmintic, anti-inflammatory, antimicrobial, antiseptic, antispasmodic, antitussive, bactericidal, balsamic, carminative, diaphoretic, emmenagogue, expectorant, fungicidal, nervine, stimulant, stomachic.

Extraction Essential oil by steam distillation from the crude. (A resinoid and absolute are also produced by solvent extraction.)

Characteristics A water-white or pale yellow liquid with a sweet-balsamic, rich, tenacious odor. It blends well with ylang ylang, jasmine, mimosa, rose, lavender, carnation, violet, cassie, and spice oils.

Perfume

Scent: Sweet, resinous, spicy. **Key qualities:** Calming, soothing, relaxing, de-stressing, promotes easy breathing, sedative. **Odor intensity:** High.

Aromatherapy use

Skin care: Cuts, ringworm, scabies, wounds. **Respiratory system:** Bronchitis, catarrh, coughs. **Nervous system:** Anxiety, stress-related conditions.

IN CHINA, IT IS TRADITIONALLY USED FOR COUGHS, COLDS, EPILEPSY, AND SKIN PROBLEMS, INCLUDING CUTS, WOUNDS, AND SCABIES.

SAFETY DATA
Nontoxic, nonirritant, possible sensitization in some individuals.

May chang

LITSEA CUBEBA FAMILY *LAURACEAE*

Description A small tropical tree with fragrant, lemongrass-scented leaves and flowers. The small fruits are shaped like peppers, from which the name "cubeba" derives.

Actions Antiseptic, deodorant, digestive, disinfectant, insecticidal, stimulant, stomachic.

Extraction Essential oil by steam distillation from the fruits.

Characteristics A pale yellow mobile liquid with an intense, lemony, fresh-fruity odor (sweeter than lemongrass but less tenacious).

SAFETY DATA
Nontoxic, nonirritant, possible sensitization in some individuals.

Perfume

Scent: Lemony, fresh-fruity, spicy.
Key qualities: Refreshing, stimulating, uplifting, tonic, cleansing, antiseptic, antiviral, astringent. **Odor intensity:** Medium.

Aromatherapy use

Skin care: Acne, dermatitis, excessive perspiration, greasy skin, insect repellent, spots. **Digestive system:** Flatulence, indigestion. **Immune system:** Epidemics, sanitation.

Tea tree

MELALEUCA ALTERNIFOLIA FAMILY MYRTACEAE

Description A small tree or shrub (the smallest of the melaleuca family), with needle-like leaves, similar to those of cypress, and heads of stalkless yellow or purplish-colored flowers.

Actions Anti-infectious, anti-inflammatory, antiseptic, antiviral, bactericidal, balsamic, cicatrizant, diaphoretic, expectorant, fungicidal, immunostimulant, parasiticide, vulnerary.

Extraction The oil is extracted by steam or water distillation from the leaves and twigs.

Extraction A pale yellowy-green or water-white, mobile liquid, with a warm, fresh, spicy-camphoraceous odor. It blends well with lavender, clary sage, rosemary, pine, ylang ylang, geranium, marjoram, and spice oils, especially clove and nutmeg.

Perfume

Scent: Medicinal, fresh, powerful, camphoraceous, pungent, slightly spicy.
Key qualities: Penetrating, medicinal, stimulating, refreshing. **Odor intensity:** High.

Aromatherapy use

Skin care: Abscess, acne, athlete's foot, blisters, burns, bruises, chicken pox rash, cold sores, dandruff, herpes, insect bites, oily skin, rashes (nappy rash), spots, verrucae, warts, wounds (infected). **Respiratory system:** Asthma, bronchitis, catarrh, coughs, sinusitis, tuberculosis, whooping cough. **Reproductive system:** Thrush (vaginal), vaginitis. **Immune system:** Colds, fever, flu, infectious illnesses. **Urinary system:** Cystitis, pruritus.

SAFETY DATA
Nontoxic, nonirritant, although there are indications of possible sensitization in some individuals.

Cajeput

MELALEUCA CAJEPUTI FAMILY MYRTACEAE

Description A tall evergreen tree, up to 100ft (30m) high, with thick, pointed leaves, and white flowers. The flexible trunk has a whitish, spongy bark that flakes easily.

Actions Mildly analgesic, antimicrobial, antineuralgic, antispasmodic, antiseptic (pulmonary, urinary, intestinal), anthelmintic, diaphoretic, carminative, expectorant, febrifuge, insecticide, sudorific, tonic.

Extraction The oil is extracted by steam distillation from the fresh leaves and twigs.

Characteristics A pale yellowy-green, mobile liquid (the green tinge derives from traces of copper found in the tree), with a penetrating, camphoraceous-medicinal odor. Compared to eucalyptus oil, it has a slightly milder, fruity body note. It blends well with herb and spice oils.

SAFETY DATA
Nontoxic, nonsensitizing, but may irritate the skin in high concentration.

Perfume

Scent: Fresh, camphoraceous, slightly medicinal, fruity-sweet. **Key qualities (mind):** Clearing, refreshing, reviving, anaphrodisiac. **Odor intensity:** Medium–high.

Aromatherapy use

Skin care: Insect bites, oily skin, spots. **Circulation, muscles, and joints:** Arthritis, muscular aches and pains, rheumatism. **Respiratory system:** Asthma, bronchitis, catarrh, colds, coughs, flu, sinusitis, sore throat. **Genitourinary system:** Cystitis, urethritis, urinary infection. **Immune system:** Colds, flu, infections.

Niaouli

MELALEUCA VIRIDIFLORA FAMILY *MYRTACEAE*

Description An evergreen tree with a flexible trunk and spongy bark, pointed linear leaves and bearing spikes of sessile yellowish flowers. The leaves have a strong aromatic scent when they are crushed.

Actions Analgesic, anthelmintic, anticatarrhal, antirheumatic, antiseptic, antispasmodic, bactericidal, balsamic, cicatrisant, diaphoretic, expectorant, regulator, stimulant, vermifuge.

Extraction Essential oil by steam distillation from the leaves and young twigs.

Characteristics A colorless, pale yellow, or greenish liquid with a sweet, fresh, camphoraceous odor.

SAFETY DATA
Nontoxic, nonsensitizing, but may irritate the skin in high concentration.

Perfume

Scent: Sharp, clear, pungent, medicinal, floral, slightly sweet, fresh, earthy, musty, harsh, spicy camphoraceous, warm. **Key qualities:** Stimulant, revitalizing, disinfecting, clarifying, antiseptic, astringent, purifying. **Odor intensity:** Medium.

Aromatherapy use

Skin care: Acne, boils, burns, cuts, insect bites, oily skin, spots, ulcers, wounds. **Circulation, muscles, and joints:** Muscular aches and pains, poor circulation, rheumatism. **Respiratory system:** Asthma, bronchitis, catarrhal conditions, coughs, sinusitis, sore throat, whooping cough. **Genitourinary system:** Cystitis, urinary infection. **Immune system:** Colds, fever, flu.

Melissa/lemon balm

MELISSA OFFICINALIS FAMILY *LABIATAE (LAMIACEAE)*

Description A sweet-scented herb about 2ft (60cm) high, soft and bushy, with bright green, serrated leaves, square stems, and tiny white or pink flowers.

Actions Antidepressant, antihistaminic, antispasmodic, bactericidal, carminative, cordial, diaphoretic, emmenagogue, febrifuge, hypertensive, nervine, sedative, stomachic, sudorific, tonic, uterine, vermifuge, insect-repellent.

Extraction The oil is extracted by steam distillation from the leaves and flowering tops.

Characteristics A pale yellow liquid, with a light, fresh, lemony fragrance. It blends well with lavender and geranium oil and with all floral, and citrus oils.

Perfume

Scent: Lemony, light, fresh, green, herbaceous, honey-sweet. **Key qualities:** Soothing, calming, uplifting, regulating, sedative, appeasing, comforting, heart tonic, strengthening, revitalizing, protecting, antidepressant. **Odor intensity:** High.

Aromatherapy use

Skin care: Allergies, insect bites. **Respiratory system:** Asthma, bronchitis, chronic coughs. **Digestive system:** Colic, indigestion, nausea. **Reproductive system:** Menstrual problems. **Nervous system:** Anxiety, depression, hypertension, insomnia, migraine, nervous tension, shock, vertigo. **Other:** Insect repellent.

WARNING
Skin irritant. Use in low dilutions (up to 1%). Narcotic in large doses, causing headaches.

Available information suggests possible sensitization and skin irritation.

Peppermint

MENTHA X PIPERITA FAMILY *LAMIACEAE (LABIATAE)*

Description A perennial herb, up to 3ft (1m) high. White peppermint has green stems and leaves; black peppermint has dark green, serrated leaves, purplish stems, and reddish-violet flowers.

Actions Analgesic, anti-inflammatory, antimicrobial, antiphlogistic, antipruritic, antiseptic, antispasmodic, antiviral, astringent, diaphoretic, carminative, cephalic, cordial, emmenagogue, expectorant, febrifuge, hepatic, nervine, stomachic, sudorific, vasoconstrictor, vermifuge.

Extraction The oil is extracted by steam distillation from the flowering herb.

Characteristics A pale yellow or greenish liquid, with a highly penetrating, grassy-minty, camphoraceous odor. It blends well with benzoin, rosemary, lavender, marjoram, lemon, eucalyptus, and bergamot.

SAFETY DATA
Nontoxic, nonirritant, but possible sensitization due to the menthol content. Do not use oil with homeopathic remedies. Use in low dilutions on the skin. Suitable for use with children (with care) as described in this book.

Perfume

Scent: Fresh, bright, minty, penetrating, clean.
Key qualities: Refreshing, restorative, nerve tonic, cephalic, aphrodisiac, stimulant (mental).
Odor intensity: High.

Aromatherapy use

Skin care: Acne, dermatitis, ringworm, scabies, toothache. **Circulation, muscles, and joints:** Neuralgia, muscular pain, palpitations. **Respiratory system:** Asthma, bronchitis, sinusitis, spasmodic cough. **Digestive system:** Colic, cramp, dyspepsia, flatulence, nausea. **Immune system:** Colds, flu, fevers. **Nervous system:** Fainting, headache, mental fatigue, migraine, nervous stress, vertigo. **Other:** Treats halitosis, insect repellent.

Mint, spearmint

MENTHA SPICATA FAMILY LAMIACEAE (LABIATAE)

Description A hardy branched perennial herb with bright green, lance-shaped, sharply toothed leaves, quickly spreading underground runners and pink- or lilac-coloured flowers in slender cylindrical spikes.

Actions Anesthetic (local), antiseptic, antispasmodic, astringent, carminative, cephalic, cholagogue, decongestant, digestive, diuretic, expectorant, febrifuge, hepatic, nervine, stimulant, stomachic, tonic.

Extraction Essential oil by steam distillation from the flowering tops.

Characteristics A pale yellow or olive mobile liquid with a warm, spicy-herbaceous, minty odor. It blends well with lavender, lavandin, jasmine, eucalyptus, basil, and rosemary, and is often used in combination with peppermint.

SAFETY DATA
Nontoxic, nonirritant, nonsensitizing.

Perfume

Scent: Crisp, minty, fresh, soft, sweet. **Key qualities:** Refreshing, cleansing, uplifting, energizing, cooling. **Odor intensity:** Low.

Aromatherapy use

Skin care: Acne, dermatitis, congested skin. **Respiratory system:** Asthma, bronchitis, catarrhal conditions, sinusitis. **Digestive system:** Colic, dyspepsia, flatulence, hepatobiliary disorders, nausea, vomiting. **Immune system:** Colds, fevers, flu. **Nervous system:** Fatigue, headache, migraine, nervous strain, neurasthenia, stress.

Champaca

MICHELIA CHAMPACA FAMILY *MAGNOLIACEAE*

Description Champaca is a large, sub-tropical tree up to 20ft (6m) high with a smooth gray bark and long, oval-shaped, glossy evergreen leaves. The flowers have 10–20 yellow, orange, or cream-colored narrow petals and an extremely heady fragrance. They bloom both in spring and fall—on a warm, humid night, the scent can be enjoyed several hundred feet away! Champaca fruit are brown, containing bright red seeds.

Actions Antidepressant, aphrodisiac, antispasmodic, antiseptic, antiviral, astringent, emollient, euphoric, emollient, febrifuge, stimulant, and tonic.

Extraction The absolute is produced by solvent extraction from the fresh flowers. (An oil is also produced by steam distillation of the petals.) The absolute requires thousands of fresh flowers to produce a tiny amount: thus its high cost.

Characteristics An intense, fresh, green-floral scent with an underlying warmth and subtle leafy notes. It blends well with jasmine, lemon, coriander, tuberose, grapefruit, bergamot, rose, ylang ylang, neroli, sandalwood, and other floral scents.

Perfume

Scent: Deep, sensual, complex, sweet, floral, warm, spicy. **Key qualities:** Revitalizing, aphrodisiac, strengthening, calming, relaxing. **Odor intensity:** High.

Aromatherapy use

Skin care: Dry, mature skin and sensitive skin, wrinkles, and general skin care.
Nervous system: Anxiety, depression, fear, grief, insomnia, nervous debility, tension headaches, mood swings, stress.

SAFETY DATA
Nontoxic, nonirritant, possible sensitization. Avoid during pregnancy.

Nutmeg

MYRISTICA FRAGRANS FAMILY *MYRISTICACEAE*

Description An evergreen tree, up to 70ft (20m) high, with dense foliage, and small, dull-yellow flowers.

Actions Analgesic, antiemetic, antioxidant, antirheumatic, antiseptic, antispasmodic, carminative, digestive, emmenagogue, orexigenic, prostaglandin inhibitor, stimulant, tonic.

Extraction The oil is extracted by steam (or water) distillation from the dried, worm-eaten nutmeg seed, or the dried, orange-brown aril or husk (mace).

Characteristics Nutmeg oil is a water-white or pale yellow, mobile liquid, with sweet, warm-spicy odor with terpeney top note. It blends well with lavender, bay, orange, geranium, clary sage, rosemary, lime, petitgrain, mandarin, coriander, and other spice oils.

> *Perfume*
>
> **Scent:** Rich, spicy, oriental, sensual, sweet, warm. **Key qualities:** Aphrodisiac, analgesic, narcotic, tonic (nerve and heart), comforting, soothing, calming, elevating, cephalic, euphoric. **Odor intensity:** High.

Aromatherapy use

Circulation, muscles, and joints: Arthritis, gout, muscular aches and pains, poor circulation, rheumatism. **Digestive system:** Flatulence, indigestion, nausea, sluggish digestion. **Immune system:** Bacterial infection. **Nervous system:** Frigidity in women, impotence in men, neuralgia, nervous fatigue.

WARNING
Used in large doses nutmeg oil shows signs of toxicity. Use in moderation. Do not use during pregnancy, or on young children.

Nutmeg is generally nontoxic, nonirritant, and nonsensitizing.

Balsam, Peru

MYROXYLON BALSAMUM VAR. PEREIRAE FAMILY *FABACEAE (LEGUMINOSAE)*

Description A large tropical tree up to 80ft (25m) high, with a straight smooth trunk, beautiful foliage and very fragrant flowers. Every part of the tree contains a resinous juice, including the fibrous fruit. The balsam is a pathological product, obtained from the exposed lacerated wood, after strips of the bark have been removed. It is a "true'"balsam, which is collected in the form of a dark brown or amber semi-solid mass.

Actions Anti-inflammatory, antiseptic, balsamic, expectorant, parasiticide, stimulant; promotes the growth of epithelial cells.

Extraction A resin-free essential oil is produced from the crude balsam by high vacuum dry distillation. (A wood oil is also produced by steam distillation from the wood chippings, which is considered of inferior quality.)

Characteristics The oil is a pale amber or brown viscous liquid with a rich, sweet, balsamic, vanilla-like scent. It blends well with ylang ylang, patchouli, petitgrain, sandalwood, rose, spices, floral, and oriental bases.

Perfume

Scent: Dry-woody, amber, balsamic, resinous.
Key qualities: Soothing, purifying, uplifting.
Odor intensity: High.

Aromatherapy use

Skin care: Dry and chapped skin, eczema, rashes, sores, and wounds. **Circulation, muscles, and joints:** Low blood pressure, rheumatism. **Respiratory system:** Asthma, bronchitis, coughs. **Immune system:** Colds. **Nervous system:** Nervous tension, stress; like other balsams it has a warming, opening, comforting quality.

SAFETY DATA
Nontoxic, nonirritant; however the balsam (not the oil) is a common contact allergen, which may cause dermatitis.

Myrtle

MYRTUS COMMUNIS FAMILY MYRTACEAE

Description A large bush or small tree, with many tough but slender branches, a brownish-red bark, and small, sharp, pointed leaves. It has white flowers, followed by small, black berries; both leaves and flowers are very fragrant.

Actions Anticatarrhal, antiseptic, astringent, balsamic, bactericidal, expectorant, regulator, slightly sedative.

Extraction The oil is extracted by steam distillation from the leaves and twigs (and sometimes the flowers).

Characteristics A pale yellow or orange liquid, with a clear, fresh, camphoraceous, sweet, herbaceous scent somewhat similar to eucalyptus. It blends well with bergamot, lavender, rosemary, clary sage, hyssop, bay, lime, ginger, clove, and other spice oils.

SAFETY DATA
Nontoxic, nonirritant, nonsensitizing.

Perfume

Scent: Clear, fresh, balsamic, camphoraceous, floral, spicy, diffusive. **Key qualities:** Mildly stimulating, tonic (nerve), antiseptic, clarifying, cleansing, uplifting, aphrodisiac, refreshing. **Odor intensity:** Medium–high.

Aromatherapy use

Skin care: Acne, hemorrhoids, oily skin, open pores. **Respiratory system:** Asthma, bronchitis, catarrhal conditions, chronic coughs, tuberculosis. Because of its relative mildness, this is a very suitable oil for children's coughs and chest complaints. **Immune system:** Colds, flu, infectious disease.

Lotus

NELUMBO NUCIFERA FAMILY *NELUMBONACEAE (NYMPHAEACEAE)*

Description The sacred lotus is a perennial aquatic plant with rhizomes that grow in the mud at the bottom of shallow ponds, lakes and marshes. Its large leaves, which rise above the water surface, can be up to 24in (60cm) in diameter, with a 10ft (3m) horizontal spread, while the showy flowers can be up to 8in (20cm) in diameter. The beautiful pink, fragrant flowers are solitary, borne at or above the leaf level, with a brilliant yellow center and white sepals. The fruits form a conical pod, with seeds contained in holes in the pod.

Actions Antibacterial, antimicrobial, antidepressant, antioxidant, refrigerant, rejuvenating, sedative, tonic (heart, immune system, nervous system), vasodilator.

Extraction An absolute by solvent extraction from fresh flowers. The CO2 extraction process achieves a cleaner end product that is true to the oil and is thicker than other extraction methods. This product is often adulterated or blended with other oils.

Characteristics A viscous liquid with an intense rich, sweet-floral scent and a spicy-leathery undertone. It blends well with tuberose, jasmine, neroli, rose, gardenia, and spice oils.

Perfume

Scent: Rich, earthy, sweet, floral, spicy, leathery.
Key qualities: Antidepressant, sedative, relaxing, cleansing, astringent, soothing, cooling, anti-aging. **Odor intensity:** High.

Aromatherapy use

Skin care: Damaged, sensitive, and mature skin: improves the condition of uneven or tired-looking skin as it helps regulate, soothe, illuminate, and rejuvenate the tissue. **Immune system:** Weak immunity. **Nervous system:** Anxiety, depression, fear, insomnia, nervous debility and tension, mood swings, poor libido, stress.

SAFETY DATA
Generally considered a safe oil.

Basil, sweet/French

OCIMUM BASILICUM FAMILY *LAMIACEAE (LABIATAE)*

Description A tender annual herb up to 2.5in (60cm) high, with dark green, ovate leaves, grayish-green beneath. It bears whorls of two-lipped, greenish or pinky-white flowers. The whole plant has a powerful aromatic scent.

Actions Antiseptic, antispasmodic, carminative, digestive, emmenagogue, expectorant, febrifuge, galactagogue, nervine, prophylactic, stimulant of adrenal cortex, stomachic, tonic, insecticide.

Extraction The oil is extracted by steam distillation from the flowering herb.

Characteristics Sweet basil oil is a colorless or pale yellow liquid, with a light, fresh, sweet-spicy scent, and balsamic undertones. It blends well with bergamot, clary sage, lime, citronella, geranium, hyssop, and other green notes.

WARNING
Possible sensitization. Use in moderation. Avoid prolonged use, and do not use during pregnancy.

Perfume

Scent: Fresh, slightly spicy, clove-like. **Key qualities:** Restorative, tonic, antidepressant, refreshing, uplifting, fortifying, purifying, clearing, warming, cephalic, stupefying (in excess). **Odor intensity:** High.

Aromatherapy use

Skin care: Insect bites (mosquito, wasp), insect repellent. **Circulation, muscles, and joints:** Gout, muscular aches and pains, rheumatism. **Respiratory system:** Bronchitis, colds, coughs, earache, sinusitis. **Digestive system:** Dyspepsia, flatulence, nausea. **Reproductive system:** Cramps, scanty periods. **Immune system:** Colds, fever, flu, infectious disease. **Nervous system:** Anxiety, depression, fatigue, insomnia, migraine, nervous tension.

Marjoram, sweet

ORIGANUM MARJORANA/MARJORANA HORTENSIS FAMILY *LAMIACEAE (LABIATAE)*

Description A tender, bushy perennial plant, up to 2ft (60cm) high, with a hairy stem, dark green oval leaves, and small grayish-white flowers growing in clusters.

Actions Analgesic, anaphrodisiac, antioxidant, antiseptic, antispasmodic, antiviral, bactericidal, carminative, cephalic, cordial, diaphoretic, digestive, diuretic, emmenagogue, expectorant, fungicidal, hypotensor, laxative, nervine, sedative, tonic, vasodilatator, vulnerary.

Extraction The oil is extracted by steam distillation from the dried flowering herb.

Characteristics A pale yellow or amber-colored, mobile liquid with a warm, woody, spicy, camphoraceous odor. Blends well with lavender, rosemary, bergamot, chamomile, cypress, tea tree, and eucalyptus.

WARNING
This oil should not be used during pregnancy.

Perfume

Scent: Warm, woody, spicy, nutty, camphoraceous, herbaceous, penetrating. **Key qualities:** Anaphrodisiac, stupefying in large doses, cephalic, sedative, nervine, restorative, warming, comforting. **Odor intensity:** Medium.

Aromatherapy use

Skin care: Chilblains, bruises, tics. **Circulation, muscles, and joints:** Arthritis, lumbago, muscular aches and stiffness, rheumatism, sprains, strains. **Respiratory system:** Asthma, bronchitis, colds, coughs. **Digestive system:** Colic, constipation, dyspepsia, flatulence. **Reproductive system:** Amenorrhea, dysmenorrhea, leukorrhea, PMS. **Nervous system:** Headache, hypertension, insomnia, migraine, nervous tension, stress-related conditions.

Geranium, rose

PELARGONIUM GRAVEOLENS FAMILY *GERANIACEAE*

Description A perennial hairy shrub, up to 3ft (1m) high, with lobed leaves, serrated at the edges, and small pink flowers. The whole plant is aromatic.

Actions Antihemorrhagic, anti-inflammatory, antiseptic, astringent, cicatrizant, deodorant, diuretic, fungicidal, hemostatic, stimulant (to adrenal cortex and lymphatic system), styptic, tonic, vermifuge, vulnerary.

Extraction The oil is extracted by steam distillation from the leaves, stalks, and flowers.

Characteristics Greenish-olive liquid with a green, rosy-sweet, minty scent. (The Bourbon oil is generally preferred in perfumery work.) It blends well with lavender, patchouli, clove, rose, sandalwood, jasmine, juniper, neroli, bergamot, and other citrus oils.

Perfume

Scent: Green, rosy-sweet, floral-minty, fresh, strong, powerful. **Key qualities:** Tonic, antidepressant, uplifting, balancing, refreshing, soothing, warming, regulating. **Odor intensity:** Medium–high.

Aromatherapy use

Skin care: Acne, bruises, broken capillaries, burns, congested skin, cuts, dermatitis, eczema, hemorrhoids, lice, oily complexion, mature skin, ringworm, ulcers, wounds.
Circulatory system: Cellulitis, engorgement of breasts, edema, poor circulation.
Respiratory system: Sore throat, tonsillitis.
Reproductive and endocrine system: Adrenocortical glands and menopausal problems, PMS. **Nervous system:** Nervous tension, neuralgia, stress-related conditions.
Other: Insect repellent (especially mosquitoes).

SAFETY DATA
Nontoxic, nonirritant, generally nonsensitizing, but may cause contact dermatitis in hypersensitive individuals (especially the Bourbon type).

Parsley seed

PETROSELINUM CRISPUM FAMILY APIACEAE (UMBELLIFERAE)

Description A biennial or short-lived perennial herb, up to 28in (70cm) high, with crinkly, bright green foliage, and small, greenish-yellow flowers producing small brown seeds (when ripe).

Actions Antimicrobial, antirheumatic, antiseptic, astringent, carminative, diuretic, depurative, emmenagogue, febrifuge, hypotensive, laxative, stimulant (mild), stomachic, tonic (uterine).

Extraction This oil is extracted by steam distillation from the seeds. (A different oil with slightly different properties is also produced from the herb.)

Characteristics A yellow, amber or brownish liquid, with a warm, woody-spicy, herbaceous odor. It blends well with rose, neroli, ylang ylang, tea tree, clary sage, and spice oils.

Perfume

Scent: Herbaceous, spicy, fresh, warm, pungent. **Key qualities (mind):** Refreshing, stimulating, warming. **Odor intensity:** Medium.

WARNING
Avoid using this oil during pregnancy.

Aromatherapy use

Circulation, muscles, and joints: Accumulation of toxins, arthritis, broken blood vessels, cellulitis, rheumatism, sciatica. **Digestive system:** Colic, flatulence, indigestion, hemorrhoids. **Reproductive system:** Amenorrhea, dysmenorrhea, to aid labor. **Urinary system:** Cystitis, urinary infection.

SAFETY DATA
Although the oil is moderately toxic and has been shown to have irritant properties, it is nonsensitizing when used in moderation.

Bay, West Indian

PIMENTA ACRIS FAMILY *MYRTACEAE*

Description A tropical evergreen tree up to 28ft (8m) high, with large, leathery leaves, and aromatic fruits.

Actions Analgesic, anticonvulsant, antineuralgic, antirheumatic, antiseptic, astringent, expectorant, stimulant, hair tonic.

Extraction The oil is extracted by water or steam distillation from the leaves.

Characteristics A dark yellow, mobile liquid with a fresh-spicy top note, and a sweet balsamic undertone. It blends well with lavender, rosemary, geranium, ylang ylang, citrus, and spice oils.

WARNING
Moderately toxic due to high eugenol content, but generally nonirritant, nonsensitizing. Use in moderation.

Perfume

Scent: Fresh, penetrating, slightly camphoraceous, spicy-medicinal.
Key qualities (mind): Reviving, warming, clearing, refreshing.
Odor intensity: Medium.

Aromatherapy use

Skin care: Scalp stimulant; treats dandruff, greasy, lifeless hair; promotes hair growth.
Circulation, muscles, and joints: Rheumatism, arthritis, aches and pains, strains, neuralgia, poor circulation. **Immune system:** Colds, flu, infectious diseases.

Aniseed

PIMPINELLA ANISUM FAMILY *APIACEAE (UMBELLIFERAE)*

Description An annual herb, less than 3ft (1m) high, with delicate leaves, and white flowers.

Actions Antiseptic, antispasmodic, carminative, diuretic, expectorant, galactagogue, stimulant, stomachic.

Extraction The oil is extracted by steam distillation from the seeds.

Characteristics
A colorless to pale yellow liquid, with a characteristic warm, spicy-sweet scent. Bay is a good masking agent. It blends well with other spice oils.

Perfume

Scent: Spicy-sweet, liquorice-like, rich, very pervasive. **Key qualities:** Warming, purifying, aphrodisiac, uplifting, reviving, soothing, comforting, stimulant (in small doses), stupefying (in excess). **Odor intensity:** Very high.

Aromatherapy use

Circulation, muscles, and joints: Muscular aches and pains, rheumatism. **Respiratory system:** Bronchitis, colds, coughs. **Digestive system:** Colic, cramp, flatulence, indigestion.

SAFETY DATA
The major component, anethole, is known to cause dermatitis in some individuals—avoid in allergic and inflammatory skin conditions. In large doses it is narcotic, slows down the circulation, and can lead to cerebral disorders.

A NISEED STIMULATES DIGESTION, SO HAS TRADITIONALLY BEEN ENJOYED AFTER A MEAL AS A FLAVORING IN DESSERTS OR DIGESTIFS.

WARNING
Use in moderation only.

Pine, longleaf

PINUS PALUSTRIS FAMILY PINACEAE

Description A tall evergreen tree with long needles and a straight trunk, grown extensively for its timber. It exudes a natural oleoresin from the trunk, which provides the largest source for the production of turpentine in the United States.

Actions Analgesic (mild), antirheumatic, antiseptic, bactericidal, expectorant, insecticidal, stimulant.

Extraction The crude oil is obtained by steam distillation from the sawdust and wood chips from the heartwood and roots of the tree (wastage from the timber mills), and then submitted to fractional distillation under atmospheric pressure to produce pine essential oil.

Characteristics A water-white or pale yellow liquid with a sweet-balsamic, pinewood scent. It blends well with rosemary, pine needle, cedarwood, citronella, rosewood, ho leaf, and oakmoss.

SAFETY DATA
Nontoxic; nonirritant (except in concentration).

Perfume

Scent: Balsamic, camphoraceous, woody, sweet, resinous, fresh, evergreen. **Key qualities:** Stimulating, strengthening, energizing, stress-relieving, uplifting, cleansing, antiseptic, anti-inflammatory. **Odor intensity:** Medium.

Aromatherapy use

Circulation, muscles, and joints: Arthritis, debility, lumbago, muscular aches and pains, poor circulation, rheumatism, stiffness, etc. **Respiratory system:** Asthma, bronchitis, catarrh, sinusitis. **Other:** Used extensively in medicine, particularly in veterinary antiseptic sprays, disinfectants, detergents, and insecticides (as a solvent carrier).

Pine needle, Scotch

PINUS SYLVESTRIS FAMILY PINACEAE

Description A tall evergreen tree, up to 130ft (40m) high. It has reddish-brown, deeply fissured bark, long, stiff needles growing in pairs, and pointed, brown cones.

Actions Antimicrobial, antineuralgic, antirheumatic, antiscorbutic, antiseptic, antiviral, bactericidal, balsamic, cholagogue, choleretic, deodorant, diuretic, expectorant, hypertensive, insecticide, restorative, rubefacient, stimulant (circulatory and nervous systems), vermifuge.

Extraction The oil is extracted by dry distillation from the needles.

Characteristics Pine needle oil is a colorless or pale yellow, mobile liquid, with a strong, dry-balsamic, turpentine-like aroma. It blends well with cedarwood, rosemary, tea tree, sage, lavender, juniper, lemon, cajeput, eucalyptus, and marjoram.

WARNING
Do not use this oil if there are allergic skin conditions. It is a skin irritant in concentration—use in low dilutions only.

Perfume

Scent: Fresh, camphoraceous, balsamic, woody, penetrating, strong. **Key qualities:** Strengthening, cleansing, restorative, reviving, refreshing, stimulant (nerve), soothing (mental). **Odor intensity:** Medium–high.

Aromatherapy use

Skin care: Cuts, lice, excessive perspiration, scabies, sores. **Circulation, muscles, and joints:** Arthritis, gout, muscular aches and pains, neuralgia, poor circulation, rheumatism. **Respiratory system:** Asthma, bronchitis, catarrh, colds, coughs, flu, sinusitis, sore throat. **Urinary system:** Cystitis, urinary infection. **Nervous system:** Fatigue, nervous exhaustion, stress-related conditions.

Pepper, black

PIPER NIGRUM FAMILY PIPERACEAE

Description A perennial woody vine, up to 16.5ft (5m) high, with heart-shaped leaves, and small white flowers. The berries turn from red to black as they mature—black pepper is the dried, unripe fruit.

Actions Analgesic, antimicrobial, antiseptic, antitoxic, aperitif, bactericidal, carminative, diaphoretic, digestive, diuretic, febrifuge, laxative, rubefacient, stimulant, stomachic, tonic.

Extraction The oil is extracted by steam distillation from the black peppercorns, which have been dried and crushed.

Characteristics A water-white to pale olive, mobile liquid, with a fresh, dry-woody, warm, spicy scent. It blends well with frankincense, sandalwood, lavender, rosemary, marjoram, spices, and florals when used in minute quantities.

WARNING
This oil is toxic and irritant in concentration—use in low dilutions only (not more than 1% in a blend).

Perfume

Scent: Spicy, camphoraceous, fresh, woody, active, masculine, oriental, sensual, warm. **Key qualities:** Aphrodisiac, stimulant (mental), tonic (nerve), restorative, strengthening, comforting, analgesic, antiseptic. **Odor intensity:** High.

Aromatherapy use

Skin care: Chilblains. **Circulation, muscles, and joints:** Anemia, arthritis, muscular aches and pains, neuralgia, poor circulation, poor muscle tone, rheumatic pain, sprains, stiffness. **Respiratory system:** Catarrh, chills. **Immune system:** Colds, flu, infections, viruses. **Digestive system:** Colic, constipation, diarrhea, flatulence, heartburn, loss of appetite, nausea.

Frangipani

PLUMERIA RUBRA FAMILY APOCYNACEAE

Description Plumeria rubra is a small tree up to 16ft (5m) tall with a "candelabrum" shape, having a single trunk and branches that spread to form an open canopy. The deciduous pointed leaves, dark green on top and a lighter shade underneath, cluster at the tips of branches. The grayish-green, scaly bark produces a milky, sticky sap that is poisonous, much like oleander. The frangipani flowers, which appear in clusters, each with five waxy petals, are most fragrant at night in order to lure moths to pollinate them.

Actions Anti-inflammatory, antioxidant, antimicrobial, antifungal, antitumoral, antiviral, aphrodisiac, astringent, nervine.

Extraction Frangipani absolute is obtained by alcoholic or solvent extraction from the concrete prepared from *P. rubra* (acutifolia).

Characteristics The absolute has a heavy, sweet, floral-green aroma, with a soft-spicy background and hints of apricot. It blends with sandalwood, rose, patchouli, tuberose, clove bud, jasmine, neroli, bergamot, ginger, ylang ylang, and most citrus oils.

Perfume

Scent: Strong, rich, heavy, sweet, floral, spicy, apricot. **Key qualities:** Romantic, relaxing, aphrodisiac, astringent, purifying. **Odor intensity:** High.

Aromatherapy use

Skin care: Inflamed and sensitive skin, mature skin, wrinkles, and general skin care.
Nervous system: Anxiety, depression, fear, insomnia, nervous debility and tension, mood swings, stress.

SAFETY DATA
Generally considered to be a safe oil, but avoid using in pregnancy and for children. May cause skin irritation in concentration.

Patchouli

POGOSTEMON PATCHOULI FAMILY LAMINACEAE (LABIATAE)

Description A perennial bushy herb, up to 3ft (1m) high, with large, fragrant, furry leaves, and white flowers tinged with purple.

Actions Antidepressant, anti-inflammatory, antiemetic, antimicrobial, antiphlogistic, antiseptic, antitoxic, antiviral, astringent, bactericidal, carminative, cicatrizant, deodorant, digestive, diuretic, febrifuge, fungicidal, nervine, prophylactic, stimulant, stomachic, tonic.

Extraction The oil is extracted by steam distillation of the dried leaves.

Characteristics An amber or dark orange, viscous liquid, with a sweet, rich, herbaceous-earthy odor that improves with age. It blends well with vetivert, sandalwood, cedarwood, geranium, clove, lavender, rose, neroli, bergamot, myrrh, frankincense, clary sage, and oriental bases.

SAFETY DATA
Nontoxic, nonirritant, nonsensitizing. However, its overuse can cause loss of appetite, insomnia, and nervous attacks.

Perfume

Scent: Earthy, musky, spicy, woody, diffusive, warm, oriental, medicinal, powerful. **Key qualities:** Stimulant in small amounts, sedative in large doses, aphrodisiac, nerve tonic, appeasing, calming, uplifting. **Odor intensity:** Very high.

Aromatherapy use

Skin care: Acne, athlete's foot, cracked and chapped skin, dandruff, dermatitis, eczema (weeping), fungal infections, hair care, impetigo, sores, oily hair and skin, open pores, wounds, wrinkles. **Nervous system:** Frigidity, nervous exhaustion, stress-related complaints. **Other:** Insect repellent (moths).

Tuberose

POLIANTHES TUBEROSA FAMILY AGAVACEAE

Description A tender, tall, slim perennial up to 20in (50cm) high, with long slender leaves, a tuberous root and large, very fragrant, white lily-like flowers.

Actions Narcotic.

Extraction A concrete and absolute by solvent extraction from the fresh flowers, picked before the petals open. (An essential oil is also obtained by distillation of the concrete.)

Characteristics The absolute is a dark orange or brown soft paste, with a heavy, sweet-floral, sometimes slightly spicy, tenacious fragrance. It blends well with gardenia, violet, opopanax, rose, jasmine, carnation, orris, Peru balsam, neroli, and ylang ylang.

Perfume

Scent: Floral, rich, intense. **Key qualities:** Aphrodisiac, relaxation, de-stressing, sedative, warming, moisturizing. **Odor intensity:** High.

Aromatherapy use

Perfume.

SAFETY DATA
No safety data available—often adulterated.

"PURE ABSOLUTE EXTRACTION OF TUBEROSE IS PERHAPS THE MOST EXPENSIVE NATURAL FLOWER OIL AT THE DISPOSAL OF THE MODERN PERFUMER."

Ravensara

RAVENSARA AROMATICA FAMILY LAURACEAE

Description The genus Ravensara includes many species of evergreen trees or shrubs native to Madagascar and the Comoro Islands. These evergreen trees can grow up to 100ft (30m) tall in rainforests, usually on all type of soils. The best-known species of this genus is *R. aromatica* used for its essential oil. It grows to a height of about 65ft (20m) with several buttress roots at the base, with reddish bark, dark green shiny leaves, and small yellow-green flowers. The fruit, a fleshy berry, is an important food source for birds. All parts of the tree are aromatic.

Actions Antiviral, antibacterial, antifungal, anti-infectious, antiseptic, antispasmodic, expectorant, immune stimulant.

Extraction Ravensara oil is steam distilled from the leaves of the plant.

Characteristics
Ravensara oil (from the leaf) has a sweet, fresh, slightly lemony, licorice-like scent with an earthy undertone.

SAFETY DATA
Generally considered a safe oil (nontoxic and nonirritant), although avoid during pregnancy.

Perfume

Scent: Slightly spicy, camphoraceous, woody, herbaceous. **Key qualities:** Uplifting, relaxing, soothing, protective, antimicrobial, disinfectant, cleansing. **Odor intensity:** Medium.

Aromatherapy use

Skin care: Chickenpox, cold sores, herpes (all types), shingles. **Circulation, muscles, and joints:** Aching limbs, arthritis, cramp, gout, muscle fatigue, rheumatism. **Respiratory system:** Bronchitis, colds, congestion, influenza, sinusitis, throat and lung infections, whooping cough. **Immune system:** Viral infections especially herpes, hepatitis, chicken pox. **Nervous system:** Anxiety, insomnia, nervous tension, stress.

Rose maroc

ROSA CENTIFOLIA/R . GALLICA FAMILY ROSACEAE

Description The rose that is generally used for oil production is a hybrid between *R. centifolia* and *R. gallica*. It grows to 8ft (2.5m) and produces pink or rosy-purple flowers.

Actions Antidepressant, antiphlogistic, antiseptic, antispasmodic, antiviral, aphrodisiac, astringent, bactericidal, choleretic, cicatrizant, depurative, hemostatic, hepatic, laxative, appetite regulator, sedative, stomachic, tonic.

Extraction The oil or otto is extracted by water or steam distillation from the fresh petals. Concrete and absolute are produced by solvent extraction from the fresh petals.

Characteristics The oil is pale yellow, while the absolute is red-orange. Blends well with jasmine, orange flower, geranium, bergamot, lavender, clary sage, sandalwood, patchouli, benzoin, chamomile, clove, and palmarosa.

WARNING
Although generally safe, this oil should be avoided during the first 4 months of pregnancy.

Perfume

Scent: Floral, rosy, rich, tenacious, sweet, tender, warm. **Key qualities:** Aphrodisiac, soothing, comforting, antidepressant, sedative (to the nervous system), uplifting, appeasing, regulating, tonic (heart). **Odor intensity:** Very high.

Aromatherapy use

Skin care: Thread veins, dry, mature, and sensitive skin, wrinkles, eczema, herpes (nonirritant, nonsensitizing). **Circulation, muscles, and joints:** Palpitations, poor circulation. **Respiratory system:** Asthma, coughs, hay fever. **Digestive system:** Cholecystitis, liver congestion, nausea. **Reproductive system:** Irregular menstruation, leukorrhea, menorrhagia, uterine disorders. **Nervous system:** Depression, impotence, insomnia, frigidity, headache, nervous tension, stress-related complaints.

Rose damask

ROSA DAMASCENA FAMILY *ROSACEAE*

Description Small prickly shrub between 3ft (1m) and 6ft (2m) high, with pink, very fragrant blooms with 36 petals, and whitish hairy leaves. It requires a very specific soil and climate.

Actions Antidepressant, antiphlogistic, antiseptic, antispasmodic, antitubercular agent, antiviral, aphrodisiac, astringent, bactericidal, choleretic, cicitrisant, depurative, emmenagogue, haemostatic, hepatic, laxative, regulator of appetite, sedative, stomachic, tonic.

Extraction Essential oil by water or steam distillation from the fresh petals.

Characteristics A pale yellow or olive yellow liquid with a very rich, deep, sweet-floral, slightly spicy scent. It blends well with most oils, and is useful for "rounding off" blends. The Bulgarian type is considered superior in perfumery work, but in therapeutic practice it is more a matter of differing properties between the various types of rose.

SAFETY DATA
Nontoxic, nonirritant, nonsensitizing.

Perfume

Scent: Deep, rosy, floral, sweet, fresh.
Key qualities: Soothing, harmonizing, relaxing, de-stressing, hydrating, uplifting, stimulating, astringent, antiseptic, healing, aphrodesiac. **Odor intensity:** High.

Aromatherapy use

Skin care: Broken capillaries, conjunctivitis (rose water), dry skin, eczema, herpes, mature and sensitive complexions, wrinkles. **Circulation, muscles, and joints:** Palpitations, poor circulation. **Respiratory system:** Asthma, coughs, hay fever. **Digestive system:** Cholecystitis, liver congestion, nausea. **Genitourinary system:** Irregular menstruation, leucorrhoea, menorrhagia, uterine disorders. **Nervous system:** Depression, impotence, headache, nervous tension, and stress-related complaints.

Rosemary

ROSMARINUS OFFICINALIS FAMILY *LAMIACEAE (LABIATAE)*

Description An aromatic, shrubby evergreen bush, up to 6ft (2m) high, with silvery-green leaves, and pale blue flowers.

Actions Analgesic, antimicrobial, antioxidant, antiseptic, antispasmodic, astringent, carminative, choleretic, cicatrizant, cordial, diaphoretic, digestive, diuretic, emmenagogue, fungicidal, hepatic, hypertensor, restorative, rubefacient, stimulant, stomachic, sudorific, tonic.

Extraction The oil is extracted by steam distillation from the fresh flowering tops, or, (more commonly in Spain), from the whole plant.

Characteristics A colorless or pale yellow, mobile liquid with a strong, minty-herbaceous, woody-balsamic scent. It blends well with frankincense, lavender, citronella, basil, thyme, pine, peppermint, elemi, cedarwood, petitgrain, and spice oils.

Perfume

Scent: Penetrating, fresh, camphoraceous, woody-balsamic, strong. **Key qualities:** Stimulant (nervous and mental), analgesic, tonic (to the nervous system), strengthening, restorative, purifying, protective, reviving, refreshing. **Odor intensity:** Medium–high.

Aromatherapy use

Skin care: Acne, dermatitis, eczema, lice, scabies, hair, and scalp. **Circulation, muscles, and joints:** Arteriosclerosis, fluid retention, gout, muscular pain, neuralgia, palpitations, poor circulation, varicose veins, rheumatism. **Respiratory system:** Asthma, bronchitis, whooping cough. **Digestive system:** Colitis, dyspepsia, flatulence, hepatic disorders, jaundice. **Reproductive system:** Dysmenorrhea, leukorrhea. **Immune system:** Colds, flu, infections. **Nervous system:** Headaches, hypotension, nervous exhaustion, stress-related disorders.

WARNING
This oil should not be used by people suffering from epilepsy, or during pregnancy.

Sage, Spanish

SALVIA LAVANDULIFOLIA FAMILY *LAMIACEAE (LABIATAE)*

Description An aromatic evergreen shrub, similar to the garden sage, but with narrower leaves, and small purple flowers. The oil is mainly produced in Spain.

Actions Antidepressant, anti-inflammatory, antimicrobial, antiseptic, antispasmodic, astringent, carminative, deodorant, depurative, digestive, emmenagogue, expectorant, febrifuge, hypotensive, nervine, stimulant, stomachic, tonic.

Extraction The oil is extracted by steam distillation from the leaves.

Characteristics A pale yellow, mobile liquid, with a fresh-herbaceous, camphoraceous, slightly pine-like odor. It blends well with rosemary, lavender, pine, eucalyptus, juniper, clary sage, and cedarwood.

WARNING
Do not use during pregnancy. Always use in moderation only.

Perfume

Scent: Camphoraceous, fresh, herbaceous, penetrating, powerful. **Key qualities (mind):** Refreshing, invigorating, clearing. **Odor intensity:** High.

Aromatherapy use

Skin care: Acne, cuts, dandruff, dermatitis, eczema, excessive sweating, hair loss, sores. **Circulation, muscles, and joints:** Arthritis, debility, fluid retention, muscular aches and pains, poor circulation, rheumatism. **Respiratory system:** Asthma, coughs, laryngitis. **Digestive system:** Jaundice, liver congestion. **Reproductive system:** Amenorrhea, dysmenorrhea, sterility. **Immune system:** Colds, fevers, flu. **Nervous system:** Headaches, nervous exhaustion, stress-related conditions. **Other:** Treats gingivitis and other gum infections.

Sage, clary

SALVIA SCLARIA FAMILY *LABIATAE (LAMIACEAE)*

Description Stout biennial or perennial herb, up to 3ft (1m) high, with large, hairy leaves, green with a hint of purple, and small blue flowers.

Actions Anticonvulsive, antidepressant, antiphlogistic, antiseptic, aphrodisiac, astringent, bactericidal, carminative, cicatrizant, deodorant, digestive, emmenagogue, hypotensive, nervine, sedative, stomachic, uterine tonic.

Extraction The oil is extracted by steam distillation from the flowering tops, and leaves.

Characteristics A colorless or pale yellowy-green liquid, with a sweet, nutty-herbaceous scent. It blends well with juniper, lavender, coriander, cardamom, geranium, sandalwood, cedarwood, pine, jasmine, frankincense, bergamot, and all the citrus oils.

Perfume

Scent: Musky-amber, mellow, rich, warm, herbaceous, sweet; imperative in eau-de-Cologne. **Key qualities:** Relaxing, rejuvenating, balancing, inspiring, sedative (to the nervous system) revitalizing, aphrodisiac, intoxicating, euphoric, warming. **Odor intensity:** Medium–high.

Aromatherapy use

Skin care: Acne, boils, dandruff, hair loss, inflamed conditions, oily skin and hair, ulcers, wrinkles. **Circulation, muscles, and joints:** High blood pressure, muscular aches and pains. **Respiratory system:** Asthma, throat infections, whooping cough. **Digestive system:** Colic, cramp, dyspepsia, flatulence. **Reproductive system:** Amenorrhea, labor pain, dysmenorrhea, leukorrhea. **Nervous system:** Depression, frigidity, impotence, migraine, nervous tension, stress-related disorders.

WARNING
Nontoxic in normal use, but avoid during pregnancy. Do not use clary sage oil while drinking alcohol, since it can induce a narcotic effect, and exaggerated drunkenness.

Sandalwood

SANTALUM ALBUM FAMILY SANTALACEAE

Description A small, evergreen, parasitic tree, up to 30ft (9m) high, with brown-gray trunk, and many smooth, slender branches. It has small, pinky-purple flowers.

Actions Antidepressant, antiphlogistic, antiseptic, antispasmodic, aphrodisiac, astringent, bactericidal, carminative, cicatrizant, diuretic, expectorant, fungicidal, insecticide, sedative, tonic.

Extraction The oil is extracted by water or steam distillation from the powdered and dried roots and heartwood.

Characteristics A pale yellow, greenish or brownish, viscous liquid, with a deep, soft, sweet-woody, balsamic scent. It blends well with rose, clove, lavender, black pepper, bergamot, rosewood, geranium, benzoin, vetivert, patchouli, myrrh, and jasmine.

SAFETY DATA
Nontoxic, nonirritant, nonsensitizing.

Perfume

Scent: Dry-woody, amber, balsamic, musky, oriental, sensual, masculine, tenacious, warm. **Key qualities:** Aphrodisiac, soothing, relaxing, uplifting, purifying, warming, grounding, opening, elevating, sedative (to the nervous system). **Odor intensity:** Low–medium.

Aromatherapy use

Skin care: Acne; dry, cracked, and chapped skin, after-shave (for barber's rash), greasy skin, moisturizer. **Respiratory system:** Bronchitis, catarrh, coughs (dry, persistent), laryngitis, sore throat. **Digestive system:** Diarrhea, nausea. **Genitourinary system:** Cystitis. **Nervous system:** Depression, insomnia, nervous tension, stress-related complaints.

Benzoin

STYRAX BENZOIN FAMILY *STYRACACEAE*

Description A large tropical tree, up to 66ft (20m) high, with hard-shelled fruit. When cut, the trunk exudes a balsamic resin.

Actions Anti-inflammatory, antioxidant, antiseptic, astringent, carminative, cordial, deodorant, diuretic, expectorant, sedative, styptic, vulnerary.

Extraction Benzoin resinoid, or resin absolute, is prepared from the crude benzoin using solvents such as benzene and alcohol, which are then removed. Commercial benzoin is usually sold dissolved in ethyl glycol, or similar solvent.

Characteristics Benzoin resinoid is an orange-brown, viscous mass, with an intensely rich, sweet-balsamic odor. It blends well with sandalwood, rose, jasmine, frankincense, myrrh, cypress, juniper, lemon, coriander, and other spice oils.

WARNING
Do not use on babies. Nontoxic, nonirritant, but can cause possible sensitization due to the solvents used.

Perfume

Scent: Sweet, balsamic, vanilla-like, resinous, rich, intense. Acts as a fixative, and preservative.
Key qualities: Warming, energizing, uplifting, comforting, purifying, elevating, stimulant, soothing, antidepressant. **Odor intensity:** Medium.

Aromatherapy use

Skin care: Cuts, chapped skin, inflamed and irritated conditions. **Circulation, muscles, and joints:** Arthritis, gout, poor circulation, rheumatism. **Respiratory system:** Asthma, bronchitis, chills, colic, coughs, flu, laryngitis.
Nervous system: Nervous tension and general stress-related problems.

Clove bud

SYZYGIUM AROMATICUM FAMILY MYRTACEAE

Description A slender evergreen tree with a smooth, gray trunk, up to 40ft (12m) high. It has large bright green leaves, standing in pairs on short stalks. At the start of the rainy season, long buds appear, with a rosy-pink corolla at the tip; as the corolla fades, the calyx slowly turns deep red.

Actions Anthelmintic, antibiotic, antiemetic, antirheumatic, antineuralgic, antioxidant, antiseptic, antiviral, carminative, expectorant, larvicidal, spasmolytic, stimulant, stomachic, vermifuge.

Extraction The oil is obtained by water distillation from the flower buds.

Characteristics Clove bud oil is a pale yellow liquid, with a sweet-spicy odor that has a fruity, fresh top note. Used in perfumery, it blends well with rose, lavender, clary sage, bergamot, bay, and ylang ylang.

Perfume

Scent: Hot, fruity, floral, fresh, fragrant, peppery, sweet-spicy, diffusive, powerful, clean, medicinal, oriental. **Key qualities:** Tonic, stimulating, revitalizing, aphrodisiac, warming, comforting, purifying, active. **Odor intensity:** High.

WARNING
Use this oil in moderation only, and in low dilution (less than 1%).

SAFETY DATA
Clove bud oil can cause skin and mucous membrane irritation, and may cause dermatitis in some individuals. See Warning box.

Aromatherapy use

Skin care: Acne, athlete's foot, bruises, burns, cuts, toothache, ulcers, wounds. **Circulation, muscles, and joints:** Arthritis, rheumatism, sprains. **Respiratory system:** Asthma, bronchitis. **Digestive system:** Colic, dyspepsia, nausea. **Immune system:** Colds, flu, minor infections. **Other:** Insect repellent (mosquitoes).

Tagetes

TAGETES MINUTA FAMILY ASTERACEAE (COMPOSITAE)

Description A strongly scented annual herb, about 1ft (30cm) high, with bright orange, daisy-like flowers, and soft green feathery leaves.

Actions Anthelmintic, antispasmodic, bactericide, carminative, diaphoretic, emmenagogue, fungicidal, stomachic.

Extraction The oil is extracted by steam distillation from the fresh flowering herb.

Characteristics A dark orange or yellow, mobile liquid, which slowly solidifies on exposure to air and light. It has a bitter-green, herby odor, and blends well with clary sage, lavender, jasmine, bergamot, and other citrus oils in very small percentages.

WARNING
Use with care, and in moderation.

It is quite possible that the main constituent, tagetone, is toxic. There have been some reported cases of dermatitis with the tagetes species.

Perfume

Scent: Bitter-green, herbaceous, fruity, powerful, citrus-like. **Key qualities:** Penetrating, hypotensive, soothing, relaxing, narcotic (in excess). **Odor intensity:** Very high.

Aromatherapy use

Skin care: Bunions, calluses, corns, fungal infections.

Thyme, white

THYMUS VULGARIS. FAMILY *LAMIACEAE (LABIATAE)*

Description A perennial evergreen sub-shrub, up to 18in (45cm) high, with small, gray-green, oval, aromatic leaves, and pale purple or white flowers.

Actions Anthelmintic, antimicrobial, antioxidant, antirheumatic, antiseptic, antispasmodic, antitussive, antitoxic, astringent, bactericidal, balsamic, carminative, cicatrizant, diuretic, emmenagogue, expectorant, fungicidal, hypertensive, nervine, rubefacient, stimulant, sudorific, aphrodisiac, tonic, vermifuge.

Extraction The oil is extracted by water or steam distillation from the fresh, or partially dried, leaves and flowering tops.

Characteristics White thyme oil is a clear, pale yellow liquid, with a sweet, green-fresh scent. It blends well with bergamot, lemon, rosemary, melissa, lavender, marjoram, pine, and spice oils.

Perfume

Scent: Warm, spicy-herbaceous, powerful, penetrating, fresh, sporty, medicinal, green.
Key qualities (mind): Stimulating, restorative, warming, reviving, refreshing, purifying, antidepressant. **Odor intensity:** High.

Aromatherapy use

Skin care: Abscess, acne, bruises, burns, cuts, dermatitis, eczema, insect bites, lice.
Circulation, muscles, and joints: Arthritis, gout, muscular aches and pains, obesity, edema, poor circulation, rheumatism, sprains.
Respiratory system: Asthma, bronchitis, catarrh, coughs, laryngitis, sinusitis, tonsillitis.
Digestive system: Diarrhea, dyspepsia, flatulence. **Immune system:** Chills, colds, flu, infectious diseases. **Urinary system:** Cystitis, urethritis. **Nervous system:** Headaches, insomnia, and stress-related complaints.

WARNING
Some thyme oils contain large amounts of toxic phenols. Use all thyme oils in moderation and in low dilution. Avoid during pregnancy.

Spruce, hemlock

TSUGA CANADENSIS FAMILY PINACEAE

Description A large evergreen tree up to 164ft (50m) tall, with slender horizontal branches, finely toothed leaves and smallish brown cones, which yields a natural exudation from its bark.

Actions Antimicrobial, antiseptic, antitussive, astringent, decongestant, diaphoretic, diuretic, expectorant, nervine, rubefacient, tonic.

Extraction Essential oil by steam distillation from the needles and twigs.

Characteristics A colorless or pale yellow liquid with a pleasing, fresh-balsamic, sweet-fruity odor. It blends well with pine, oakmoss, cedarwood, galbanum, benzoin, lavender, lavandin, and rosemary.

Perfume

Scent: Fresh, crisp, evergreen, woody, earthy, balsamic. **Key qualities:** Invigorating, energizing, calming, clearing, elevating, grounding, stimulating, fortifying. **Odor intensity:** Medium.

SAFETY DATA
Nontoxic, nonirritant, nonsensitizing.

Aromatherapy use

Circulation, muscles, and joints: Muscular aches and pains, poor circulation, rheumatism. **Respiratory system:** Asthma, bronchitis, coughs, respiratory weakness. **Immune system:** Colds, flu, infections. **Nervous system:** Anxiety, stress-related conditions.

Fenugreek

TRIGONELLA FOENUM-GRAECUM FAMILY *FABACEAE*

Description
An annual plant reaching a height of 20in (50cm) with trifoliate, bright green leaves. It blossoms during the summer season and produces beautiful small white flowers. The leaves' fragrance slightly resembles lovage and the brownish-yellow seeds are a distinctive cuboid shape.

Actions
Antioxidant, anti-inflammatory, antiviral, aphrodisiac, bactericidal, carminative, demulcent, expectorant, laxative, nervine, stomachic.

Extraction
Essential oil by steam distillation from the seeds. A fixed oil is also pressed from the seeds.

Characteristics
Pale yellow to light brown liquid with a bitter, spicy scent. It blends well with sandalwood, clove, cinnamon, cardamom, and other spice oils.

SAFETY DATA
The oil may cause skin irritation: dilute well before use. Avoid use during pregnancy, since it has the potential to induce labor.

Perfume

Scent: Potent, sweet-spicy, earthy.
Key qualities: Rejunvenating, aphrodesiac, strengthening. **Odor intensity:** High.

Aromatherapy use

Skin care: Boils, burns, boils, eczema, hair care (dandruff and hair loss), scars, wrinkles.
Circulation, muscles, and joints: Aching limbs, arthritis, cramp, gout, high blood pressure, muscle spasm. **Digestive system:** Indigestion, heartburn. **Respiratory system:** Bronchitis, colds, congestion, fever, sinusitis.
Genitourinary system: Menstrual cramps, PMS, hot flushes and mood fluctuations.
Immune system: Helps fight infections.
Nervous system: Anxiety, insomnia, hypertension, stress, soothes the heart.

Valerian

VALERIANA OFFICINALIS, FAMILY VALERIANACEAE

Description A perennial herb, up to 5ft (1.5m) high, with a hollow, erect stem, deeply dissected dark leaves, and many purplish-white flowers. It has short, thick, grayish roots, showing above ground; these have a strong odor.

Actions Anodyne (mild), antidandruff, antidiuretic, antispasmodic, bactericidal, carminative, depressant of the central nervous system, hypnotic, hypotensive, regulator, sedative, stomachic.

Extraction The oil is extracted by steam distillation from the roots.

Characteristics An olive to brown liquid, darkening with age, with a warm-woody, balsamic, musky odor; fresh oils have a green top note. It blends well with patchouli, pine, lavender, cedarwood, mandarin, petitgrain, and rosemary.

Perfume

Scent: Warm, woody, balsamic, musky, earthy, green. **Key qualities (mind):** Sedative (mental and nervous), depressant of the central nervous system, mildly hypnotic, regulator, calming, soothing, grounding. **Odor intensity:** Very high.

Aromatherapy use

Nervous system: Insomnia, nervous indigestion, migraine, restlessness, tension states.

WARNING
In large amounts, valerian can cause headaches, mental agitation, and delusions. Use in moderation, and do not use over long periods of time (more than a month) without a break. Nontoxic, nonirritant, but can cause possible sensitization.

Vanilla

VANILLA PLANIFOLIA FAMILY *ORCHIDACEAE*

Description A perennial herbaceous climbing vine up to 80ft (25m) high, with green stems and large white flowers that have a deep narrow trumpet. The green capsules or fruits are ready to pick after eight or nine months on the plant, and then have to be "cured." The immature vanilla pod (or bean) which is 5.5in (14cm) to 8.5in (22cm) long, has to be fermented and dried to turn it into the fragrant brown vanilla pods of commerce—a process that can take up to six months to complete. During the drying process vanillin can accumulate as white crystals on the surface of the bean.

Actions Balsamic.

Extraction A resinoid (often called an oleoresin) by solvent extraction from the "cured" vanilla beans. (An absolute is occasionally produced by further extraction from the resinoid.)

Characteristics A viscous dark brown liquid with a rich, sweet, balsamic, vanilla-like odor. It blends well with sandalwood, vetiver, opopanax, benzoin, balsams, and spice oils.

Perfume

Scent: Rich, sweet, balsamic, vanilla-like. **Key qualities:** Aphrodesiac, comforting, calming. **Odor intensity:** High.

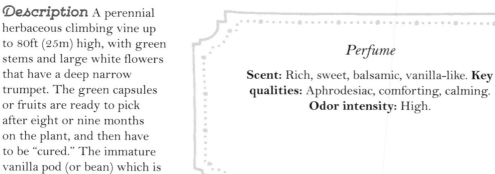

Aromatherapy use

None.
Other: Used in pharmaceutical products as a flavoring agent. Used as a fragrance ingredient in perfumes, especially oriental types. Widely used to flavor tobacco and as a food flavoring, mainly in ice cream, yogurt, and chocolate.

SAFETY DATA
Nontoxic, common sensitizing agent. Widely adulterated.

WHEN VANILLA IS GROWN, THE DEEP, TRUMPET-SHAPED FLOWERS HAVE TO BE HAND-POLLINATED—EXCEPT IN MEXICO WHERE NATIVE HUMMINGBIRDS DO MOST OF THE WORK!

Vetivert

VETIVERIA ZIZANOIDES/ANDROPOGON MURICATUS FAMILY POACEAE (GRAMINEAE)

Description A tall, tufted, perennial, scented grass, with a straight stem, long, narrow leaves, and an abundant, complex lacework of undergound white rootlets.

Actions Antiseptic, antispasmodic, depurative, rubefacient, sedative (to the nervous system), stimulant (circulatory, and to blood itself), tonic, vermifuge.

Extraction The oil is extracted by steam distillation from the roots and rootlets—which have been washed, chopped, dried, and soaked.

Characteristics A dark brown, olive, or amber, viscous oil, with deep, smoky, earthy-woody odor, and a sweet, persistent undertone. The color and scent can vary according to the source. It blends well with sandalwood, rose, jasmine, patchouli, lavender, clary sage, and ylang ylang.

SAFETY DATA
Nontoxic, nonirritant, nonsensitizing.

Perfume

Scent: Smoky, rich, earthy, dry-woody, sweet, green, diffusive, masculine, sporty, warm.
Key qualities: Sedative (nervous and mental), soothing, calming, tonic (nervous), grounding, uplifting, protective. **Odor intensity:** High.

Aromatherapy use

Skin care: Acne, cuts, oily skin, wounds.
Circulation, muscles, and joints: Arthritis, muscular aches and pains, rheumatism, sprains, stiffness. **Nervous system:** Debility, depression, insomnia, nervous tension—known as the oil of tranquillity.

Violet

VIOLA ODORATA FAMILY VIOLACEAE

Description A small, tender, perennial plant with dark green, heart-shaped leaves, fragrant violet-blue flowers, and an oblique underground rhizome.

Actions Analgesic (mild), anti-inflammatory, antirheumatic, antiseptic, decongestant (liver), diuretic, expectorant, laxative, soporific, stimulant (circulation).

Extraction A concrete and absolute from fresh leaves and flowers.

Characteristics The leaf absolute is an intense dark green viscous liquid with a strong green-leaf odor and a delicate floral undertone. The flower absolute is a yellowish-green viscous liquid with a sweet, rich, floral fragrance, characteristic of the fresh flowers. It blends well with tuberose, clary sage, boronia, tarragon, cumin, hop, basil, hyacinth, and other florals.

SAFETY DATA
Nontoxic, nonirritant, possible sensitization in some individuals.

Perfume

Scent: Earthy, green notes, sweet, delicate, floral. **Key qualities:** Comforting, calming, relaxing, soothing, inspirational. **Odor intensity:** High.

Aromatherapy use

Skin care: Acne, eczema, refines the pores, thread veins, wounds. **Circulation, muscles, and joints:** Fibrosis, poor circulation, rheumatism. **Respiratory system:** Bronchitis, catarrh, mouth and throat infections.
Nervous system: Dizziness, headaches, insomnia, nervous exhaustion—the scent was traditionally believed to comfort and strengthen the heart.

Plai

ZINGIBER CASSUMUNAR FAMILY *ZINGIBERACEAE*

Description The root of this tropical perennial plant is tuberous, with long fleshy fibers and jointed appendages, much like ginger but slightly larger. The fresh rhizome, which is yellow inside, has a cool, green, camphoraceous, spicy-warm scent. The stem is made of green leaf sheaths which are grass-like with brownish-purple pointed shoots bearing pale yellow flowers.

Actions Analgesic, antioxidant, antibacterial, antimicrobial, antihistamine, antineuralgic, antifungal, anti-inflammatory, antiseptic, antispasmodic, antitoxic, antiviral, carminative, digestive, diuretic, febrifugal, laxative, rubefacient, rejuvenating, stimulant, tonic, vermifuge.

Extraction Steam distilled from the fresh rhizome (roots) of the Plai plant (*Zingiber cassumunar*).

Characteristics The oil is a pale amber color with a fresh, herbaceous, spicy-green scent and a resinous, slightly floral undertone. It will blend well with black pepper, bergamot, ginger, grapefruit, lemongrass, lime, jasmine, lavender, neroli, petitgrain, rosemary, sandalwood, and tea tree.

Perfume

Scent: Herbaceous, fresh, earthy, spicy, bright, peppery. **Key qualities:** Energizing, balancing, grounding, protective, soothing, cooling, anti-aging, uplifting. **Odor intensity:** Medium.

Aromatherapy use

Skin care: Acne, cuts, stretch marks, scars, wounds. **Circulation, muscles, and joints:** All types of aches and pains caused by inflammation, including arthritis and rheumatism, cramp, gout, joint problems, muscle spasm, sprains and strains, torn muscles and ligaments, as well as post-operative pain. **Digestive system:** Cramps, colic, constipation, diarrhea, flatulence, indigestion, heartburn. **Respiratory system:** Asthma, catarrh, chronic colds, bronchitis, congestion, fever, flu, sinusitis. **Genitourinary system:** Menstrual cramps. **Immune system:** Stimulates the immune system and boosts vitality. **Nervous system:** Anxiety, nervous tension, stress.

SAFETY DATA
Nontoxic, nonirritating, and nonsensitizing.

Ginger

ZINGIBER OFFICINALE FAMILY ZINGIBERACEAE

Description An erect perennial herb, up to 3ft (1m) high, with a thick, spreading, tuberous rhizomatous root, which is very pungent. The green, reed-like stalk, with narrow, spear-shaped leaves, and white or yellow flowers grows up from the root.

Actions Analgesic, antioxidant, antiseptic, antispasmodic, aperitif, aphrodisiac, bactericidal, carminative, cephalic, expectorant, febrifuge, laxative, rubifacient, stimulant, stomachic, tonic.

Extraction The oil is extracted by steam distillation from the unpeeled, dried, ground root.

Characteristics A pale yellow, amber, or greenish liquid, with a warm, slightly green, fresh, woody-spicy scent. It blends well with sandalwood, vetiver, patchouli, frankincense, rosewood, cedarwood, coriander, rose, lime, neroli, orange, and lemon.

SAFETY DATA
Nontoxic, nonirritant (except in high concentration), but may cause some sensitization—use in low dilutions only. Slightly phototoxic.

Perfume

Scent: Fresh, woody-spicy, rich, slightly green, peppery, fiery, penetrating, diffusive, exotic. **Key qualities:** Tonic, aphrodisiac, stimulating, warming, cephalic, comforting. **Odor intensity:** High.

Aromatherapy use

Circulation, muscles, and joints: Arthritis, fatigue, muscular aches and pains, poor circulation, rheumatism, sprains, strains. **Respiratory system:** Catarrh, congestion, coughs, sinusitis, sore throat. **Digestive system:** Diarrhea, colic, cramp, flatulence, indigestion, loss of appetite, nausea, travel sickness. **Immune system:** Chills, colds, flu, fever, infectious disease. **Nervous system:** Debility, nervous exhaustion.

Sourcing oils

It's a good idea to buy essential oils from a practicing aromatherapist when you are still learning. Once you are familiar, you can source many oils online. See the resources listed on page 395.

PART FIVE

♡

Index of Carrier Oils

Index of carrier oils

CARRIER OILS ARE USED in aromatherapy practice as standard bases for making blends in combination with essential oils, in making massage lotions, facial serums, or other aromatic products. But what exactly is a "carrier oil" or "base oil" as they are known in aromatherapy practice? This can be a confusing matter because the term "oil" is often used indiscriminately for several distinct types of product.

In this chapter we are not talking about essential oils (such as lavender oil) or aromatic absolutes (such as jasmine oil), as these are volatile substances, whereas all the carrier oils are "fixed" in nature. This means that if you spill a little of a fixed oil on your sleeve it will stain your garment, whereas an essential oil, which is naturally volatile, will gradually evaporate leaving no mark.

Nevertheless both essential oils and fixed oils are "hydrophobic," meaning they both repel water, so they are very compatible with each other. This is why fixed oils are commonly used as carriers for essential oils in products like massage oil blends or facial serums. The fixed oils can be divided into several different types:

♡ Vegetable oils (such as sweet almond oil)
♡ Liquid wax (such as jojoba oil)
♡ Infused herbal oils (such as calendula oil)

VEGETABLE OILS

The vegetable oils, which are made up of liquid lipids or fats, are further divided into two main types: those containing mainly saturated fats and those containing mainly nonsaturated fats.

Saturated oils, sometimes called "vegetable fats," tend to be solid at room temperature, such as coconut oil. In terms of the healing benefits, saturated fats (and especially the "trans" fats which refer to those found in processed foods) are usually considered to be bad for the health. However, the naturally occurring saturated fats found in coconut oil actually have some amazing health benefits, including lowering cholesterol, increasing metabolism as well as having superb skin and hair conditioner properties. Coconut also has a very long shelf life.

Unsaturated oils tend to be liquid at room temperature and are well known for their nutrition-rich, health-giving properties. The highest quality unsaturated vegetable oils are cold-pressed from the fatty fruits, nuts, and seeds whose names they bear. Oils such as olive, apricot kernel, grapeseed, and avocado are not only commonly used for their culinary and nutritional benefits, but are also frequently used in herbal preparations, natural cosmetics, and skin products due to their healing qualities.

LIQUID WAX

Jojoba "oil" belongs in a class of its own: a liquid wax produced from the seed of the Jojoba plant (*Simmondsia chinensis*), which is a shrub native to the southern regions of North America. The terms jojoba "oil" and jojoba "wax" are often used interchangeably because the wax visually appears to be like a mobile oil. It is a very valuable healing substance, especially for skin care, where its unique composition accounts for its amazing shelf-life stability compared with true vegetable oils. It also displays an extraordinary resistance to high temperatures.

INFUSED HERBAL OILS

In the context of aromatherapy, "infused oils" are another important form of herbal preparation, usually intended primarily for use on the skin. To make infused herbal oils like calendula or St. John's wort, a traditional process called "digestion" is used: this involves a very low heat, prolonged extraction technique designed to draw out the plant's bioactive compounds. In this process, the herb is steeped in a vegetable oil base (the "menstruum"), such as olive oil or sunflower oil, over a period of time. Gradually, the active therapeutic compounds of the herb dissolve into the base oil, so the resulting infused oil represents a whole herb extract of the plant, where the individual herbs impart their healing properties to the resulting infused oil.

In aromatherapy practice, the use of specific carrier oils, when used skillfully, can add tremendous nutritional value and a whole range of health benefits alongside those of the essential oils, when employed in blends. This is especially valuable in the context of skin care, due to the fact that many of the fixed oils contain high levels of vitamins, minerals, and fatty acids that are essential for keeping the skin looking radiant and youthful.

FATTY ACIDS

Fatty acids are lipid components that play a major role in the construction of cell membranes throughout the human body, including the skin. There are many types of fatty acids: saturated fatty acids, monounsaturated fatty acids, and polyunsaturated fatty acids.

Saturated fatty acids are mainly of animal origin, and are found in butter and cream as well as in vegetable oils, like palm oil. They facilitate cholesterol deposits in the arteries and, as a consequence, cardiovascular disease.

Unsaturated fatty acids are mainly found in vegetable products including vegetable oils, as well as oily fish like salmon, sardines, or tuna. They are especially healthy and help protect the cardiovascular system as well as playing a vital role in the health of the skin. A list of the principal fatty acids and their benefits can be found on page 384.

Key to symbols

Icons in the top right corner of every page in this section indicate the parts of plants that each oil is extracted from. There is also a symbol to indicate oils that are recommended for children.

TREE

FRUIT

FLOWERS

SEEDS

PARTS OF PLANTS

ROOTS

RESIN

WHOLE PLANT

LEAVES

GOOD FOR CHILDREN

Argan oil

ARGANIA SPINOSA

Description This precious oil, which is extracted from the nut of a small tree native to Morocco, has long been recognized throughout the Middle East for its cosmetic value.

Actions Anti-aging, antibacterial, antidandruff, anti-inflammatory, antioxidant, antisebum (regulates sebum levels), cicatrizant (wound-healing), emollient, hypo-allergenic.

Extraction A premium quality oil is 100% organically produced, and cold pressed from the kernels of the argan tree.

Characteristics This pale yellow oil has a luxurious, silky texture, which makes the skin feel smooth and soft, even after a single application! It is quickly absorbed by the skin, imparting a visible moisturizing effect, but without leaving behind any oily residue.

Skin Types Beneficial for all skin types: dry, cracked skin; oily or blemished skin; mature and aging skin, sensitive skin (children and babies), as well as combination skin.

Nutritional Value It is very rich in antioxidants, vitamins A and E, squalane, phytosterols, and essential fatty acids, including linoleic acid and oleic acid, plus it contains many bioactive, micronutrients.

Aromatherapy Use

Argan oil is renowned for its skin moisturizing and repairing properties. It is a perfect oil to use in body or massage oils or in a facial serum for reducing fine lines and wrinkles. Argan is also a natural anti-inflammatory and helps to balance sebum production in oily skins, reducing acne. Used in body oils, it increases dermal elasticity leaving the skin feeling firmer with an overall smoother appearance. Argan is also beneficial for promoting hair health and growth, leaving it silky, shiny and soft.

Skin Care: This oil is particularly rich in Vitamins A and E, as well as being packed with powerful antioxidants, such as linoleic acid, which help hold back the aging process. It also promotes cellular regeneration, which is vital for mature skin by reducing the appearance of fine wrinkles. At the same time, its healing qualities help eliminate scars, stretch marks, age spots, and blemishes.

Argan oil balances excessive sebum levels, thus helping to regulate oily skin and prevent the occurrence of acne, blackheads, or spots. As an anti-inflammatory, the oil can also help soothe skin infections and rashes, such as after shaving, and sunburn. Being very gentle and pure, it is also suited to sensitive skin, so can be applied even to the most delicate areas, such as around the eyes, and be used for children. In this sense, it is a truly all-purpose skin-care oil, which is suitable and beneficial for all skin types!

Hair Care: The nutritional effect of this oil makes it an excellent hair conditioner and being nongreasy, the oil can even be left in to further "feed" the scalp, giving the hair shine and body. Argan oil can promote hair growth when massaged into the scalp on a regular basis. To make a quick-fix hair conditioner, just put a single drop into the palm after washing and towel dry the hair, then massage it thoroughly into the roots and scalp. For dry or brittle hair, it is best to give the hair a more intensive and in-depth treat by using a few drops of oil applied as an overnight treatment.

It is also excellent as a beard conditioning treatment and to help eliminate shaving rashes.

SAFETY DATA
Avoid contact with eyes. Argan oil should be avoided by those with nut allergies.

Tips

♥ To give the complexion a natural daily glow, simply put a couple of drops into the palm and then apply the oil to the entire facial area and neck using gentle circular stokes.

♥ Apply generously to cracked heels or brittle nails to repair them fast.

FCC Statement:

CAUTION: Changes or modifications not expressly approved by the party responsible for compliance could void the user's authority to operate the equipment

NOTE: This equipment has been tested and found to comply with the limits for a Class B digital device, pursuant to part 15 of the FCC Rules. These limits are designed to provide reasonable protection against harmful interference in a residential installation. This equipment generates, uses and can radiate radio frequency energy and, if not installed and used in accordance with the instructions, may cause harmful interference to radio communications. However, there is no guarantee that interference will not occur in a particular installation. If this equipment does cause harmful interference to radio or television reception, which can be determined by turning the equipment off and on, the user is encouraged to try to correct the interference by one or more of the following measures:

- Reorient or relocate the receiving antenna.
- Increase the separation between the equipment and receiver.
- Connect the equipment into an outlet on a circuit different from that to which the receiver is connected.
- Consult the dealer or an experienced radio/TV technician for help.

FCC Statement:

CAUTION: Changes or modifications not expressly approved by the party responsible for compliance could void the user's authority to operate the equipment

NOTE: This equipment has been tested and found to comply with the limits for a Class B digital device, pursuant to part 15 of the FCC Rules. These limits are designed to provide reasonable protection against harmful interference in a residential installation. This equipment generates, uses and can radiate radio frequency energy and, if not installed and used in accordance with the instructions, may cause harmful interference to radio communications. However, there is no guarantee that interference will not occur in a particular installation. If this equipment does cause harmful interference to radio or television reception, which can be determined by turning the equipment off and on, the user is encouraged to try to correct the interference by one or more of the following measures:

• Reorient or relocate the receiving antenna.

• Increase the separation between the equipment and receiver.

• Connect the equipment into an outlet on a circuit different from that to which the receiver is connected.

• Consult the dealer or an experienced radio/TV technician for help.

Borage oil

BORAGO OFFICINALIS

Description Borage, or "starflower," is an annual plant native to the Mediterranean region. All parts of the plant, including the beautiful blue flowers, have been used in food and drink for centuries.

Actions Anti-arthritic, antidandruff, anti-inflammatory, antioxidant, cicatrizant (wound-healing), emollient, hypo-allergenic, immune stimulant.

Characteristics A light orange, slightly viscous oil with a relatively strong odor.

Skin Types Excellent for very dry, sun-damaged, aged and mature skins; also good for skin conditions such as dermatitis, cradle cap, and eczema.

Nutritional Value Borage seed oil contains 17–28% gamma-linoleic acid (GLA), the richest known source. The oil also contains several other beneficial fatty acids, mainly oleic acid (16–20%) and linoleic acid (35–38%).

Aromatherapy Use

A valuable anti-inflammatory oil for conditions such as rheumatoid arthritis when applied topically on a regular basis, especially when combined with essential oils in an aromatherapy massage. Particularly useful added to body oil blends where stress is also implicated, and makes an excellent ingredient in facial serums due to its powerful regenerative properties.

Skin Care: Borage oil is invaluable for promoting cellular skin regeneration due to its high gamma-linoleic acid (GLA) content. In fact, it has the highest concentration of the omega-6 essential fatty acids including GLA of any oil, making it the richest plant source of essential fatty acids! As such, it can be used as an effective anti-aging treatment all on its own, or can be added to facial oils or serums as a "booster" oil, especially for its rejuvenating effect. It can also quickly restore moisture and elasticity to dry or sun-damaged skin as well as having a healing effect on inflammatory skin disorders such as eczema and dermatitis, which are caused by deficiencies in skin lipids or natural oils.

Hair Care: An excellent restorative hair conditioner, imparting moisture to dried or over-treated hair. Massaging borage oil into the scalp can help reduce follicular inflammation, thus helping to prevent hair loss and encourage new growth. It can also help to eliminate dandruff, itchy scalp conditions, and seborrhoeic dermatitis, a common condition in infants known as "cradle cap," when massaged into the scalp regularly.

SAFETY DATA
Avoid contact with eyes.

Tips

♡ Apply a few drops of borage oil directly to patches of sun-damaged skin, scaly skin (including cradle cap), and to sunspots for its healing effect.

Calendula oil
CALENDULA ARVENSIS

Description Calendula oil is derived from the marigold, a common herbaceous plant grown in gardens throughout the world due to its bright orange or yellow flowers. An annual herb, it is naturalized across western Europe, south-eastern Asia and the Mediterranean.

Actions Anti-aging, antifungal, anti-inflammatory, antioxidant, cicatrizant (wound-healing), antiseptic, emollient, nourishing.

Extraction A good-quality oil should be infused in a base, or "menstruum," and then filtered without the use of solvents. The resulting product is an oily extract containing the lipid soluble active principals of the marigold flowers in the base oil. Sunflower oil makes a particularly good menstruum, as it has been shown that the healing acids within calendula display greater antimicrobial and antiviral effects when combined with sunflower oil.

Characteristics A bright yellow, oily liquid with a consistency that depends on the base oil, or menstruum, used for the infusion.

Skin types Excellent for dry, mature skin types. Also for the treatment of a wide range of skin conditions including blemishes, burns, bruises, rashes, sunburn, minor cuts, insect bites, scars, and stretch marks.

Nutritional Value Rich in calendulin, beta-carotene, waxes, and Vitamins A, C, and E; the fatty acid "linoleic acid" is also found in high concentrations. The petals contain especially high levels of anti-oxidants in the form of carotenoids and flavonoids.

Tips

♥ Apply to the skin directly after sun exposure to prevent damage.

Aromatherapy Use

A popular skin-care oil, which is particularly helpful for irritated or inflamed conditions. It helps soothe and reduce the pain of muscle spasm, sprained muscles, or bruises when applied locally, while helping lessen any swelling.

Skin Care: Traditionally known as a good wound healer, calendula has been used for centuries to treat scarred or damaged skin, due to its excellent healing effect. It does this by increasing the blood flow and oxygen to wounds or infected areas, so the skin grows new tissue in response and thus heals more rapidly.

Calendula oil is a great moisturizer for all types of dry skin conditions. As such, it is especially valuable for severely chapped areas such as on the hands or feet, or to soften patches of rough skin. Being mild and gentle, it is particularly recommended for healing eczema, dermatitis, nappy rash, or other irritated skin conditions for those with delicate or sensitive skin, including children. It has anti-fungal properties too, so can help clear up infections like ringworm and athlete's foot.

Calendula is also used to improve skin firmness and hydration. As a potent anti-oxidant and having rejuvenating properties, calendula is valuable in the care and treatment of aging skin, by repairing skin tissue rapidly. Calendula's restorative properties deeply hydrate the skin and make it look younger and more supple. It can also be used on the delicate areas around the eyes to treat puffiness.

Hair Care: Calendula oil, when applied regularly, helps hydrate the scalp and eliminate dandruff. Its regenerative properties enable the hair follicles to grow more quickly, encouraging healthier hair.

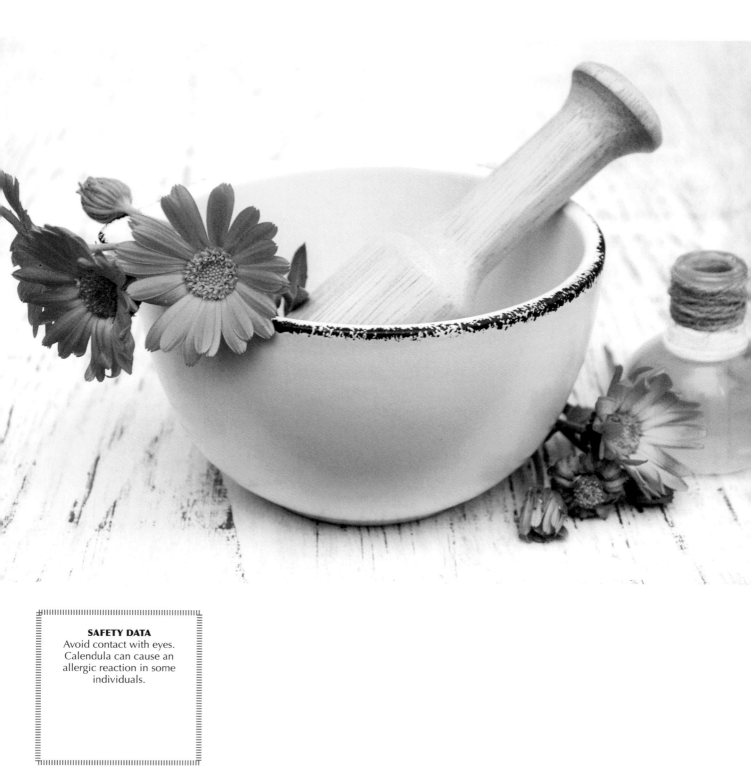

Coconut oil

COCOS NUCIFERA

Description The coconut is a common tropical palm tree with large leathery leaves, found in warm regions throughout the world. The coconut (truly a "drupe"), which has a rough hairy shell, is produced in clusters and is used to produce several different edible products including coconut milk, water, flesh, and oil.

Actions Anti-aging, antibacterial, antidandruff, antifungal, anti-inflammatory, antioxidant, antisebum (regulates sebum levels), antiviral, cicatrizant (wound-healing), emollient, hypoallergenic, immune stimulant, moisturizing.

Extraction Coconut oil is made from the dried fleshy part of the coconut called "copra," which is cold-pressed to extract the pure coconut oil. Organic virgin coconut oil is the least refined of all the graded oils. However, because it solidifies at cool temperatures, the fraction of the oil that remains mobile at room temperature can also be poured off to create another product, known as light coconut oil.

Characteristics Virgin coconut oil is solid at temperatures below 75°F (24°C), but it remains a liquid at higher temperatures, having a pleasing coconut aroma. Light coconut oil remains mobile at room temperature and is odorless. For consumption, most nutritionists recommend using organic virgin coconut oil, but light coconut oil provides most of the health benefits found in virgin coconut oil and is a more generally versatile product for cosmetic use.

Skin Types Dry, mature, sun-damaged skin as well as for oily skin, acne, and dermatitis. Coconut oil is also good for sensitive skin and is safe for babies.

Nutritional Value Coconut oil contains over 80% saturated fats where 45–55% of this is lauric acid; also rich in caprylic acid and other natural fats plus squalane and Vitamin E.

Tips

♡ Light coconut oil is colorless, odorless, and will not stain or go rancid, so it makes an ideal base for making up home blends or perfumes. As it is absorbed easily and quickly, it also makes a perfect quick, all-in-one cleanser, moisturizer, and makeup remover.

SAFETY DATA
Avoid contact with eyes. Coconut is not a true nut, but a "drupe," so coconut products are usually safe for those with nut allergies.

Aromatherapy Use

Coconut oil melts on the skin and is easily absorbed without leaving a greasy residue. It therefore makes a fantastic all-purpose moisturizer, which is high in Vitamin E and healthy fatty acids. It has been used for centuries, traditionally to nourish and condition both skin and hair. The powerful anti-oxidants in coconut have good anti-aging properties, while its anti-inflammatory action can help relieve arthritis when applied locally in massage or body oils. The high percentage of lauric acid in coconut oil also increases the body's natural immunity.

Skin Care: The plentiful healthy fatty acids in coconut oil enable the skin to heal and repair itself fast, which is of great value in preventing premature signs of aging, such as fine lines, wrinkles, or sunspots. These often occur as a result of over exposure to UV rays, environmental pollution, and the use of harsh chemical products. Coconut oil is very gentle on the skin, acting as a physical barrier to environmental pollutants, while sealing in moisture. Its anti-oxidant action also helps reduce damage from external stress, plus it keeps the skin elastic, smooth, and supple by promoting collagen formation. Used regularly, coconut oil can thus protect the skin from the signs of aging by protecting and healing it from damage caused by sun exposure and other environmental factors.

Due to its healing effects, coconut oil can also be used to soothe a range of skin conditions, such as atopic dermatitis, eczema, and rashes. The oil has natural antibacterial properties, making it valuable for oily skin and acne. The feather-light emollient property of light coconut oil especially provides a soothing barrier without clogging the pores in the case of blemished skin. In addition, the antimicrobial properties of coconut help fight fungal skin conditions such as ringworm, athlete's foot, or nail infections.

Hair Care: Coconut oil provides protection for the hair against the sun's ultraviolet rays, and is able to penetrate deep into the hair shaft making it an efficient hair conditioner. Used regularly, coconut oil improves overall hair health as well as helping to eliminate dandruff or dry scalp problems. Simply massage one tablespoon of coconut oil into the hair roots and leave it on for 2-3 hours before shampooing.

St. John's wort oil

HYPERICUM PERFORATUM

Description A small, shrubby perennial plant with bright yellow 5-petaled flowers, which according to folklore was named after St. John the Baptist. Native to Europe, Asia, and North Africa, it is now common in many temperate regions of the world.

Actions Anti-aging, antifungal, anti-inflammatory, antioxidant, cicatrizant (wound-healing), antiseptic, antiviral, astringent, emollient, nourishing, vulnerary.

Extraction A high-quality oil should be made from the flowering tops infused in a base oil, or menstruum, (such as sunflower oil) and then cold-pressed and filtered without the use of solvents. The resulting product is an oily extract containing the soluble active principals of St. John's wort in the base oil.

Characteristics A bright red oil with an oily texture and a herbal odor, which takes on a strong blood-red color when exposed to sunlight.

Skin Types Recommended for dry, sensitive, and mature skin, particularly damaged or scarred skin, as well as for piles, varicose veins, or thread veins.

Nutritional Value The main active ingredient is "hypericin" which is found in the flowers. It has plentiful amounts of oleic acid (64.8%), linoleic acid (26.3%), as well as palmitic, linolenic, and stearic fatty acids. It also contains Vitamins A, B1, B2, B6, and D, plus tannins and minerals.

Tips

♡ Apply St. John's wort oil directly to the site of the problem in cases of capillary damage to delicate skin, including piles, varicose veins, or thread veins.

Aromatherapy Use

St. John's wort oil makes a valuable massage oil applied locally, as it helps ease muscular strain and tension. Massaged directly onto aching muscles and joints, it helps ease pain, including from gout, over-activity at sports, or due to growing pains. It is commonly used in herbal medicine in the treatment of nerve pain, such as sciatica, as well as for depression and anxiety. Its unique chemical composition has also been shown to help regulate hormonal imbalance in menopausal women, thus reducing mood swings, irritability, depression, and stress.

Skin Care: Used in body and facial oils, it can help ease a range of skin problems due to its natural healing and anti-inflammatory properties. St. John's wort oil has a strong vulnerary action, which means it helps the skin to regenerate and heal itself. Traditionally used as a wound-healing salve, this oil is good for the treatment of all types of inflamed and damaged skin conditions including sunburn, bruises, cuts, minor burns, and scrapes. St. John's wort can be used to help remedy fragile skin problems such as thread veins or varicose veins. Applied to existing wounds or scars, including stretch marks, it can also reduce scarring.

Anti-oxidant and having rejuvenating properties, St. Johns wort oil is valuable in the care and treatment of aging skin, repairing skin tissue rapidly. It is especially suited to dry, delicate, and mature complexions, helping the skin look smoother and plumper by hydrating the skin from within, thus reducing the appearance of fine lines and wrinkles.

Hair Care: St. John's wort is known to defend the hair against sun damage: apply directly to the hair to provide protection before sun exposure.

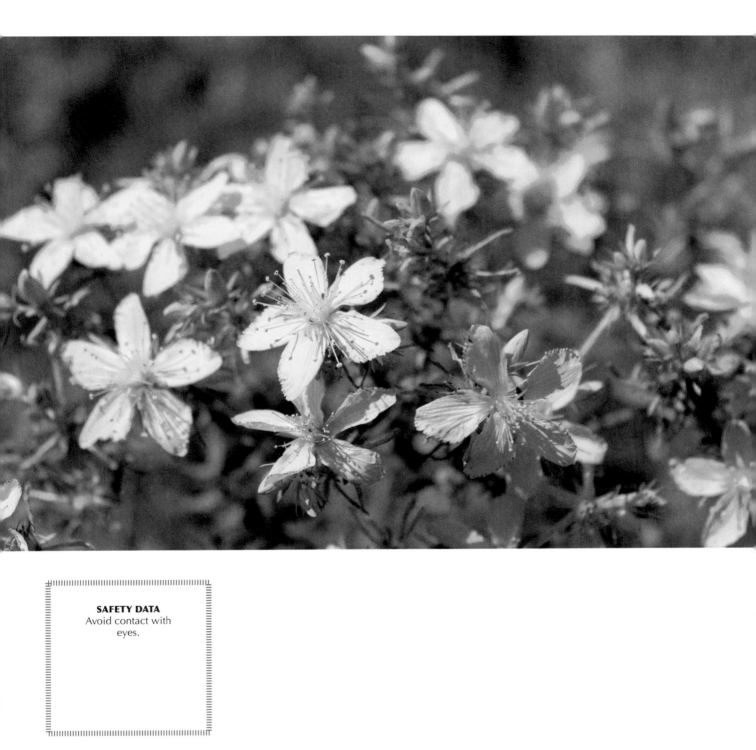

Evening primrose oil

OENOTHERA BIENNIS

Description Evening primrose is a biennial plant with attractive, bright yellow flowers, which have a slight lemony scent. Oblong seedpods contain many small seeds from which the oil is extracted. Originating from Mexico, it can now be found growing all over the world in temperate climates including Europe and America.

Actions Anti-aging, anti-inflammatory, antioxidant, cicatrizant (wound-healing), antiseptic, emollient, nourishing.

Extraction A good-quality oil should be cold-pressed and naturally filtered, without the use of solvents, from the seeds of the flowers.

Characteristics A pale yellow, exceptionally finely textured oil with superb moisturizing properties, being quickly and easily absorbed. It has a relatively short shelf life compared to other carrier oils.

Skin Types Dry, mature, or sun-damaged skin; also especially valuable in the treatment of acne, eczema, psoriasis, rosacea, and dermatitis.

Nutritional Value This oil is particularly plentiful in essential omega-6 fatty acids: linoleic (70%) and gamma-linoleic acid (10%), plus others including alpha-linoleic acid, beta-linoleic acid, stearic acid, and aspartic acid. It is also rich in Vitamin C and the minerals: potassium, magnesium, manganese, ammonia, copper, boron, iron, zinc, calcium, and phosphorus.

Tips

♡ Massage a few drops of the oil into the cuticles regularly: the rich fatty acids in evening primrose not only prevent brittle nails from cracking but also make them strong and healthy.

Aromatherapy Use

Evening primrose contains a high concentration of the fatty acid gamma-linoleic acid (or GLA) along with other fatty acids, and it is this factor that is largely responsible for the remarkable healing properties of this oil. Used in massage or body oil blends, these plentiful fatty acids are beneficial in helping to rebuild and renew the cellular structure of the skin. They are also active in improving the firmness of the skin and promoting elasticity, so this oil is especially good for aging or sun-damaged skin. In addition, evening primrose oil can help overcome the pain and morning stiffness caused by rheumatoid arthritis when applied locally.

Skin Care: Evening primrose is particularly effective in helping to stabilize hormonal imbalances, due to the rich array of nutrients present in the oil. For example, the plentiful omega-6 fatty acids in evening primrose oil can help to regulate hormone levels during puberty and deal with outbreaks of acne. This oil is likewise valuable for those suffering from psoriasis, since the cause of psoriasis can include hormonal changes, alongside other factors such as poor diet. The essential fatty acids present in evening primrose oil actively re-establish hormonal balance, thus helping eliminate the root of the problem. Eczema often flares up due to a deficiency of GLA, one of the most important fatty acids for maintaining healthy skin. Evening primrose oil is very rich in GLA, making it effective in relieving many symptoms associated with eczema, rosacea, or dermatitis, including itching and redness. Applying the oil to the affected area in all these types of skin conditions can therefore aid in the healing process.

Hair Care: This oil makes a fantastic hair conditioner as it nourishes both the scalp and hair. The omega-6 fatty acid GLA is essential for promoting hair growth: use evening primrose oil as a natural growth stimulant by massaging one tablespoon of warm oil into the scalp and leaving on for 2–3 hours before washing out.

SAFETY DATA
Avoid contact with eyes.

Avocado oil

PERSEA AMERICANA

Description The avocado tree is native to the western hemisphere, from southern Mexico to the Andes. The fruits have a greenish or yellowish flesh with a buttery consistency and a very rich, nutty taste.

Actions Anti-aging, antidandruff, anti-inflammatory, anti-oxidant, antiseptic, cicatrizant (wound-healing), emollient, nourishing.

Extraction The oil is derived from the flesh (not the kernel) of the fruit, which is cold-pressed naturally. A high-quality oil should contain a high proportion of wax and, if refined, be simply filtered without using solvents.

Characteristics The unfiltered oil is thick and dark green in color with a rich, fatty odor. If the oil is refined or filtered, then it has a finer texture with a greenish-yellow color and a less pungent scent.

Skin Types Mature, dry, and sun-damaged skin; particularly suited to very dry or parched skin conditions.

Nutritional Value Contains a very high concentration of monounsaturated fatty acids (especially oleic acid), Vitamin E, and other antioxidants. It also contains Vitamins A, D, B1, B2, pantothenic acid, lecithin, lutein, chlorophyll, and high levels of potassium.

Aromatherapy Use

The minimal refinement of cold-pressed avocado oil preserves the important nutrients it contains, which despite its thick consistency, it delivers deep into the skin. The most abundant fatty acid in avocado oil is oleic acid, a nutrient that provides numerous health benefits. Therefore, it is one of the richest, most highly nourishing skin- and hair-conditioning oils available. Avocado oil has an even higher quantity of beneficial monounsaturated fats than olive oil, which makes it one of the most nutritional vegetable oils!

Skin Care: Avocado oil is extremely good at hydrating and softening the skin, at the same time preventing the skin from drying out, thus allowing the tissues to be hydrated for longer. Mature complexions especially benefit from avocado oil as it helps to diminish age spots and fine lines. The beta-carotene, protein, lecithin, fatty acids, and Vitamins A, D, and E found in avocado oil also help protect the skin from damaging UV rays and increase collagen metabolism, thus protecting against the causes of aging. The oil can also aid in the treatment of acne, eczema, psoriasis, and other forms of skin irritation, and promotes the healing of wounds.

Hair Care: The extremely high content of monounsaturated fatty acids present in avocado oil, together with high levels of Vitamins A and E, make avocado a superb hair conditioner. When applied directly, it both nourishes and strengthens hair strands, thereby improving their health while protecting them from further damage. Massaging avocado oil into the scalp also prompts blood flow to the hair follicles, encouraging new hair growth and a glossy shine. It also helps to remove dandruff.

SAFETY DATA
Avoid contact with eyes.

Tips

♡ Avocado oil has excellent lubricant qualities: apply avocado oil direct to areas of cracked skin, such as rough patches on hands, elbows, or heels.

Peach kernel oil

PERSICA VULGARIS

Description The peach is a small tree native to Asia. The white or pink flowers appear in the early spring before the leaves. The edible fruit contains a single kernel from which the oil is extracted.

Actions Analgesic, anti-aging, antibacterial, antidandruff, anti-inflammatory, antioxidant, antiseptic, cicatrizant (wound-healing), emollient, hypo-allergenic.

Extraction High-quality oil is obtained from the dried kernels or seeds of the fruit using the cold-pressing method. Cold-pressed oil is better than the oil produced by solvent extraction, as cold-pressing does not alter the nutritional value of the oil.

Characteristics A light, textured oil which is pale yellow in color. It has a delicate, slightly nutty aroma.

Skin Types Sensitive skin (babies and children); eczema, dermatitis, psoriasis, and irritated skin conditions; sun-damaged skin; dry, flaky, and mature skin. Best avoided by those with oily, combination skin, or acne due to high oleic acid content.

Nutritional Value Vitamin E and A along with the Vitamin B group. Contains the mineral boron plus plentiful amounts of oleic acid and gamma-linoleic acid (GLA).

Aromatherapy Use

A versatile massage or body oil, somewhat similar to sweet almond or apricot kernel oil, which spreads easily on the skin. Peach kernel oil has a lipid content similar to that of the skin. When the skin's lipid content becomes too low, then dry or irritated skin conditions can result. This oil's naturally fine texture allows a rapid skin penetration, which promotes prompt healing of dry or rough skin. A massage using peach kernel oil is therefore especially good for dry, parched skin conditions.

Skin Care: Peach kernel oil has a light texture that is valuable for use in facial treatments or as a body oil, leaving the skin feeling smooth and soft. This oil is particularly good for people with sensitive skin as it is mild, gentle, non-irritant, and soothing: thus it is recommended for babies and young children. It is rich in linoleic and oleic fatty acids, along with Vitamin E and A, which have anti-aging properties that promote the elasticity and suppleness of skin. The high GLA content in peach kernel oil also helps the skin to maintain the correct moisture balance and plays a role in firming and toning the skin.

Hair Care: Used as a conditioning agent, peach kernel oil helps to promote hair growth and improves its overall health because of the high level of nutrients in it. For a deep conditioning treatment, warm one tablespoon of oil and apply it to the hair and scalp, then leave it on for 2-3 hours before washing it off.

SAFETY DATA
Avoid contact with eyes. Those with nut allergies should avoid.

Tips

♡ Recommended for use by those with delicate skin as a daily gentle moisturizer, but can also be used as an everyday makeup remover. Peach kernel oil is suitable for use on the delicate, sensitive skin of babies as well as on the lips as a moisturizer and to help heal chapped lips.

Almond oil, sweet

PRUNUS AMYGDALUS VAR. DULCUS

Description The sweet almond is a deciduous tree, bearing ornamental white or pale pink flowers, appearing before the leaves in early spring. Sweet almond trees grow best in Mediterranean-type climates and produce a delicious edible nut.

Actions Analgesic, anti-dandruff, anti-inflammatory, antioxidant, cicatrizant (wound-healing), emollient, hypo-allergenic, immune stimulant, muscle relaxant.

Extraction High-quality oil is made from the dried sweet almond kernels, which are cold-pressed and filtered without the use of solvents. The cold-pressed quality is recognizable by its slightly thicker consistency. It is more costly than the chemically extracted product, which is often misleadingly sold as cold-pressed. The chemical extraction process damages the natural fatty acids and significantly reduces the vitamin content.

Characteristics A pale yellow oil of medium viscosity with a light, sweet, nutty aroma. It is absorbed relatively slowly by the skin, which is why it is favored as a versatile massage oil.

Skin Types Sensitive skin (babies and children); eczema, dermatitis, psoriasis, and irritated skin conditions; sun-damaged skin; dry, flaky, and mature skin. Best avoided by those with oily, combination skin or acne, as it is not absorbed readily.

Nutritional Value Rich in Vitamins E, K, and B complex, plus traces of A, C, and D. Also contains plentiful amounts of oleic acid and linoleic acid, plus the minerals manganese, calcium, zinc, iron, and selenium.

> *Tips*
>
> ♡ This oil is particularly rich in zinc, the deficiency of which causes brittle nails and white spots to appear. Apply a drop of warm oil on the nails and rub it into the cuticle every day (or once a week) to improve nail health.

Aromatherapy Use

The most popular massage oil used in aromatherapy, making the ideal medium-light skin-care base. Relieving muscular pain is one of the main traditional uses of sweet almond oil for massage purposes, especially when it is applied warm.

Skin Care: Almond oil is an excellent lubricant for the skin, keeping it soft and supple. Revitalizing, soothing, and nourishing, it is well suited for use as an everyday body moisturizer, best blended with an essential oil added to suit your skin type. Regular external application of the oil can prevent dehydration, and as the oil is especially rich in proteins, can provide the amino acids required for the formation of collagen, which helps reverse the signs of aging. Applied regularly to the area beneath the eyes, it can also help to remove unsightly dark circles.

Hair Care: Use almond oil on a regular basis to control hair loss, flaky scalp and dandruff. Warm one tablespoon of oil and apply it to the hair and scalp, then leave it on for 2–3 hours before washing it off.

SAFETY DATA
Avoid contact with eyes. Those with nut allergies should avoid.

Apricot kernel oil

PRUNUS ARMENIACA

Description
The apricot is a small tree with a spreading canopy, which originates from Asia. The white or pink flowers appear in the early spring before the leaves. The edible fruit contains a hard nut or shell containing a single kernel from which the oil is extracted.

Actions
Analgesic, anti-aging, antibacterial, antidandruff, anti-inflammatory, antioxidant, antiseptic. cicatrizant (wound-healing), emollient, hypo-allergenic.

Extraction
High-quality oil is obtained from the dried kernels of the fruit using the cold-pressed method. Cold-pressed oil is better than the oil produced by solvent extraction as cold-pressing does not alter the nutritional value of the oil.

Characteristics
A viscous oil which is pale yellow in color. It can also be a slightly darker yellow depending on the variety of apricots and the extraction process used. It has a sweet, slightly nutty aroma.

Skin Types
Sensitive skin (babies and children); eczema, dermatitis, psoriasis, and irritated skin conditions; sun-damaged skin; dry, flaky, and mature skin. Best avoided by those with oily, combination skin, or acne due to high oleic acid content.

Nutritional Value
Very rich in Vitamin E, plus A, C, K, and D; plus plentiful amounts of oleic acid and linoleic acid (GLA).

Aromatherapy Use

A light-weight massage or body oil, somewhat similar to sweet almond and peach kernel oil, which spreads easily on the skin. Apricot oil has a lipid content similar to that of the skin. When the skin's lipid content becomes too low, then dry or irritated skin conditions can result. This oil's naturally fine texture allows more rapid skin penetration, which promotes more prompt healing of dry or rough skin. A massage using apricot kernel oil is therefore especially good for dry, parched skin conditions.

Skin Care: Skin-care benefits of this oil include lubricating, nourishing, and moisturizing the skin. Apricot kernel oil is particularly good for people with sensitive skin as it is mild, gentle, non-irritant, and soothing: thus it is recommended for babies and young children. Apricot oil is very rich in Vitamin E, which helps nourishes the skin from deep within, thus helping to improve skin tone and reduce the signs of aging. The high GLA content in apricot kernel oil also helps the skin to maintain the correct moisture balance and plays a role in firming and toning the skin. It helps to calm inflammation or irritation associated with eczema and dermatitis. When combined with an equal amount of St. John's wort oil, it acts as an anti-inflammatory and has a cooling effect.

Hair Care: Used as a conditioning agent, apricot oil helps to detangle the hair, making it softer and more manageable. It also promotes hair growth and improves the overall health because of the high level of nutrients in it. Warm one tablespoon of oil and apply it to the hair and scalp, then leave it on for 2–3 hours before washing it off.

SAFETY DATA
Avoid contact with eyes. Those with nut allergies should avoid.

Tips

♡ Apricot kernel oil is suitable for use on the delicate, sensitive skin of the lips as a moisturizer and to help heal chapped lips.

Rosehip seed oil

ROSA RUBIGINOSA

Description Rosehip seed oil is extracted from the bright red hips (the fleshy fruit left behind after a rose has flowered) of a specific variety of rose: *Rosa rubiginosa* or *Rosa moschata*, both having pinky-red flowers, now predominately cultivated in Chile.

Actions Anti-aging, anti-inflammatory, anti-irritant, antioxidant, antiseptic, cicatrizant (wound-healing), emollient, immune stimulant, very nourishing.

Extraction The premium-quality oil is cold-pressed from the rose hips, and when used for cosmetic usage, is best filtered without the use of solvents. Cold-pressed rosehip oil also retains more nutrients than oil, which has been processed using heat in the extraction process.

Characteristics This oil has a rich reddish-orange color and is called a "dry" oil, as it is absorbed quickly by the skin. Rosehip oil is also quite sensitive to oxidation, meaning it can easily go rancid, so it's important to store it in a cool place, in a dark-colored glass bottle.

Skin Types Particularly good for dry, itchy, sun-damaged, and mature skin conditions, including the treatment and prevention of scars, fine lines, and sunspots. It should not be applied directly to active acne (although it is perfect for treating acne scars), and is best avoided for regular use by those with oily skin, despite the fact it does not leave a greasy residue. It is also good for normal skin.

Nutritional Value
A very rich source of Vitamin C, plus Vitamins A (particularly retinoic acid), D, E, F, and B-carotene. The oil also contains high levels of essential fatty acids, specifically oleic, palmitic, linoleic, and gamma-linolenic acid (GLA). Overall, a very nutritious oil.

Tips

♡ Apply the oil twice daily directly to the face using gentle upward strokes, being careful not to drag on the skin, especially to the area around the eyes. Also ideal for use in facial serums. Apply this oil daily to treat and prevent stretch marks, during pregnancy and after birth.

SAFETY DATA
Avoid contact with eyes.

Aromatherapy Use

Rosehip seed oil is packed full of vitamins, antioxidants, and essential fatty acids and is one of the richest plant sources of Vitamin C. The oil contains an amazing 77% of fatty acids (linoleic and linolenic), which play a very important role in the regeneration of skin cells and repair of damaged tissues. This makes it a primary choice for skin rejuvenation and nutrition, while also providing a range of anti-aging benefits. It stimulates skin cell growth and renewal, promotes collagen production, helps maintain the elasticity of the tissue, thus helping it to stay soft, smooth, and young-looking. And since Vitamin C helps boost the immune system, it also acts to keep the skin in optimum health when used as a body or massage oil ingredient.

Skin Care: Traditionally, this oil has been used for centuries to treat scarring, wounds, and inflammation, especially to counter redness or skin irritation, including rosacea. The essential fatty acids found in rosehip oil can also reduce the effects of eczema by promoting skin regeneration. Above all, rosehip oil can protect skin cells from premature aging when used regularly and can act as a preventive measure against stretch marks or long term scarring. Rosehip oil's anti-aging properties combined with its super light and non-greasy texture make it the ideal ingredient in facial serums. And because Vitamin A has naturally small molecules, this allows deeper penetration into the skin, thus improving the skin's moisture levels from within, reducing wrinkles, blemishes, and fine lines. The antioxidants found in rosehip oil also help combat free radicals that cause sun damage to the skin, resulting in sunspots and uneven pigmentation.

Hair Care: The essential fatty acids in rosehip seed oil can reduce dry scalp and itchiness when used topically.

Jojoba oil

SIMMONDSIA CHINENSIS

Description A small shrub native to the warm, dry regions of south-western North America, with broad, thick waxy leaves and small greenish-yellow flowers. It was originally named *Buxus sinensis* due to a misunderstanding that it came from China.

Actions Anti-aging, antibacterial, antidandruff, antifungal, anti-inflammatory, antioxidant, antisebum (regulates sebum levels), antiviral, cicatrizant (wound-healing), emollient, hypo-allergenic, moisturizing.

Extraction Cold-pressed from the jojoba bean or nut. Premium-quality jojoba oil for cosmetic usage is best filtered without the use of solvents. This process also removes any odor.

Characteristics A pale yellow liquid that is actually a liquid wax rather than a "real" vegetable oil: it has no smell and does not go rancid, so it makes an ideal base for body lotions, natural perfumes, or facial oils. It is also light and easily absorbed.

Skin Types All skin types: excellent for oily or acne-prone skin by helping unclog the pores. It is also beneficial for damaged, dry, aging, and inflamed skin conditions, including eczema and psoriasis. Suitable for sensitive skin and children.

Nutritional Value It contains high amounts of Vitamin E, B complex, and the minerals: silicon, chromium, copper, and zinc, plus a very high percentage of iodine at 82%. It also contains plentiful amounts of gadoleic acid and oleic fatty acids.

Tips

♡ As a liquid wax, jojoba can create a smooth surface applied to the skin prior to shaving, and then used afterwards, imparts moisture, heals cuts quickly, and helps to prevent shaving rash. It can also be applied as a natural cleanser or makeup remover and makes a great lip balm.

Aromatherapy Use

A very versatile aromatherapy skin-care product with a long shelf life, jojoba oil enjoys enduring popularity for use in massage or body lotions as well as facial serums. It is very similar in consistency to the skin's own sebum, so is one of the best natural moisturizers. A few drops of jojoba oil massaged gently into the face on a daily basis leaves it feeling soft and smooth, reducing the appearance of fine lines. It is also high in proteins and minerals, so simultaneously nourishes, soothes, and heals the skin from within.

Skin Care: Soaps tend to strip the skin of the sebum that the skin glands produce to provide natural lubrication and protection. Keeping the skin hydrated by locking in the moisture constitutes a basic skin-care principle. Being a waxy substance, jojoba oil seals in moisture, and since it is so structurally similar to the skin's own sebum, it is readily absorbed. Oily skin is the result of overactive sebaceous glands in the skin, which can result in seborrheic dermatitis or acne. Acne develops when the hair follicles become blocked by the accumulation of sebum, keratin, and other cell debris. Being a mobile liquid wax, jojoba is able to penetrate deep into the hair follicle where it acts as a cleanser by dissolving the sebum deposits and dislodging blockages. When the skin remains well hydrated, the sebaceous glands also respond to it by reducing sebum production, which helps to clear acne when used regularly.

The moisturizing, anti-inflammatory, and antibacterial properties of jojoba are also valuable in helping to counter the irritation and dryness characteristic of eczema and psoriasis. Applied locally, it helps soothe redness caused by sunburn, as well as healing sun-damaged, cracked, or peeling skin. It stimulates collagen production, making it ideal for dehydrated and aging skin, and since it is also non-toxic when used on the skin, it is also suitable for sensitive complexions.

Hair Care: Jojoba has been used for centuries as a nourishing hair conditioner, giving it a glossy shine and helping remedy split ends, brittle, dry, or damaged hair. Jojoba oil can also help control hair loss by deep cleansing the hair follicles of excessive sebum, facilitating the growth of new hair. Jojoba oil is naturally rich in zinc and selenium, which help control dandruff and scalp psoriasis. To use as a quick-fix conditioner, simply rub into damp hair for 20 minutes before shampooing out.

SAFETY DATA
Avoid contact with eyes. Those with nut allergies should consult a medical practitioner before using jojoba.

Wheat germ oil

TRICUM VULGARE

Description Wheat germ oil is derived from the germ or "heart" of the wheat, a type of grass grown as a crop across the world and used as a food staple. The wheat germ is the most nutritious component of the wheat kernel, or seed, and contains over 23 different nutrients.

Actions Anti-aging, anti-inflammatory, antioxidant, cicatrizant (wound-healing), emollient, nourishing, noncomedogenic (does not clog the pores).

Extraction Cold-pressed and then filtered from the wheat germ kernel. Organic cold-pressed wheat germ oil is of superior nutritional quality.

Characteristics A rich, reddish oil with a thick texture and a strong odor, which is readily absorbed by the skin.

Skin Types Excessively dry or damaged skin, especially cracked or scarred skin, where regular application can completely banish existing scars. It can also prevent scarring used regularly over a period of time, making it valuable during pregnancy.

Nutritional Value Wheat germ oil is loaded with essential nutrients: Vitamins E, A, D, and B complex; plus the minerals: phosphorus, zinc, iron, selenium, and potassium, as well as being rich in omega-3 fatty acids, all of which are very beneficial for the skin, hair, and overall health.

Aromatherapy Use

Wheat germ oil has a high Vitamin E content, so exhibits good anti-aging properties and is especially valuable for treating damaged skin. Wheat germ oil also contains high levels of the omega-3 fatty acids, which help in regulating the nervous system. It is therefore indicated for stress-related conditions especially in combination with aromatherapy massage.

Skin Care: Overall, wheat germ oil has a pronounced regenerative effect on skin tissue, being healing and nourishing. The oil is loaded with vitamins and minerals, which specifically improve skin elasticity, while nourishing and moisturizing the skin cells from deep within, providing natural long-lasting hydration. It is readily absorbed by the skin, has excellent lubricant qualities and can help maintain even skin tone.

The oil also helps in building collagen, the most abundantly found protein in the body that provides the skin with strength and tone. It is therefore valuable for aging skin and during pregnancy as a pre-birth lubricant. Applied directly to the skin tissue, it provides elasticity, encourages natural cellular regeneration, and helps heal scars and stretch marks.

Wheat germ oil used in moderation in facial oils can also help balance excess sebum levels, which can lead to other skin problems like acne and pimples. The nourishing and healing qualities of the oil can also prevent many skin problems like psoriasis, eczema, and dry, cracked skin, applied in blends.

Hair Care: Being rich in linoleic acid, wheat germ is a useful oil for nourishing the hair and imparting shine. Use it in the ratio 10:1 with other carrier oils such as almond oil, avocado oil, or argan oil, and apply to the hair and scalp, then leave it on for 2–3 hours before washing it off.

SAFETY DATA
Avoid contact with eyes. Those with a wheat or gluten allergy or sensitivity should avoid using wheat germ oil.

Tips

♡ Adding 5–15% of wheat germ oil to a body or facial oil acts as a natural preservative, lengthening the life of the blend, plus adding valuable nutrients.

Grapeseed oil ⊙ ♀

VITIS VINIFERA

Description Grape vines are grown the world over for their delicious and popular fruit, as well as for the production of wine. Nevertheless, the berries or pips of grapes have also long been valued, due to their high nutritional value. In fact, grapeseed oil is very similar to olive oil in nutrition, calories, and fat content, but unlike olive oil, grapeseed oil does not contain any saturated fat.

Actions Anti-aging, antibacterial, anti-inflammatory, antimicrobial, antioxidant, astringent, cicatrizant (wound-healing), emollient, moisturizing, noncomedogenic, nourishing.

Extraction Grapeseed oil is obtained from the seeds of the grape (as a by-product of the wine industry), which are either cold-pressed or extracted using a solvent, after which it is refined for cosmetic use. The oil that is cold-pressed and then naturally filtered from the dried seeds of the grape (ideally from organically produced fruit) exhibits a greater nutritional skin-care benefit than the solvent-extracted oil.

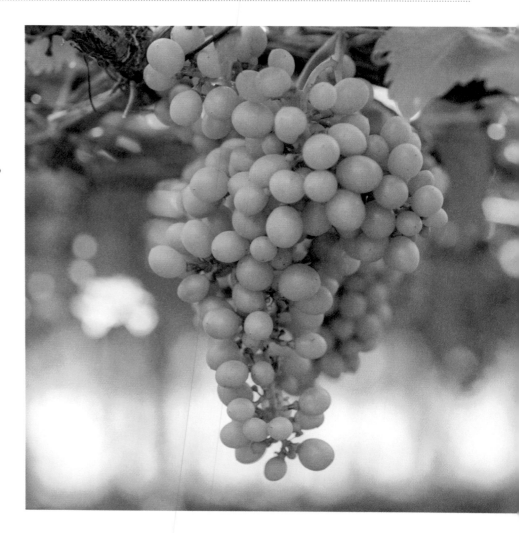

SAFETY DATA
Avoid contact with eyes.

Characteristics A pale yellow mobile liquid, with little odor, which is light-weight to apply and is easily absorbed. It is a very nutritional oil, often compared with the health-giving powers of olive oil.

Skin Types Suitable for all skin types, but especially oily skin, combination skin, and acne-prone complexions, as well as aging and scarred skin.

Nutritional Value This oil is rich in beta-carotene (known to prevent aging) plus Vitamins D, C, and E, and ceramides. It is an excellent source of essential fatty acids, especially oleic and linoleic acids, which both have outstanding regenerative properties, important for protecting skin cell membranes.

Aromatherapy Use

This oil makes a versatile and economical body oil base, with excellent emollient or skin-softening properties. It has a fine texture with little odor, so it is ideal for aromatherapy massage used in combination with essential oils or for making home blends. A useful oil for those with nut allergies, as it is a safe, nutritional ingredient, including for those with sensitive skin.

Skin Care: Grapeseed oil is non-comedogenic, which means it doesn't clog the pores of the skin, so is good for complexions that are prone to greasiness as well as being useful in the treatment of acne. As a moisturizer it is non-greasy, and can also help treat unsightly scars, such as those resulting from previous outbreaks of acne. The polyphenols and antioxidants in the oil help treat acne as well. Since the fine structure of the oil can penetrate the pores and cleanse the skin from within, it can also prevent breakouts from occurring. In fact, this oil can help balance both dry and oily patches on the skin so it is well suited to combination skin types.

Many cosmetic products use grapeseed oil as their base, being naturally rich in Vitamins C, D, and E, all of which help in the fight against the signs of aging. Applied locally it can also reduce wrinkles, scars, and stretch marks, help to tighten sagging skin, and diminish dark circles around the eyes. Being very high in Vitamin E and antioxidants it can also restore collagen, making it valuable for mature skin. Vitamins C and E and fatty acids make the oil a wonderful skin conditioner, while the high linoleic acid content can also aid in treating eczema.

Hair Care: Grapeseed oil moisturizes and conditions the hair without leaving it feeling greasy. It also reduces dandruff and hair loss by strengthening the hair, enabling it to grow faster. Being high in ceramides, grapeseed oil is also great for making the hair feel soft: apply as a conditioner for 20 minutes before shampooing off.

Tips

♡ Despite the fear of "adding oil to oil," grapeseed oil can be a great aid in overcoming acne when applied sparingly on a daily basis to affected areas. It also makes an effective makeup remover.

PART SIX

Safety Guidelines

Safety guidelines

IN GENERAL, all the essential oils listed in this book are safe to use for aromatherapy or household purposes. However, it is necessary to be aware of the following safety measures.

Safety data
Always check with specific safety data before using a new oil (see information on individual oils, pages 239–371).

Internal use
Do not take essential oils internally. Essential oils may damage the lining of the digestive tract and some essential oils are toxic if taken internally.

Toxicity
Essential oils that should be used in moderation because of toxicity levels when absorbed through the skin are: aniseed, West Indian bay, white camphor, clove bud, coriander, eucalyptus blue gum, hyssop, nutmeg, sweet fennel, parsley seed, Spanish sage, tagetes, thyme. Penny royal, mustard, sassafras, rue, and mugwort should not be used at all and are not included in this book.

Neat application
In general, essential oils should not be applied neat to the skin. Exceptions are lavender and tea tree, for applications described in this book. Nonirritant oils such as jasmine, ylang ylang, or sandalwood may be applied neat for use as a perfume.

Patch test
Before applying any new oil to the skin, do a patch test. Put a few drops on the back of your wrist, cover with a plaster, and leave for an hour. If irritation or redness occurs, bathe with cold water. For future use, reduce the recommended concentration level by half or avoid using the oil altogether.

Sensitive skin
Neat tea tree may cause skin irritation in people with very sensitive skins. These people should dilute it first in a nonoily cream or gel. Oils that may cause an adverse reaction on very sensitive skin, even when diluted, include benzoin, lemon eucalyptus, melissa, tagetes, valerian, yarrow, and skin-irritant oils.

Skin irritation
Oils that may irritate the skin, especially in high concentrations, are: aniseed, sweet basil, black pepper, cajeput, white camphor, Virginian cedarwood, cinnamon leaf, clove bud, eucalyptus blue gum, ginger, juniper, lemon, lemongrass, parsley seed, peppermint, pine needle, and thyme. Do not use more than 3 drops of these oils in the bath.

Phototoxicity
Oils that can cause adverse reaction if used before exposure to sunlight or ultraviolet light (e.g. sunbeds) are: angelica root, bergamot, lime, bitter orange, lemon, grapefruit, sweet orange, and tangerine.

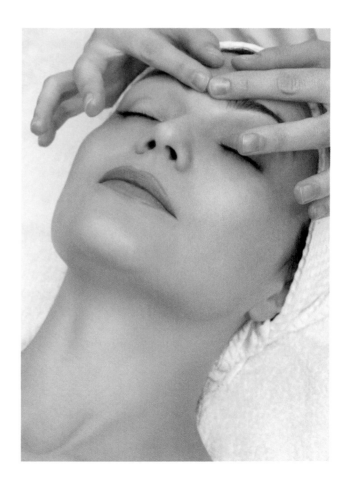

Babies and children

Always increase the dilution for babies and infants to at least half the recommended amount. For babies, avoid the possibly toxic and irritant oils altogether. For babies 0–12 months: use only 1 drop of lavender, rose, or chamomile oil, diluted in 1 tsp/5ml carrier oil for massage or bathing (do not use other oils).

For infants 1–5 years: use only 2–3 drops of any of the nontoxic and nonirritant oils, diluted in 1 tsp/5ml carrier oil for massage or bathing.

For children 6–12 years: use as for adults but in half the stated concentration.

Pregnancy

During pregnancy, use essential oils in half the stated amount. Do not use oils that are potentially toxic or have emmenagogue properties. Avoid altogether: basil, Virginian cedarwood, celery seed, clary sage, clove, cinnamon leaf, citronella, hyssop, juniper, marjoram, myrrh, nutmeg, Spanish sage, thyme. Avoid during the first four months: angelica root, Atlas cedarwood, sweet fennel, rose, rosemary.

High blood pressure

Avoid using the following oils in any form in cases of high blood pressure: rosemary, Spanish sage, thyme.

Epilepsy

Avoid using the following oils in cases of epilepsy: fennel, hyssop, rosemary, Spanish sage.

Alcohol

Clary sage should not be used in any form within a few hours (before or after) of drinking alcohol. It can cause nausea and exaggerated drunkenness.

Homeopathy

Homeopathic treatment is not compatible with the following oils, due to their strength: black pepper, camphor, eucalyptus, peppermint.

Storage

Store essential oils and blends in dark, well-stoppered bottles, kept away from light and heat, and well out of reach of children. Label bottles clearly.

Chemical constituents

THIS APPENDIX SHOWS the chief chemical constituents of the most common essential oils described in this book. For each oil, the major chemical groups and their approximate proportions are shown, linked to the principal effects of the oil. Constituents that are mainly stimulating in their effect are shown in red, those that are mainly relaxing/sedating are shown in blue, and those that are mainly balancing are shown in purple. These are for standard samples, but it must be borne in mind that the chemical makeup of essential oils can vary enormously, depending on the source. Small quantities of trace elements may also be present.

	RELAXING			BALANCING			STIMULATING		
	ESTERS	ALDEHYDES	KETONES	SEQUISTERPENES	OXIDES	ACIDS	MONOTERPENES	ALCOHOLS	PHENOLS
YARROW *Achillea millefolium*				34%	11%		25%	9%	
DILL *Anethum graveolens*			UP TO 55%	UP TO 21%			UP TO 69%	UP TO 4%	UP TO 18%
ANGELICA ROOT *Angelica archangelica*	UP TO 15%			UP TO 34%	14%		UP TO 80%	UP TO 19%	
ROSEWOOD *Aniba rosaeodora*								70%	
CELERY SEED *Apium graveolens*				21%			75%		
FRANKINCENSE *Boswellia carteri*	UP TO 10%						UP TO 50%	UP TO 12%	
YLANG YLANG *Cananga odorata forma genuina*	UP TO 16%			16%			UP TO 47%	20%	
ELEMI *Canarium luzonicum*							UP TO 85%		
CEDARWOOD, ATLAS *Cedrus atlantica*			3%	86%				10%	
CHAMOMILE, ROMAN *Chamaemelum nobilis, Anthemis nobilis*	UP TO 70%			4%			10%	35%	
CHAMOMILE, GERMAN/BLUE *Chamomilla matricaria Matricaria recutita*				47%	19%				
CAMPHOR *Cinnamomum camphora*			37%				UP TO 58%	10%	
CINNAMON LEAF *Cinnamomum zeylanicum*				6%				5%	74%
LIME *Citrus aurantifolia*					3%		UP TO 84%	11%	
PETITGRAIN ORANGE *Citrus aurantium var. amara*	75%							UP TO 40%	
NEROLI *Citrus aurantium var. amara*	13%						29%	UP TO 40%	
BERGAMOT *Citrus bergamia*	28%						UP TO 52%	13%	
LEMON *Citrus limon*							80%		
GRAPEFRUIT *Citrus x paradisi*							88%	3%	

CHEMICAL CONSTITUENTS

	ESTERS	ALDEHYDES	KETONES	SEQUISTERPENES	OXIDES	ACIDS	MONOTERPENES	ALCOHOLS	PHENOLS
MANDARIN *Citrus reticulata*							89%		
ORANGE, SWEET *Citrus sinensis, Citrus aurantium var. dulcis*	3%	UP TO 39%	5%				UP TO 95%	UP TO 15%	
MYRRH *Commiphora myrrh*				UP TO 32%				43%	
CORIANDER *Coriandrum sativum*	2%		4%				9%	81%	
CYPRESS *Cupressus sempervirens*				3%			UP TO 77%	10%	
LEMONGRASS, WEST INDIAN *Cymbopogon citratus*		74%					3%	10%	
PALMAROSA *Cymbopogon martinii,*	10%			2%				83%	
CITRONELLA *Cymbopogon nardus*		UP TO 49%		2%			UP TO 11%	UP TO 25%	1%
CARROT SEED *Daucus carota*	UP TO 19%		10%	UP TO 30%	UP TO 31%		UP TO 35%	UP TO 85%	
CARDOMOM *Elettaria cardamomum*	52%				31%		4%	5%	
LEMON EUCALYPTUS *Eucalyptus citriodora*	3%	82%			2%			9%	
EUCALYPTUS BLUE GUM *Eucalyptus globulus*					96%		4%		
GALBANUM *Ferula gumosa*							70%		
FENNEL, SWEET *Foeniculum vulgare*		2%	14%				2%		77%
HYSSOP *Hyssopus officinalis*			48%	16%			13%		
JASMINE *Jasminum officinale*	70%							8%	
JUNIPER *Juniperus communis*				2%			70%		
CEDARWOOD, VIRGINIAN *Juniperus virginiana*				56%				33%	
LAVENDER, TRUE *Lavandula angustifolia/L.officinalis*	43%			2%	6%		37%		
TEA TREE *Melaleuca alternifolia*				2%	3%		36%	48%	
CAJEPUT *Melaleuca cajeputi*				11%	35%		23%	21%	2%

CHEMICAL CONSTITUENTS

	ESTERS	ALDEHYDES	KETONES	SEQUISTERPENES	OXIDES	ACIDS	MONOTERPENES	ALCOHOLS	PHENOLS
MELISSA *Melissa officinalis*	UP TO 6%	UP TO 92%	UP TO 9%	UP TO 10%		UP TO 9%		UP TO 3%	
PEPPERMINT *Mentha x piperata*			UP TO 40%				6%	UP TO 48%	
NUTMEG *Myristica fragrans*				2%			UP TO 88%	8%	7%
MYRTLE *Myrtus communis*	25%				37%		31%	3%	
BASIL, SWEET/ FRENCH *Ocimum basilicum*	8%				7%			64%	3%
MARJORAM, SWEET *Origanum majorana/ Marjorana hortensis*				2.4%			30%	52%	
GERANIUM, ROSE *Pelargonium graveolens*	30%		6%				2%	54%	
PARSLEY SEED *Petroselinum crispum*							45%		UP TO 59%
BAY, WEST INDIAN *Pimenta acris*	4%						21%	2%	64%
ANISEED *Pimpinella anisum*		UP TO 2%					2%		UP TO 96%
PINE NEEDLE, SCOTCH *Pinus sylvestris*	27%			2%			UP TO 61%	3%	
PEPPER, BLACK *Piper nigrum*				7%			77%		
PATCHOULI *Pogostemon patchouli*				UP TO 60%				25%	
ROSE MAROC *Rosa centifolia*		UP TO 38%						UP TO 93%	3%
ROSEMARY *Rosmarinus officinalis*			13%				69%		
SAGE, SPANISH *Salvia lavandulifolia*	9%		26%				30%	23%	
SAGE, CLARY *Salvia sclarea*	72%			3%				14%	
SANDALWOOD, EAST INDIAN *Santalum album*				3%				68%	
BENZOIN *Styrax benzoin*	80%	2%			17%				
CLOVE *Syzygium aromaticum*	5%			4%					84%
TAGETES *Tagetes minuta*			UP TO 95%				UP TO 35%		
THYME, WHITE (COMMON) *Thymus vulgaris*							40%	50%	
VALERIAN *Valeriana officinalis*	30%			5%			12%	2%	
VETIVERT *Vetiveria zizanoides*			12%	6%		5%		20%	
GINGER *Zinziber officinale*		3%		60%	5%		15%		

Vitamins and dietary sources

VITAMINS AND OTHER NUTRIENTS are essential for health and well-being. They aren't found in essential oils, due to the process of distillation and the volatile nature of the oils, but carrier oils are a rich source (see pp. 345–371). Here are some key vitamins, all of which are found in commonly used carrier oils.

VITAMIN A (RETINOL)

- Needed for vision, skin health, resistance to infection, growth, reproduction. Needs oils and fats for absorption into body. Not affected by heat.
- Found in meat, fish, dairy produce, fortified spreads, carrots, greens, sweet potatoes, endive, tomatoes, green beans, dried apricots, cantaloup, prunes.
- Found in argan oil (p. 350), calendula oil (p. 352), St. John's wort oil (p. 356), avocado oil (p. 360), peach kernel oil (p. 361), apricot kernel oil (p. 363), rosehip seed oil (p. 364), wheat germ oil (p. 368).

VITAMIN B1 (THIAMINE)

- Needed for release of energy from food. Aids appetite and digestion.
- Found in unrefined foods, cereals (wheat germ, soy flour, whole wheat flour, brown rice), nuts, seeds, brewer's yeast, molasses, fortified foods.
- More may be needed by pregnant or breastfeeding women, the elderly, drinkers, smokers.
- Found in St. John's wort oil (p. 356), avocado oil, (p. 360), peach kernel oil (p. 361), sweet almond oil (p. 362), jojoba oil (p. 366), wheat germ oil (p. 368).

VITAMIN B2 (RIBOFLAVIN)

- Needed for vitality, release of energy from food, healthy eyes, and skin.
- Found in meat (liver, lamb, beef, pork, chicken, kidney), cereals (wheat germ), nuts and seeds, molasses, brewer's yeast.
- Found in St. John's wort oil (p. 356), avocado oil (p. 360), peach kernel oil (p. 361), sweet almond oil (p. 362), jojoba oil (p. 366), wheat germ oil (p. 368).

B3 (NIACIN/NICOTINIC ACID)

- Needed for production of energy.
- Found in: meat, fish, cereal, nuts, seeds, molasses, brewer's yeast.
- Extra may be needed by pregnant and breastfeeding women, those suffering from stress, and the elderly.
- Found in peach kernel oil (p. 361), sweet almond oil (p. 362), jojoba oil (p. 366), wheat germ oil (p. 368).

B5 (PANTOTHENIC ACID)

- Needed for cell growth and utilization of energy from foods. Needed for synthesis of hormones by adrenal glands.
- Found in meat (especially offal), cereals, vegetables, yeast. Lost in cooking, canning, exposure to light, and storage.
- Those suffering from stress, allergies, or injury may have increased need.
- Found in peach kernel oil (p. 361), sweet almond oil (p. 362), jojoba oil (p. 366), wheat germ oil (p. 368).

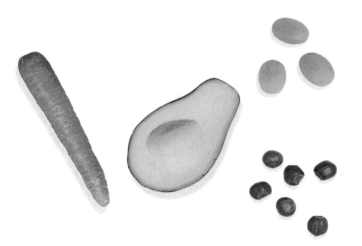

LEFT A balanced diet of vitamins, fats, and other nutrients is essential for overall health and well-being.

B6 (PYRIDOXINE)

• Needed for normal functioning of brain and nerves, in utilization of essential fatty acids, production of many enzymes; regulating magnesium levels.
• Found in meat (especially offal), yeast, cereals (wheat bran and germ), molasses.
• Extra needed in pregnancy, when taking oral contraceptives; may help with epilepsy, diabetes, anemia, kidney stones.
• Found in St. John's wort oil (p. 356), peach kernel oil (p. 361), sweet almond oil (p. 362), jojoba oil (p. 366), wheat germ oil (p. 368).

B7 (BIOTIN)

• Needed for fat metabolism; deficiency of biotin may be involved in dermatitis and hair loss.
• Found in egg yolk and liver; also made in the intestine.
• Found in peach kernel oil (p. 361), sweet almond oil (p. 362), jojoba oil (p. 366), wheat germ oil (p. 368).

B9 (FOLATE OR FOLIC ACID)

• Needed for cell division; production of red blood cells; growth and healing; utilization of pantothenic acid.
• Found in meat (especially liver), nuts, green vegetables, yeast.
• Important in and before pregnancy.
• Found in peach kernel oil (p. 361), sweet almond oil (p. 362), jojoba oil (p. 366), wheat germ oil (p. 368).

B12 (COBALAMINE)

• Needed by rapidly dividing cells, such as those in the bone marrow that form red blood cells.
• Found in meat (especially liver), dairy produce, fortified products (e.g. breakfast cereals). (Only in animal foods.)
• Vegetarians, vegans, the elderly, and those pregnant or breastfeeding should check they have adequate B12.
• Found in peach kernel oil (p. 361), sweet almond oil (p. 362), jojoba oil (p. 366), wheat germ oil (p. 368).

BETA-CAROTENE

• Needed for good vision, strong immunity, and general good health.
• Found in carrots (where it's responsible for the orange color), sweet potatoes, squash, and kale.
• Found in calendula oil (p. 352), rosehip seed oil (p. 364), and grapeseed oil (p. 370).

RIGHT Vitamin D is essential for the absorption of calcium. This is especially important for growing children.

VITAMIN C (ASCORBIC ACID)

• Needed for resistance to infection and allergies, healing, strong gums, teeth, and bones, skin elasticity, strong connective tissue. Detoxifies harmful substances. Aids iron absorption.
• Found in fruit (high in strawberries, oranges, lemons), greens, raw sweet pepper, meat (especially liver).
• Vitamin C cannot be stored in the body. Extra needed in illness. Destroyed in food preparation and storage.
• Found in calendula oil (p. 352), evening primrose oil (p. 358), apricot kernel oil (p. 363), rosehip seed oil (p. 364), and grapeseed oil (p. 370).

CHOLINE

• Used to form lecithin with inositol.
• Found in meat (including brains, liver, kidneys), egg yolk, wheat germ, yeast. Can be made in the blood, given adequate folic acid and B12.
• Those with high blood pressure or high cholesterol levels may need more.

VITAMIN D

• Needed for absorption, retention, and utilization of calcium (essential for strong bones and teeth, relaxes nerves, decreases pain sensitivity, aids sound sleep). Vitamin D is fat-soluble and can only be absorbed if fat is present in the diet. Excessive amounts can be toxic.
• Found in oily fish, fish-liver oils, fortified products; also formed by the action of sunlight on the skin.
• Important for those with low exposure to sunlight, children, vegetarians, vegans.
• Found in St. John's wort oil (p. 356), avocado oil (p. 360), apricot kernel oil (p. 363), rosehip seed oil (p. 364), wheat germ oil (p. 368), and grapeseed oil (p. 370).

VITAMIN E

• Prevents oxidation of unsaturated fatty acids, Vitamin A, various hormones; for glands, hormones, reproduction. Prevents thrombosis in legs. Aids liver function. Fat and bile need to be present in the intestine for absorption.
• Found in oils of all cereals, nuts, and seeds, stoneground flour, cold-pressed oils. Destroyed by cooking and storage.
• Found in argan oil (p. 350), calendula oil (p. 352), coconut oil (p. 354), avocado oil (p. 360), peach kernel oil (p. 361), sweet almond oil (p. 362), apricot kernel oil (p. 363), rosehip seed oil (p. 364), jojoba oil (p. 366), wheat germ oil (p. 368), and grapeseed oil (p. 370).

VITAMIN F

• Repairs and creates tissue in the body, helps with metabolism, healing, reproductive health, skin regeneration, and hair growth.
• Found in oils, nuts, seeds, some fish, and soybeans.
• Found in rosehip seed oil (p. 364).

INOSITOL

• Combines with choline to make lecithin in the liver. This keeps cholesterol in small particles to prevent clogging of blood vessels. Inositol also aids the digestion.
• Found in meat, cereals, molasses, yeast.
• Those with high blood pressure or high cholesterol levels, and smokers may need extra inositol and choline.

VITAMIN K

• Needed for blood clotting and healing.
• Found in green leafy vegetables like broccoli and spinach, vegetable oils, cereal grains.
• Found in sweet almond oil (p. 362), apricot kernel oil (p. 363).

Vitamins and minerals are an important part of a balanced lifestyle. Eating fresh vegetables and fruits, and using nutritious carrier oils as directed on pages 345–371 is a great way to get the nutrients your body needs. You can also take additional supplements, but consult your doctor or health care practitioner for recommendations.

Fatty acids and their benefits

FATTY ACIDS ARE found in plentiful quantities in vegetable oils, and as such, provide one of the best sources for these important nutrients, which are essential for keeping the skin in an optimum condition. The healthy, unsaturated fatty acids are divided into two main sub-categories: omega-3 and -6 are both polyunsaturated fatty acids, whereas omega-9 is a monounsaturated fatty acid.

OMEGA-3 FATTY ACIDS

Omega-3 fatty acids are lipid components that the body is unable to produce for itself, so must be obtained from an external source: thus they are called "essential" fatty acids. Although they are valuable for preventing cardiovascular disease and inflammation, omega-3 fatty acids often require the assistance of omega-6 fatty acids to be effective.

OMEGA-6 FATTY ACIDS

Omega-6 fatty acids play an important role in constructing immune cells, improving the skin healing process, reducing inflammatory reactions, and protecting the cardiovascular system. In order for omega-6 fatty acids to be effective, they must be combined with a sufficient supply of omega-3. There are two very important omega-6 fatty acids which are plentifully found in certain vegetable oils, such as borage oil: linoleic acid (the only essential omega-6 fatty acid) and gamma-linoleic acid (GLA). GLA has been shown to prevent deficiency in skin lipids, preventing flare-ups, including those typical of eczema.

OMEGA-9 FATTY ACIDS

Omega-9 fatty acids can be synthesized in sufficient amounts using the saturated fats generally found in food. Omega-9 fatty acids are composed of several acids including oleic acid, the most commonly known, which is also found plentifully in vegetable oils such as argan oil. Oleic acid helps prevent cardiovascular diseases, reduces cholesterol and hypertension, as well as improving the health of the skin.

ALPHA-LINOLEIC ACID

In the omega-3 family, alpha-linoleic acid is the only acid considered "essential" since it cannot be synthesized by the body. In the cosmetic industry, alpha-linoleic acid is known for its hydrating power, which adds suppleness to the skin. It is anti-inflammatory and thus soothes redness and irritations in the skin.

CAPRYLIC ACID

A saturated fatty acid naturally present in dairy products, and also in breastmilk, caprylic acid is also found in coconut oil and palm kernel oil. In cosmetics, it is used for its emollient and hydrating properties, as well as its antifungal properties.

GADOLEIC ACID

In the omega-9 family, gadoleic acid is an unsaturated fatty acid present in several vegetable oils, including jojoba. Similar to human sebum, it has a high absorption power in the skin and can therefore moisturize without a greasy effect.

MYRISTIC ACID

Myristic acid is a saturated acid naturally found in dairy products, and in coconut oil. It is used in cosmetics for its cleansing, smoothing, and protective properties.

LAURIC ACID

Lauric acid is a saturated fatty acid mainly found in coconut oil and used in cosmetics for its cleansing and emulsifying properties. Lauric acid also has antimicrobial action and helps harden balms, soaps, and body butters.

LINOLEIC ACID

Linoleic acid is found in several vegetable oils, such as borage oil, and is one of the essential fatty acids in the omega-6 family. The human body is unable to synthesize this acid so it must be obtained from an external source. Linoleic acid helps produce cell membranes, and in the skin it is found in ceramides, which form a truly protective epidermal barrier. Omega-6 deficiency results in severe skin dryness, a dull complexion, and brittle, lackluster hair, among other things. Grapeseed oil is especially high in ceramides.

OLEIC ACID

In the omega-9 family, oleic acid makes up 55–80% of the fatty acids found in olive oil. Found in high levels in the human body, it protects the cardiovascular system and lowers cholesterol. In cosmetics, oleic acid is a very frequently used ingredient, and is plentiful in jojoba oil as well as other carrier oils. Known for its nourishing properties, it helps strengthen the hydro-lipid film, which helps the skin preserve its elasticity and suppleness. It also has skin-healing properties.

PALMITIC ACID

Palmitic acid is a saturated fatty acid found in some vegetable oils such as rosehip seed oil and coconut oil. An important part of the skin barrier and the acidic epidermal layer, it has emollient, emulsifying, and cleansing properties.

PALMITOLEIC ACID

Especially present in macadamia nut oil, palmitoleic acid is a monounsaturated fatty acid with extremely high absorption power in the skin. Similar to human sebum, it hydrates and strengthens the epidermis without being harsh on the skin.

STEARIC ACID

Naturally present in butter and vegetable oils, stearic acid is a saturated fatty acid that is found in St. John's wort oil. Its emollient properties allow it to hydrate and protect the epidermis.

Further Reference

General glossary

A

Abortifacient: capable of inducing abortion.

Absolute: a highly concentrated, semi-solid, or solid perfume material, usually obtained by alcohol extraction from the concrete.

Acrid: leaving a burning sensation in the mouth.

Adaptogen: a substance that causes beneficial adaptive change to take place in the body.

Allergy: hypersensitivity to a foreign substance.

Alliaceous: garlic- or onion-like.

Alterative: corrects disordered bodily function.

Amebicidal: having the power of destroying amebae.

Analgesic: remedy or agent that deadens pain.

Anaphrodisiac: reduces sexual desire.

Anemia: deficiency of red corpuscles in the blood.

Anesthetic: loss of feeling or sensation; substance that causes such a loss.

Annual: a plant that completes its life cycle in one year.

Anodyne: stills pain and quiets disturbed feelings.

Anorexia: condition of being without appetite.

Anthelmintic: a vermifuge, destroying or expelling intestinal worms.

Antianemic: an agent that combats anemia.

Antiarthritic: an agent that combats arthritis.

Antibilious: an agent that helps remove excess bile.

Antibiotic: prevents the growth of, or destroys, bacteria.

Anticatarrhal: helps remove excess catarrh.

Anticonvulsant: helps arrest or prevent convulsions.

Antidepressant: helps alleviate depression.

Antidiarrheal: efficacious against diarrhea.

Antiemetic: an agent which reduces the incidence and severity of nausea or vomiting.

Antihemorrhagic: an agent that prevents or combats hemorrhage or bleeding.

Antihistamine: counteracts effects of histamine.

Anti-inflammatory: alleviates inflammation.

Antilithic: prevents the formation of a calculus or stone.

Antimicrobial: an agent that resists or destroys pathogenic micro-organisms.

Antineuralgic: relieves or reduces nerve pain.

Antioxidant: prevents or delays oxidation.

Antiphlogistic: checks or counteracts inflammation.

Antipruritic: relieves or prevents sensation of itching.

Antiputrescent: prevents and combats decay.

Antipyretic: reduces fever; see also febrifuge.

Antirheumatic: helps prevent and relieve rheumatism.

Antisclerotic: helps prevent the hardening of tissue.

Antiscorbutic: a remedy for scurvy.

Antiscrofula: combats the development of tuberculosis of lymph nodes (scrofula).

Antiseborrheic: helps control the products of sebum.

Antiseptic: destroys and prevents the development of microbes.

Antispasmodic: prevents and eases spasms or convulsions.

Antitoxic: counteracts the effects of poison.

Antitussive: relieves coughs.

Antiviral: substance that inhibits the growth of a virus.

Aperient: a mild laxative.

Aperitif: a stimulant of the appetite.

Aphonia: loss of voice.

Aphrodisiac: increases or stimulates sexual desire.

Aril: the husk or membrane covering the seed of a plant.

Aromachology: the study of the use of aromas, both natural and synthetic.

Aromatic: a substance with a strong aroma or smell.

Asthenia: see debility.

Astringent: causes contraction of organic tissues.

Atony: lessening or lack of muscular tone or tension.

Axil: upper angle between a stem and leaf or bract.

B

Bactericidal: an agent that destroys bacteria.

Balsam: a resinous semi-solid mass or viscous liquid exuded from a plant, characterized by its high content of benzoic acid, benzoates, cinnamic acid, or cinnamates.

Balsamic: a soothing medicine or application having the qualities of a balsam.

Bechic: anything that relieves or cures coughs; or referring to coughs.

Biennial: a plant which completes its life cycle in two years, without flowering in the first year.

Biliousness: condition caused by excessive secretion of bile.

Bitter: a tonic component which stimulates the appetite and promotes the secretion of saliva and gastric juices.

Blenorrhea: abnormally free secretion and discharge of mucus, sometimes from the genitals (as in gonorrhea).

Blepharitis: inflammation of the eyelids.

C

Calculus: a solid pathological concentration (or "stone"), formed in any part of the body.

Calmative: a sedative.

Calyx: the sepals or outer layer of floral leaves.

Cardiac: pertaining to the heart.

Cardiotonic: having a stimulating effect on the heart.

Carminative: settles the digestive system, relieves flatulence.

Catarrh: inflammation of mucous membranes, usually associated with an increase in secretion of mucus.

Cathartic: a purgative.

Cellulite: "orange-peel" skin.

Cephalic: remedy for disorders of the head; referring or directed toward the head.

Cerebral: pertaining to the largest part of the brain, the cerebrum.

Chemotype: the same botanical species occurring in other forms due to different conditions of growth.

Chlorosis: a rare form of anemia.

Cholagogue: stimulates the secretion and flow of bile.

Cholecystokinetic: agent that stimulates the contraction of the gall bladder.

Choleretic: aids excretion of bile by the liver, so there is a greater flow of bile.

Cholesterol: a naturally occurring steroid alcohol. Excess can lead to gallstones.

Cicatrizant: an agent that promotes healing by the formation of scar tissue.

Cirrhosis: degenerative change in any organ (specially liver), resulting in fibrous tissue overgrowth.

Colic: pain due to contraction of the involuntary muscle of the abdominal organs.

Colitis: inflammation of the colon.

Compress: a lint or substance applied hot or cold to an area of the body, for relief of swelling and pain, or to produce localized pressure.

Concrete: a concentrate, waxy, solid, or semi-solid perfume material prepared from previously live plant matter, usually using a hydrocarbon type of solvent.

Constipation: congestion of the bowels; incomplete or infrequent action of the bowels.

Contagious disease: a disease spreading from person to person by direct contact.

Cordial: a stimulant and tonic.

Corolla: the petals of a flower considered as a whole.

Counterirritant: applications to the skin that relieve deep-seated pain, usually applied in the form of heat.

Cutaneous: pertaining to the skin.

Cytophylactic: increasing the activity of leucocytes in defense of the body against infection.

Cytotoxic: toxic to all cells.

D

Debility: weakness, lack of tone.

Decoction: a herbal preparation, where the plant material (usually hard or woody) is boiled in water and reduced to make a concentrated extract.

Decongestive: an agent for the relief or reduction of congestion, e.g. mucus.

Demulcent: a substance that protects mucous membranes and allays irritation.

Depurative: helps combat impurity in the blood and organs; detoxifying.

Deodorant: an agent that corrects, masks, or removes unpleasant odors.

Dermal: pertaining to the skin.

Diaphoretic: see sudorific.

Digestive: substance that promotes or aids the digestion of food.

Disinfectant: prevents and combats spread of germs.

Diuretic: aids production of urine, promotes urination.

Dropsy: excess of fluid in the tissues.

Drupe: a fleshy fruit, with one or more seeds, each surrounded by a stony layer.

Dysmenorrhea: painful and difficult menstruation.

Dyspepsia: difficulty with digestion associated with pain, flatulence, heartburn, and nausea.

E

Edema: a painless swelling caused by fluid retention.

Elliptical: shaped like an ellipse, or regular curve.

Emetic: induces vomiting.

Emmenagogue: induces or assists menstruation.

Emollient: softens and soothes the skin.

Engorgement: congestion of a part of the tissues, or fullness (as in the breasts).

Enteritis: inflammation of the mucous membrane of the intestine.

Enzyme: complex proteins that are produced by the living cells, and catalyze specific biochemical reactions.

Erythema: a superficial redness of the skin due to excess of blood.

Essential oil: a volatile and aromatic liquid (sometimes semi-solid), which generally constitutes the odorous principles of a plant, and is obtained by a process of expression or distillation.

Estrogen: a hormone produced by the ovary, necessary for development of female secondary sexual characteristics.

Expectorant: helps promote the removal of mucus from the respiratory system.

Febrifuge: combats fever.

Fixative: a material that slows down the rate of evaporation of the more volatile components in a perfume.

Fixed oil: vegetable oil obtained from plants that, unlike essential oils, are fatty, dense, and nonvolatile.

Florets: the small individual flowers in the flower heads of the Compositae family.

Follicle: a dry, one-celled, many seeded fruit.

Fungicidal: prevents and combats fungal infection.

G

Galactagogue: increases secretion of milk.

Gastritis: inflammation of stomach lining.

Genitourinary: referring to both genital and reproductive systems.

Germicidal: destroys germs or micro-organisms.

Gingivitis: inflammation of the gum.

Gout: a disease that involves excess uric acid in the blood.

Gums: the term is often applied to "resins," specially with relation to turpentines. Strictly speaking, gums are natural or synthetic water-soluble materials, such as gum arabic.

Halitosis: offensive breath.

Hallucinogenic: causes visions or delusions.

Heartwood: the central portion of a tree trunk.

Hematuria: blood in the urine.

Hemorrhoids: piles, dilated rectal veins.

Hemostatic: arrests bleeding.

Hepatic: relating to liver; tones and aids its function.

Herpes: inflammation of the skin or mucous membrane with clusters of deep-seated vesicles.

Hormone: a product of living cells that produces a specific effect on the activity cells remote from its point of origin.

Hybrid: a plant originating by fertilization of one species or subspecies by another.

Hypertension: raised blood pressure.

Hypertensive: agent which raises blood pressure.

Hypnotic: causing sleep.

Hypocholesterolemia: lowering the cholesterol content of the blood.

Hypoglycemia: lowered blood sugar levels.

Hypotension: low blood pressure.

Hypotensive: agent that lowers blood pressure.

Hysteria: a psychoneurosis manifesting itself in various disorders of the mind and body.

I

Inflorescence: flowering structure above the last stem leaves (including bracts and flowers).

Infusion: a herbal remedy prepared by steeping the plant material in water.

Insecticide: repels insects.

Insomnia: inability to sleep.

Lanceolate: lance-shaped, oval, and pointed at both ends (usually a leaf shape).

Larvicidal: an agent that prevents and kills larvae.

Laxative: promotes evacuation of the bowels.

Legume: a fruit consisting of one carpel, opening on one side, such as a pea.

Leucocyte: white blood cells responsible for fighting disease.

Leucocytosis: an increase in the number of white blood cells above the normal limit.

Leucorrhea: white discharge from the vagina.

Ligulet: a narrow protection from the top of a leaf sheath in grasses.

Linear: of leaves, narrow and more or less parallel-sided.

Lipolytic: causing lipolysis, the chemical disintegration or splitting of fats.

Lithuria: a morbid condition marked by the presence of excessive amounts of uric acid in the urine.

Lumbago: a painful rheumatic affliction of the muscles and fibrous tissue of the lumbar region of the back.

Lymphatic: pertaining to the lymph system.

Macerate: soak until soft.

Metrorrhagia: uterine bleeding outside the menstrual cycle.

Microbe: a minute living organism, specially pathogenic bacteria, viruses, etc.

Mucilage: a substance containing gelatinous constituents that are demulcent.

Mucolytic: dissolving or breaking down mucus.

N

Narcotic: a substance that induces sleep; intoxicating or poisonous in large doses.

Nervine: strengthening and toning to the nerves and nervous system.

Nephritis: inflammation of the kidneys.

Neuralgia: a stabbing pain along a nerve pathway.

Neurasthenia: nervous exhaustion.

O

Oleo gum resin: a natural exudation from trees and plants that consists mainly of essential oil, gum, and resin.

Oleoresin: a natural resinous exudation from plants, or an aromatic liquid preparation, extracted from botanical matter using solvents. Consists almost entirely of a mixture of essential oil and resin.

Olfaction: the sense of smell.

Ophthalmia: inflammation of the eye, a term usually applied to conjunctivitis.

Orexigenic: appetite stimulant.

Ovate: egg-shaped.

Panacea: a cure-all.

Pappus: the calyx in a composite flower having feathery hairs, scales, or bristles.

Parasiticide: prevents and destroys parasites such as fleas, lice, etc.

Parturient: aiding childbirth.

Pathogenic: causing or producing disease.

Pathological: unnatural or destructive process on living tissue.

Pediculicide: an agent that destroys lice.

Peptic: applied to gastric secretions and affected areas.

Perennial: a plant that lives for more than two years.

Petiole: the stalk of a leaf.

Pharmacology: medical science of drugs that deals with their actions, properties, and characteristics.

Pharmacopoeia: an official publication of drugs in common use, in a given country.

Physiological: describes the natural biological processes of a living organism.

Phytohormones: plant substances that mimic the action of human hormones.

Phytotherapy: the treatment of disease by plants; herbal medicine.

Pinnate: a leaf composed of more than three leaflets arranged in two rows along a common stalk.

Pomade: a prepared perfume material obtained by enfleurage.

Poultice: the therapeutic application of a soft moist mass (such as fresh herbs) to the skin.

Prophylactic: preventive of disease or infection.

Psychosomatic: the manifestation of physical symptoms resulting from a mental state.

Pulmonary: pertaining to the lungs.

Purgative: a substance stimulating an evacuation of the bowels.

Pyelitis: inflammation of the kidney.

R

Raceme: an inflorescence, usually conical in outline, in which the lowest flowers open first.

Receptacle: the upper part of the stem from which the floral parts arise.

Rectification: the process of redistillation applied to essential oils to rid them of certain constituents.

Refrigerant: cooling—reduces fever.

Regulator: an agent that helps balance and regulate the functions of the body.

Relaxant: soothing, causing relaxation, relieving strain or tension.

Renal: pertaining to the kidney.

Resin: a natural or prepared product, either solid or semi-solid in nature. Natural resins are exudations from trees, such as mastic; prepared resins are oleoresins from which essential oil has been removed.

Resinoid: a perfumery material prepared from natural resinous matter, such as balsams, gum resins, etc., by extraction with a hydrocarbon type of solvent.

Resolvent: an agent that disperses swelling, or effects absorption of a new growth.

Restorative: an agent that helps strengthen and revive the body systems.

Revulsive: relieves pain by means of the diversion of blood or disease from one part of the body to another.

Rhinitis: inflammation of nasal mucous membrane.

Rhizome: a root-like underground stem.

Rosette: leaves that are closely arranged in a spiral.

Rubefacient: a substance that causes redness of the skin.

S

Sclerosis: hardening of tissue due to inflammation.

Scrofula: an outdated name for tuberculosis.

Seborrhea: increased secretion of sebum.

Sedative: an agent that reduces functional activity; calming.

Sessile: without a stalk.

Sialogogue: an agent that stimulates the secretion of saliva.

Soporific: a substance that induces sleep.

Spike: an inflorescence in which the sessile flowers are arranged in a raceme.

Splenic: relating to the spleen, the largest endocrine gland.

Splenitis: inflammation of the spleen.

Stimulant: an agent that quickens the physiological functions of the body.

Stomachic: digestive aid and tonic; improving appetite.

Styptic: an astringent agent that stops or reduces external bleeding.

Sudorific: an agent that causes sweating.

Synergy: agents working together harmoniously.

T

Tannin: a substance that has an astringent action, and helps seal the tissue.

Thrombosis: formation of a thrombus or blood clot.

Thrush: an infection of the mouth or vaginal region caused by a fungus (candida).

Tincture: a herbal remedy, or perfumery material prepared in an alcohol base.

Tonic: strengthens and enlivens the whole or specific parts of the body.

Tracheitis: inflammation of the windpipe.

Trifoliate: a plant having three distinct leaflets.

Tuber: a swollen part of an underground stem of one year's duration, capable of new growth.

U

Umbel: umbrella-like; a flower where the petioles all arise from the top of the stem.

Uterine: pertaining to the uterus.

V

Vasoconstrictor: an agent that causes narrowing of the blood vessels.

Vasodilator: an agent that dilates the blood vessels.

Vermifuge: expels intestinal worms.

Vesicant: causing blistering to the skin; a counterirritant.

Vesicle: a small blister or sac containing fluid.

Volatile: unstable, evaporates easily, as in "volatile oil;" see essential oil.

Vulnerary: an agent that helps heal wounds and sores by external application.

Further reading

Aqua Oleum, *The Essential Oil Catalogue*, Aqua Oleum, 1994

Arber, *A. Herbals, Their Origin and Evolution*, Cambridge University Press, 1912

Arctander, S., *Perfume and Flavor Materials of Natural Origin*, published by the author, Elizabeth, New Jersey, 1960

Baerheim, S.A. & Scheffer, J.J.C., *Essential Oils and Aromatic Plants*, Dr.W. Junk Publications, 1989

de Bairacli, Levy, J., *The Illustrated Herbal Handbook*, Faber & Faber, 1982

Beckett, S., *Herbs to Soothe Your Nerves*, Thorsons, 1977

Beresford-Cooke, C., *Massage for Healing and Relaxation*, Arlington, 1986

Bianchini, F. & Corbetta. F., *Health Plants of the World — Atlas of Medicinal Plants*, Newsweek Books, New York, 1977

Boulos, C. & Danin, A., *Medicinal Plants of North Africa*, Reference Publications, 1983

British Herbal Pharmacopoeia, British Herbal Medicine Association, 1983

Buchman, D.D., *Feed Your Face*, Duckworth, 1973, 1980

— *Herbal Medicine*, Rider, 1984

Carrington, H., *Perfumes, Their Sensual Lure and Charm*, Haldeman-Julius Publications, 1947

Ceres, *Herbs for Healthy Hair*, Thorsons, 1977

Chiej, R., *The Macdonald Encyclopedia of Medicinal Plants*, Arnoldo Mondadori Editore, Milan, 1984

Conway, D., *The Magic of Herbs*, Mayflower, 1973

Coon, N., *The Dictionary of Useful Plants*, Rodale, Emmaus, Pa.,1974

Cribb, A.B. & J.W., *Useful Wild Plants in Australia*, Fontana/Collins, 1982

Culpeper, N., *Culpeper's Complete Herbal*, W. Foulsham & Co. Ltd, 1952

Dastur, J.F., *Useful Plants of India and Pakistan*, D.B. Taraporevala Sons & Co. Ltd, India, 1985

Davies, W.C., *New Zealand Native Plant Studies*, A.H. & A.W. Reed, Wellington, 1961

Davis, P., *Subtle Aromatherapy*, C.W. Daniel, 1991

— *Aromatherapy An A–Z*, C.W. Daniel, 1988

Day, I., *Perfumery with Herbs*, Darton, Longman & Todd, Ltd, 1979

Dodd, G.H. & Van Toller, S., *Perfumery: The Psychology and Biology of Fragrance I*, Chapman & Hall, 1990

— *Perfumery: The Psychology and Biology of Fragrance II*, Elsevier Science, 1992

Douglas, J.S., *Making Your Own Cosmetics*, Pelham Books, 1979

Downing, G., *The Massage Book*, Penguin, 1974

Fischer-Rizzi, S., *Complete Aromatherapy Handbook*, Sterling 1990

Franchomme, P., *Phytoguide*, International Phytomedical Foundation, La Courtête, France, 1985

— and Penoël, D., *L'Aromathérapie Exactement*, Roger Jollois, Limoges, 1990

Gardner, J., *Healing Yourself During Pregnancy*, The Crossing Press, California, 1987

Gattefossé, R., *Gattefossé's Aromatherapy*, C.W. Daniel, 1993

Genders, R., *Natural Beauty*, Webb & Bower, 1986

Grieve, M., *A Modern Herbal*, Penguin, 1982

Griggs, B., *The Home Herbal*, Pan, 1983

Groom, N., *The Perfume Handbook*, Chapman & Hall, 1992

Guenther, E., *The Essential Oils*, Van Nostrand, New York, 1948

Hall, R., Klemme, D. & Nienhaus, J., *The H & R Book: Guide to Fragrance Ingredients*, Johnson Publishing, 1985

Hepper, C., *Herbal Cosmetics*, Thorsons, 1987

Heriteatu, J., *Potpourris and other Fragrant Delights*, Penguin, 1975

Hoffman, D., *The Complete Illustrated Holistic Herbal*, Element Books, 1996

Huxley, A., *Natural Beauty With Herbs*, Darton, Longman and Todd, Ltd, 1977

Jessee, J.E., *Perfume Album*, Robert E. Krieger, 1974

Jellinek, P., *The Practice of Modern Perfumery*, Leonard Hill, 1959

Kahn, I., *The Development of Spiritual Healing*, Sufi Publishing Co., 1974

Lassak, E.V. & McCarthy, T., *Australian Medicinal Plants*, Methuen, Australia, 1983

Launert, E., *Edible and Medicinal Plants of Britain and Northern Europe*, Hamlyn, 1981

Lautie, R. & Passebecq, A., *Aromatherapy; the Use of Plant Essences in Healing*, Thorsons, 1982

Lavabre, M., *Aromatherapy Workbook*, Healing Arts Press, Vermont, 1990

Lawless, J., *The Illustrated Encyclopedia of Essential Oils*, Element Books, 1995

— *Home Aromatherapy*, Kyle Cathie, 1993

— *Aromatherapy and the Mind*, Thorsons, 1994

— *Lavender Oil*, Thorsons, 1994

— *Tea Tree Oil*, Thorsons, 1994

— *Rose Oil*, Thorsons, 1995

— *Rosemary Oil*, Thorsons, 1996

Lawrence, B.M., *Essential Oils*, Allured Publishing Co., Wheaton, USA, 1978

Le Gue, A., *Scent: The Mysterious Power of Smell*, Chatto & Windus, 1993

Leung, A.Y., *Encyclopedia of Common Natural Ingredients*, John Wiley, New York, 1980

Lewis, R. *Natural Data Base UK: Aromatherapy*, Vols I-V (1993-1997), Chessington, Surrey

Lis-Balchin, Dr. M., *Aromascience*, Amberwood, 1995

Little, K., *Kitty Little's Book of Herbal Beauty*, Penguin, 1980

Maury, M., *Marguerite Maury's Guide to Aromatherapy*, C.W. Daniel, 1989

Mabey, R., *The Complete New Herbal*, Elm Tree Books, 1988

Maxwell-Hudson, C., *Aromatherapy Massage Book*, Dorling Kindersley, 1994

McIntyre, A., *Herbs for Pregnancy and Childbirth*, Sheldon Press, 1988

Metcalfe, J., *Herbs and Aromatherapy*, Webb & Bower, 1989

Meunier, C., *Lavandes et Lavandins*, Charles-Yves Chaudoreille, Edisud, Aix-en-Provence, France, 1985

Mills, S.Y., *The A–Z of Modern Herbalism*, Thorsons, 1989

Mitchell, S., *The Complete Illustrated Guide to Massage*, Element Books, 1997

Morris, E.T., *Fragrance, The Story of Perfume from Cleopatra to Chanel*, Charles Scribner & Sons, New York

Muller, P.M. & Lamparsky, D., *Perfumes, Art, Science, Technology*, Elsevier Applied Science, 1991

Naves, Y.R. & Mazuyer, G., *Natural Perfume Materials*, Reinhold Publishing, New York, 1947

Page, M., *The Observer's Book of Herbs*, Frederick Warne, 1980

Parvati, J. Hygieia, *A Woman's Herbal*, Wildwood House, 1979

Poucher, W.A., *Perfumes, Cosmetics and Soaps* Vol. II, Chapman and Hall, 1932

Price, S., *Practical Aromatherapy*, Thorsons, 1983

Rapgay, L., *Tibetan Therapeutic Massage*, published by the author, India, 1985

Roudnitska, E., *The Art of Perfumery*, Cabris, France

Ryman, D., *The Aromatherapy Handbook*, Century, 1984

Sellar, Wanda, *The Directory of Essential Oils*, C.W. Daniel, 1992

Stead, C., *The Power of Holistic Aromatherapy*, Javelin Books, 1986

Stobart, T., *Herbs, Spices and Flavourings*, Penguin, 1979

Stoddart, D.M., *The Scented Ape*, Cambridge University Press, 1990

Le Strange, R., *A History of Herbal Plants*, Angus and Robertson, 1977

Suskind, P., *Perfume, the Story of a Murderer*, Hamish Hamilton, London, 1986

Temple, A.A., *Flowers and Trees of Palestine*, SPCK, Macmillan, 1978

Thomson, W.A.R., *Healing Plants – A Modern Herbal*, Macmillan, 1978

Tisserand, R., *Aromatherapy for Women*, Thorsons, 1985

Tisserand, R., *The Essential Oil Safety Data Manual*, The Association of Tisserand Aromatherapists, 1985

Tisserand, R., *The Art of Aromatherapy*, C.W. Daniel, 1985

Valnet, J., *The Practice of Aromatherapy*, C.W. Daniel (English translation), 1982

Weiss, R.F., *Herbal Medicine*, Arcanum, 1988

Whitmont, E.C., *Psyche and Substance*, North Atlantic Books, 1980

Williams, D., *Lecture Notes on Essential Oils*, Eve Taylor Ltd, 1989

Worwood, V.A., *The Fragrant Pharmacy*, Macmillan, 1990

Wren, R.C., *Potters New Cyclopaedia of Botanical Drugs and Preparations*, C.W. Daniel, 1988

Yearbook of Pharmacy and Transactions of the British Pharmaceutical Conference, The Pharmaceutical Press, Bloomsbury, London, 1907

Wright, R., *The Science of Smell*, Allen & Unwin, 1964

Younger, D., *Household Gods*, E.W. Allen, 1898

Useful addresses

For high-quality essential oils, aromatherapy products, and for international enquiries, please contact Julia Lawless at:

Aqua Oleum Essential Oils
Unit 9, Griffin Mill Industrial Estate,
London Road, Thrupp,
Stroud, Gloucestershire
GL5 2AZ, UK
Tel: 01453 885 908
E-mail: info@aqua-oleum.co.uk
www.aqua-oleum.co.uk

also available from:

Canada & USA: Natura Trading
Box 263 1857 West 4th Avenue
Vancouver, BC, Canada, V6J 1M4
Tel: 001 604 732 7531
Toll Free: 1-800-932-7531
Email: nigel@naturatrading.ca
www.naturatrading.ca

Norway: Au Naturel (UK) Inc Norway
Kjelsasveien 168, NO-0884, Oslo
Tel: 0047 22 026580
Email: PMBerg@nutracorp.com
www.solaray.no

Japan: Kunio Inoue
Uni-World Enterprise Co Ltd
5-17-6 Kami-imaizumi Ebina 243-0431
Tel: 50-3328 0843
Email: kinoue.uwe@dream.com
www.uwe-jp.com

Finland: Aduki Oy
Sorvaajankatu 13, 00880 Helsinki
Tel: +358-9-784646
Email: adu@aduki.fi
www.aduki.fi

Information regarding qualified aromatherapists, training courses, and herbal studies can be obtained from:

International Federation of Aromatherapists (IFA)
146 South Ealing Road,
Ealing, London,
W5 4QJ, UK
Tel: +44(0)208 567 2243
www.ifaroma.org

National Association of Holistic Aromatherapy (NAHA)
PO BOX 27871
Raleigh, NC
27611-7871
Email: info@naha.org
Office: (919) 917-7491 (EST)
www.naha.

Aromatherapy Registration Council (ARC)
To find a qualified aromatherapist in your area, visit:
Aromatherapy Registration Examination
www.aromatherapycouncil.org

American Massage Therapy Association (AMTA)
500 Davis Street, Suite 900
Evanston, IL 60201-4695
Tel: 847/864-0123
Email: info@amtamassage.org
www.amtamassage.org

Californian School of Herbal Studies (CSHC)
9309 Highway 116, Forestville, CA
Tel: (707) 887-7457
Email: cshs@cshs.com
www.cshs.com

American Botanical Council
6200 Manor Road
Austin, TX 78723
Tel: 512-926-4900
www.abc.herbalgram.org

Index of oils

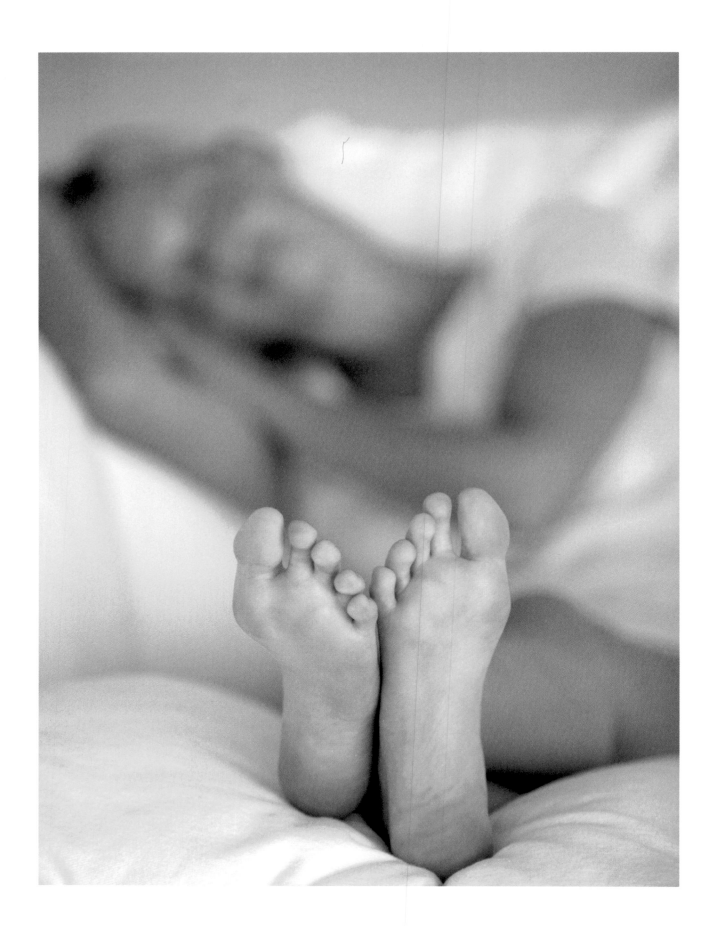

Index of ailments

General Index

bones, muscles, joints 171, 173, 174

circulatory system/heart 181, 184

digestive system 198, 202

genitourinary/endocrine systems 207, 209, 216

hair/scalp 166

nervous system 232, 235

perspiration 35, 165

grapeseed oil 31, 36, 54, 370

greasy hair 166

gum-resins 25

gums 39, 194–7

H

hair 49, 166–70

conditioner 61

rinse 61

tonic 61

halitosis 197

hand bath 35

hay fever 190

hazelnut 54

head lice 170

headaches 229

healing ointments 51

heart 177, 180

heat rash 150

hemlock see spruce

hemorrhoids 182

hip bath 35

ho wood 33, 262

holistic approach 13, 30

honey 35, 57

household fragrance 40–1

hyssop 33, 37, 289

amenorrhea 208

bruises 135

respiratory system 185, 187, 188, 189, 190, 191, 193

whooping cough 222

I

immortelle 33, 288

immune system 220–7, 243, 245–6, 251, 257, 261–5, 269, 270, 274, 278, 280, 283–4, 288, 292, 294, 297, 300–3, 305–6, 308–12, 316, 320, 324, 327–8, 332, 334–6, 341–2

impetigo 151

Indian lavender oil see linaloe

infectious disease 34, 126, 220–7

inflammation 171, 174

influenza 226

infused herbal oil 348

inhalation 23, 37, 38

insects 37, 38, 40, 41

insomnia 230

invaluable oils 32

irritable bowel syndrome 203

J

jasmine 22, 25, 29, 32, 40, 41, 129, 291

genitourinary/endocrine systems 207, 209, 215, 216, 218

high blood pressure 169

nervous system 231, 234, 236

sensitive skin/thread veins 164

stress 79

jetlag 235

joints 171–6, 243, 245–6, 250, 252, 258–9, 260–3, 265, 269–70, 273–8, 281, 284, 286–8, 290–3, 295, 297–8, 302–9, 312–13, 315–20, 324–9, 331–2, 334–42

jojoba 31, 54, 366

juniper 32, 35, 292

acne vulgaris 145

bones, muscles, joints 171, 173, 174, 175

circulatory system/heart 177, 181, 184

constipation 198

genitourinary/endocrine systems 208, 212

hair/scalp 166, 167

oily skin 160

juniper berry 140

K

King, J.R. 66

L

labdanum 33, 264

laurel 33, 294

lavandin 33, 296

lavender 22, 23, 25, 31, 32, 34, 35, 37, 48, 49, 61, 69, 126, 129, 131, 295

allergies 46

beauty care 35, 50, 159, 160, 161, 163, 164, 165

bones, muscles, joints 171, 172, 173, 174, 175

circulatory system/heart 177, 178, 180, 184

digestive system 199, 201, 202, 203, 204

disinfectant 40

first aid 40, 135, 136, 137, 138

genitourinary/endocrine systems 205, 206, 207, 209, 210, 212, 213, 214, 215, 216, 218

hair/scalp 166, 167, 168, 169, 170

immune system/infectious disease 220, 221, 222, 223, 224, 226, 227

insect repellent 41

nervous system 228, 229, 230, 231, 232, 233, 234, 235, 236, 237

respiratory system 185, 187, 188, 189, 190, 191, 192, 193

skin disorders 140, 142–5, 147–57

stings/bites 139

stress 35, 79

toothache/tooth abscess 194

lemon 25, 32, 47, 129, 131, 269

bones, muscles, joints 171, 174

childbirth 218

circulatory system/heart 177, 181

digestive system 198, 202

hair/scalp 166

immune system/infectious disease 221, 227

nervous system 232, 235

perspiration 35, 165

respiratory system 185, 190

skin disorders 142–4, 146, 155–6

lemon balm see melissa/lemon balm

lemon eucalyptus 32, 283

genitourinary/endocrine systems 210, 213, 218

tea tree 22, 31, 32, 35, 37, 126, 301
  allergies 46
  bacterial infection 47
  beauty care 35, 160, 162, 165
  bones, muscles, joints 171
  digestive system 199, 202
  disinfectant 40
  first aid 40, 135, 136, 137, 138,
    139
  fungal infection 47
  genitourinary/endocrine systems
    210, 212, 213, 214
  hair/scalp 166, 168, 169, 170
  immune system/infectious
    disease 220, 221, 222, 223, 224,
    226, 227
  mouth, teeth, gums 194, 195, 196,
    197
  respiratory system 185, 187, 191,
    192, 193
  skin 50, 51
  skin disorders 140, 142–57
teeth 194–7
tension 39
therapeutic aromatic massage 36
thread veins 164
throat infections 38, 193
thrush 35, 47, 210–11
thyme 32, 37, 39
  bacterial infection 47
  bones, muscles, joints 172
  circulatory system/heart 179,
    181, 184
  cystitis/urethritis 212
  digestive system 199, 202
  halitosis 197
  head lice 170
  immune system/infectious
    disease 220, 222, 226, 227
  perspiration 35, 165
  respiratory system 185, 187, 190,
    191, 193
  scabies 155
thyme, white 32, 334
tinea 47
Tisserand, Robert 66

toilet water 58
toiletries 60–1
toner 58
toothache/tooth abscess 194
tuberose 25, 33, 323
turmeric 33, 277

U

ulceration 152
urethritis 212
urinary system 123, 205–19, 245,
    252, 301–302, 315, 319, 334

V

valerian 32, 35, 337
  asthma 189
  circulatory system/heart 177,
    178, 180
  dysmenorrhea 205
  dyspepsia 201
  nervous system 228, 230, 236
Valnet, Dr. Jean 123
valuable oils 50–1
vanilla 33, 42, 338
vaporizer 37
varicose veins 183
vegetable oils 348
verbena, lemon 33, 247
verrucae 146
vetivert 22, 33, 339
  genitourinary/endocrine systems
    209, 216
  high blood pressure 178
  nervous system 228, 230
violet 33, 340
Virginian cedarwood see cedarwood,
    Virginian
vitamins 30, 46, 135
vomiting 204

W

warts 146
West Indian bay see bay, West
    Indian
West Indian lemongrass see
    lemongrass, West Indian
wheat germ 31, 54, 60, 368
whooping cough 38, 222
wounds 137

Y

yarrow 33, 245
  bones, muscles, joints 171, 174,
    176
  circulatory system/heart 177,
    178, 182, 183
  first aid 135, 136, 137, 138
  genitourinary/endocrine systems
    206, 212, 214
  hair/scalp 166, 167, 169
  immune system/infectious
    disease 223, 226, 227
  liver congestion 202
  sensitive skin/thread veins 164
  skin disorders 140, 152
ylang ylang 32, 35, 40, 131, 255
  aphrodisiac 131
  circulatory system/heart 178,
    180
  genitourinary/endocrine systems
    207, 209, 215, 216, 218
  hair scalp 169
  nervous system 228, 233, 234
  stress 79
yogurt 57

References

1 Davis, P., *Aromatherapy An A–Z*, p. 173
2 Cited in J. Lawless, *Aromatherapy and the Mind*, p. 114
3 Maury, M., *Marguerite Maury's Guide to Aromatherapy*, p. 51
4 Anderson, Extract from files of Museum of Applied Arts and Sciences, Sydney 1974, cited in C.W. Olsen, *Australian Tea Tree Oil*, p. 25
5 Weintraub, P., cited in "Sentimental Journeys," *Omni*, p. 52
6 Stoddard, M., *The Scented Ape*, pp. 135–141
7 Ehrlichman, H. and Bastone, L., "The use of odour in the study of emotion," in G.H. Dodds and S. Van Toller, *Perfumery: the Psychology and Biology of Fragrance*, pp. 143, 156
8 Schwartz, G., cited in "Sentimental Journeys," *Omni*, p. 116
9 Cited in H. Carrington, *Perfumes, Their Sensual Lure and Charm*, p. 4
10 Maury, op. cit., p. 82
11 Ibid., pp. 95–6
12 Maxwell-Hudson, C., *Aromatherapy Massage Book*, p. 7
13 Tisserand, R., "Success with Stress," *International Journal of Aromatherapy*, Vol. 4, No. 2, 1992, p. 14
14 Coxon, Ann, cited in *Aromatherapy Quarterly*, No. 31, p. 9
15 Rovesti, cited in R. Tisserand, *The Art of Aromatherapy*, p. 98
16 Tisserand, R., *Safety Data Manual*, p. 36
17 Valnet, J., *The Practice of Aromatherapy*, p. 48
18 Blackwell, R., *Health Independent*, 30 January 1996
19 Smith, ibid.
20 Lis-Balchin, M., *Aromascience: The Chemistry and Bioactivity of Essential Oils*, p. 26
21 Gattefossé, R.M., *Gattefossé's Aromatherapy*, p. 70

Picture credits

The publishers wish to thank the following for use of pictures:

A–Z Botanical: pp. 184B, 192B (Sylvia O'Toole), 196T (W. Broadhurst), 204B
ARDEA: p. 197B (Donald Burgess)
The Bridgeman Art Library: pp. 2 (Bibliothèque Nationale), 14, 30B
(Royal Albert Memorial Hospital, Exeter)
e.t.archive: pp. 43TR, 44T
Fine Art Photographic Library: pp. 9, 15
Holt Studios: p. 186
The Hutchison Library: p. 16B (Felix Greene)
The Image Bank: pp. 20B (L.D. Gordon), 98, 101T (Paul McCormick), 108T (David de Lossy), 110B, 124B

(Tim P. Kelly), 149 (John Love), 167 (B. Lambert), 170 (Tim Beider)
NHPA: p. 197T (Ted Hutchison)
Oxford Scientific Films: pp. 181B (Deni Bown), 202T (Deni Bown)
The Science Photo Library: pp. 29TR (M.Wurtz/ Biozentrum), 89T
(CNRI), 89M (Dr. K. Louantman), 104, 111T (K.H. Kjeldsen), 121
(D.J.F. Burgess), 143M (D. Phillips), 157 (LDC)
Zefa: pp. 19, 20T, 27BL, 29L, 30, 100B, 146B, 152, 171

Acknowledgements

Special thanks to
Philip Auchnivole, Adam Carne, Rebecca Drury, Rachel Gould,
Wendy Grantley-Oxberry, Julia Holden, Simon Holden, Carolyn
Jikiemi-Roberts, Kay Macmullan, Chloe McCausland, Jack Martin,
Debbie and Max Oliver, Sunny Pitcher, Bethany Sword *for help
with photography*

Special thanks to
Peter Coleman (ceramics); Courts plc, Shoreham; The Plinth
Company, Stowmarket, Suffolk; The Wilbury School, Centre for
Natural Therapies, Hove *for help with properties*

AUTHOR'S ACKNOWLEDGEMENTS
I would like to thank all the following people who have contributed
to the completion of this book, especially for their patience and
collaboration during the final stages of the project: Caro Ness,
Katie Worrall and Allie West at Element Books; Peter Bridgewater,
Margaret Crowther, Kevin Knight, Anne Townley and all those
at the Bridgewater Book Company; Guy Ryecart and Ian Parsons,
the photographers, and the studio models; Rosalind Hadley, beauty
therapist at the Retreat; Eileen Lawless for advice on nutrition; and
Ann Cooper and all at Aqua Oleum for compiling chemical profiles of
all the essential oils.

I would also like to thank all my friends and family who have
supported and encouraged me over the last year, especially my
husband Alec and daughter Natasha, for their ongoing help and
support—without them I would never have completed the task!

Your notes

KEEPING A RECORD of your own experiences can be hugely beneficial in learning about your personal relationship with each of the individual oils. Different scent types can correlate differently with varying personality types, so make a note of your own preferences. It may also be useful to keep a record of the preferences of others in your household in order to stock a complete home medicine chest.